普通高等教育"十一五"国家级规划教材

 全国高等医药院校药学类专业第二轮实验双语教材

药物分析实验与指导

（第4版）

主　　编　宋　敏

副 主 编　赵云丽

编　　者　（以姓氏笔画为序）

　　　　　许慧君（河北医科大学）

　　　　　苏梦翔（中国药科大学）

　　　　　宋　瑞（中国药科大学）

　　　　　徐新军（中山大学）

　　　　　高晓霞（广东药科大学）

　　　　　曹志娟（复旦大学）

英文审校　张桂军（中国药科大学）

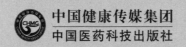

中国健康传媒集团

中国医药科技出版社

内容提要

本教材是"全国高等医药院校药学类专业第二轮实验双语教材"之一。药物分析是一门实践性很强的学科,而实验课是培养学生掌握药物分析基本实验技能必不可少的。本教材采用中英文双语编写,共分为7章,包括一般性实验指导,药物的性状、鉴别和检查,药物的含量测定,药物质量的全检验,生物样本中药物的分析,设计性实验和药物分析方法验证等。本教材为书网融合教材,即纸质教材有机融合电子教材、教学配套资源(PPT和视频)。

本教材可供药学类本科师生使用,也可供从事药品研究、生产和检验的相关专业人员参考。

图书在版编目(CIP)数据

药物分析实验与指导/宋敏主编.—4版.—北京:中国医药科技出版社,2020.1

全国高等医药院校药学类专业第二轮实验双语教材

ISBN 978-7-5214-1368-7

Ⅰ.①药… Ⅱ.①宋… Ⅲ.①药物分析-实验-双语教学-医学院校-教学参考资料-汉、英 Ⅳ.①R917-33

中国版本图书馆 CIP 数据核字(2019)第 296951 号

美术编辑 陈君杞
版式设计 南博文化

出版 **中国健康传媒集团** | 中国医药科技出版社
地址 北京市海淀区文慧园北路甲 22 号
邮编 100082
电话 发行:010-62227427 邮购:010-62236938
网址 www.cmstp.com
规格 889×1194mm $^{1}/_{16}$
印张 16 ¾
字数 372 千字
初版 2003 年 8 月第 1 版
版次 2020 年 1 月第 4 版
印次 2024 年 2 月第 3 次印刷
印刷 大厂回族自治县彩虹印刷有限公司
经销 全国各地新华书店
书号 ISBN 978-7-5214-1368-7
定价 46.00 元

获取新书信息、投稿、为图书纠错,请扫码联系我们。

教学是学校人才培养的中心环节，实验教学是这一环节的重要组成部分。"全国高等医药院校药学类专业实验双语教材"是中国药科大学坚持药学实践教学改革，突出提高学生动手能力、创新思维，通过承担教育部"世行贷款21世纪初高等教育教学改革项目"等多项教改课题，逐步建设完善的一套与药学各专业学科理论课程紧密结合的高水平双语实验教材。

本轮修订，适逢"全国高等医药院校药学类专业第五轮规划教材"及《中国药典》（2020年版）、新版《国家执业药师资格考试大纲》出版，整套教材的修订强调了与新版理论教材知识的结合，与《中国药典》（2020年版）等新颁布的法典法规结合。为更好地服务于新时期高等院校药学教育与人才培养的需要，在上一版的基础上，进一步体现了各门实验课程自身独立性、系统性和科学性，又充分考虑到各门实验课程之间的联系与衔接，主要突出了以下特点。

1. 适应医药行业对人才的要求，体现行业特色，契合新时期药学人才需求的变化，使修订后的教材符合《中国药典》（2020年版）等国家标准及新版《国家执业药师资格考试大纲》等行业最新要求。

2. 更新完善内容，打造教材精品。在上版教材基础上进一步优化、精炼和充实内容。紧密结合"全国高等医药院校药学类专业第五轮规划教材"，强调与实际需求相结合，进一步提高教材质量。

3. 为适应信息化教学的需要，本轮教材全部打造成为书网融合教材，即纸质教材与数字教材、配套教学资源、题库系统、数字化教学服务有机融合，为读者提供全免费增值服务。

4. 坚持双语体系，强调素质培养教材以实践教学为突破口，采用双语体系编写有利于加快药学教育国际接轨，提高学生的科技英语水平，进一步提升学生整体素质。

"全国高等医药院校药学类专业第二轮实验双语教材"历经15年4次建设，在各个时期广大编者的努力下，在广大使用教材师生的支持下日臻完善。本轮教材的出版，必将对推动新时期我国高等药学教育的发展产生积极而深远的影响。希望广大师生在教学实践中对本套教材提出宝贵意见，以便今后进一步修订完善，共同打造精品教材。

吴晓明

全国高等医药院校药学类专业第五轮规划教材常务编委会主任委员

2019年10月

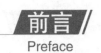

药物分析是运用经典的化学、物理学及生物学等方法和现代仪器分析研究药物性质、制订药物质量标准标准、控制药物质量的一门综合性应用学科，广义上包括了药物的化学检验、质量控制以及体内药物分析等内容。药物分析是一门实践性很强的学科，药物分析实验课培养学生掌握药物分析研究中的基本实验技能和方法，使其具备基本的科学实验思路。通过典型的药物分析实验实践，学生能掌握药物分析的基本程序和内容，熟悉并掌握药物检验的操作规范与要求。

《药物分析实验与指导》是药物分析课程的配套教材之一，本书采用中英文双语编写，由一般性实验指导，药物的性状、鉴别和检查，药物的含量测定，药物质量的全检验，生物样本中药物的分析，设计性实验和药物分析方法验证等七个部分组成。在药物质量评价方面，选取具有代表性的化学原料药及其制剂、中药及其制剂，分别采用容量分析和仪器分析方法，从鉴别、检查和含量测定三个方面设计实验内容。在体内药物分析方面，针对常见药物及毒物的常用生物样本前处理和测定方法进行编写。本书药物类别多，方法手段齐全，可使实验者的实践能力得到多方面锻炼，难度包括验证性和设计性实验两个层次，可供不同能力的实验者选用，以便于培养实验者进行药物分析研究的基本实验技能和独立从事药物分析研究的科研思路。实践教学可以根据学时和实验条件选择分项检测、测定或全检验进行。

本实验分析方法是在保留前三版教材中经典方法的基础上，依据《中国药典》2020 版进行补充，并将药物分析的操作规范及通用方法贯穿于各实验指导中，以便实验者掌握多种分析方法和手段，既增强实验者对药物分析理论知识的理解，又锻炼和规范了实验操作。

本书在中国药科大学药物分析系及兄弟院校的药物分析教学积累基础上，参照《中国药典》2020版的标准和相关文献，对第三版《药物分析实验与指导》进行了修订。感谢中国药科大学教务处和参编院校对本教材编写给予的关心和支持。

本书可供药学类本科学生药物分析实验教学使用，同时可供从事药品研究、生产和检验的相关专业人员参考。

因时间有限，对书中疏漏错误之处，敬请读者批评指正。

编　者
2019 年 12 月

第一章 一般性实验指导

Chapter 1　General Instructions

第一节　实验室安全守则

1. 时刻注意眼睛防护（佩戴防护目镜）。

2. 实验室内禁止饮食。

3. 实验室内严禁吸烟。

4. 接触具有腐蚀性的、有毒的、易燃的及其他危险的化学品必须戴手套、穿着实验服。

5. 尽量避免单独工作。

6. 吸取试剂时避免用嘴吸移液管。

7. 及时提醒他人终止危险的实验操作。

8. 务必清楚各种安全设备（洗眼喷淋、淋浴水龙头、灭火器等）的位置。

9. 使用新试剂前仔细阅读化学品安全说明书（MSDS）。

10. 掌握常见化学试剂污染的清理方法，熟悉防泄漏推车的位置、容量以及使用方法。

11. 接触化学试剂后和进食前请洗手。

12. 实验室内禁止穿着短裙、短裤、凉鞋。

13. 不应在实验室以外场所穿着实验服。

14. 实验操作过程中禁止听音乐，尤其是佩戴耳机。

Section 1　Laboratory Safety

1. Goggles must be worn at all times.

2. Eating or drinking is not allowed in laboratories where chemicals are used/stored.

3. Smoking is prohibited in the laboratory.

4. Lab coats must be worn while handling corrosive, toxic, or flammable materials. Gloves must be worn when necessary, especially when handling corrosives, toxic and dangerously reactive materials.

5. Do not work alone.

6. Avoid using a pipette with your mouth to absorb liquid.

7. If you see a colleague doing something dangerous, point it out to him or her.

8. Be sure to know where safe facilities (eyewash, shower hydrant and fire extinguisher) is

located.

9. Always reading material safety data sheet(MSDS) before handling new chemicals.

10. Knowing how to clean up spills of common chemicals you see. Be familiar with the locations and contents of Leak – proof carts and the way to use them.

11. Always wash your hands after handling chemicals and before eating.

12. Mini-skirts, shorts, and sandals are forbidden in the lab.

13. Lab coats must not be worn outside laboratories or in public areas.

14. Avoid listening to music especially wearing a walkman or other portable music devices while working in the lab.

第二节 天平使用规程

一、天平的种类

实验时，常需进行各种不同的称量操作。认识这些称量要求的准确度对于实验操作者来说是很重要的。不同的准确度要求应该使用合适的天平来称量。通常可供使用的天平分为以下两大类。

1. 托盘天平

托盘天平的准确度可以达到 ±1mg，适用于只要求保留 2~3 个有效数字的大多数称量。

2. 分析天平

分析天平的准确度通常可以达到 ±0.1mg，适用于要求保留 4 位甚至更多有效数字称量时使用。

二、称量的不同类型

在实验过程中，质量数值的表示形式通常有以下几种。

1. "称出约2g的……"这种表述是指应当称取近似2g，其质量的准确度要求不高，托盘天平就可以满足要求。

2. "准确称量约0.2g的……"这种表述是指应当使用分析天平称量接近0.2g的该物质，确切称样量必须达到 ±0.1mg 的准确度。注意，这并不要求称样量准确至0.2000g，在0.1900g 至0.2100g 之间都符合要求。无论怎样，必须知道最接近0.1mg 的量。重复称量3次样品时，并不要求3次称量结果完全相同，实际上也没有必要。

三、电子分析天平使用规则

称量是实验室最常进行的操作之一，使用的仪器是分析天平。有各厂商生产的不同型号的分析天平可供选择使用。下面以 Sartorius 天平为例说明电子分析天平的使用规则。

1. 电子分析天平简介

电子分析天平最主要的部件包括称量盘、天平箱门、显示屏、控制面板、水平脚和水平仪（图 1-1）。

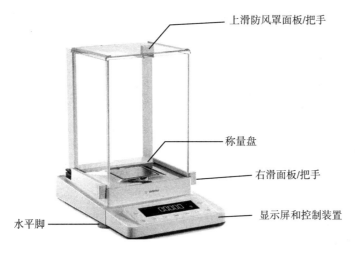

上滑防风罩面板/把手

称量盘

右滑面板/把手

水平脚

显示屏和控制装置

图 1 − 1　电子分析天平

2. 天平放置

称量结果的准确度（或可靠性）与天平所处的环境密切相关。实验台应该水平、防震。必要时可将天平置于一较重的抗磁材料上，如石头上（不可以是金属板）；天平应远离静电电荷（无塑料或玻璃），应与墙壁保持一定距离（防止由于墙体或地板震动对天平产生影响）。

3. 称量容器选择

（1）称量待加热的液体时通常选择烧杯，如在反应时产生气体物质则应使用锥形瓶进行称量。塑料称量盘（蒸发皿）只适用于称量固体，称量少量固体时也可使用称量纸。

（2）尽量使用较小的容器进行称量。

（3）应确保称量器皿干燥清洁，因为容器附着物可能引起称量结果偏高。

4. 天平开启

（1）检查天平称量盘上及周围有无散落物质，用专用的天平清理刷清扫称量盘及天平箱内部。将称量盘垂直提起，检查有无散落物质，用清理刷清理后，小心地将称量盘安置回原位。

（2）水平仪上的空气泡应处于中央，必要时可通过旋转水平脚来校正。

（3）插好天平插头。

（4）关好天平门，轻按 control 键后松开，控制面板将显示如下，并持续几秒钟。

$$8.8.8.8.8.8.8.8. \text{ g}$$

接下来，天平显示如下。

$$0.0000 \qquad \text{g}$$

0.0000 通常在开启天平时显示，如果没有如上显示或者数字出现缓慢，应确认天平是否处于防震、防气流环境下以确保稳定的零点。

（5）使用前，保持天平接通电源并开启一段时间，使系统达到热平衡。

5. 去皮和读数

（1）选择合适的量程，称量容器置于称量盘上，关闭天平门。

（2）按下红色的 Tare 键去皮，可进行多次，直到显示数字为零。

（3）将待称量样品置于称量盘中央或者称量容器中。

（4）待显示器读数稳定并显示出质量单位 g（mg）时可以读数。

（5）读数后移出样品。

6. 天平清理并关闭

（1）离开天平前，使用清理刷清扫散落的物质并擦干液体。

（2）清理结束后，关闭天平门，清零，使天平处于备用状态，方便其他操作者使用。

7. 注意事项

（1）称量过程中多称的物质应回收到一个废液缸，不可放回原容器，以免造成整瓶试剂的污染。

（2）称量物体时，为了防止气流干扰读数，务必关上天平门。完成称量后，为了防止灰尘进入，操作者应该关上天平门。

（3）称量时不要用手直接接触待测物，因手指上的湿气、油脂和灰尘会影响待测物的质量。

（4）为了称量准确，所有物品的温度应当是室温。温度较高的物体会提高天平外壳的运流电流，从而导致测定结果偏低。天平内的热空气密度小于原本室温下空气的密度，这是产生负误差的原因之一。

（5）不要让待测的化学物质直接接触天平托盘。使用容器称量，如烧杯、容量瓶，或者称量瓶。

（6）从干燥器里取出的物体会吸湿而使质量增加，操作者应当养成在相同的时间间隔进行称量的习惯。例如，如果进行称量坩埚至恒重的操作，操作者每次读数的时间都应当保持在将坩埚放入天平盘后 5 秒的时间点，以此最大程度减少因吸湿产生的影响。

（7）勿将化学物质溅入天平内。如果不慎溅入，立刻清理。

Section 2　Regulations for Using Balance

1. Types of balances

During the experiment, you need to make a variety of weighings. It is important for you to realize with what sort of accuracy these weighings should be made. Depending on the desired accuracy, you should use the proper balance to make your weighings. There are two types of balances available:

1.1　Top-loading balances

These will weigh to an accuracy of ±1mg and are suitable for most weighings of amounts that are specified to only two or three significant figures.

1.2　Analytical balances

These will weigh to an accuracy of ±0.1mg and must be used whenever you desire four or more significant figures accuracy.

2. Various types of weighing

When mass amounts are specified in experiment procedures, the following terms are commonly used.

2.1 "Weigh out about 2g of" means that you are required to weigh an amount of approximately two grams. The accuracy to which this mass amount needs is not high and the top-loading balance will suffice.

2.2 "Accurately weigh out about 0.2g of……" means that you should, with the aid of the analytical balance, weigh out an amount that is close to 0.2g, but you must know the exact amount to an accuracy of ±0.1mg. Note that it does not mean that you must weigh out exactly 0.200 0g. An amount between 0.190 0g and 0.210 0g is perfectly acceptable. However, you must know the exact amount to the nearest tenth of a milligram. When weighing out triplicate samples, it is not necessary that all three weights be exactly the same, indeed, it is poor procedure to attempt to do so.

3. Regulations for using the electronic analytical balance

Weighing is one of the most frequently performed procedures in the lab. Several different types of balance exist to accomplish this operation and may be obtained from their respective manufacturers. But this regulations will specifically refer to Sartorius as an example(Figure 1 – 1).

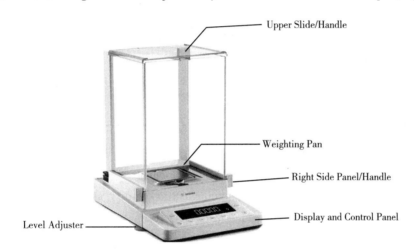

Upper Slide/Handle

Weighting Pan

Right Side Panel/Handle

Display and Control Panel

Level Adjuster

Figure 1 – 1   The electronic analytical balance of Sartorius

3.1   Description of the electronic analytical balance

The most important parts of the balance include a weighing pan, a balance door, a display, a control panel, the level indicator and leveling screws.

3.2   Location

The accuracy or reliability of weighing results is closely associated with the location of the balance. The weighing bench should not sag and should transmit as few vibrations as possible. If necessary, place the balance on a heavy block of antimagnetic material, such as stone(NOT a steel plate). The balance should be protected against electrostatic charges(no plastic or glass), and kept a certain distance from the wall(to prevent the impact of the balance due to wall or floor vibration).

3.3   Choosing a weighing vessel

A beaker may be appropriate for weighing liquids to be heated, and a conical flask may be appropriate for weighing substances that will generate a gas in subsequent reactions. A plastic weighing pan(evaporating dish) can only be used for weighing solids. Weighing paper may also be used for small quantities of solids.

Always use the smallest possible weighing vessel.

Be sure that the weighing vessel is clean and dry. Contaminants adhering to the vessel will cause its weighing result to be abnormally high.

3.4　Start-up

Inspect the balance for scattered chemicals on or near the balance. Using a dedicated balance cleaning brush to clean the weighing pan and the inside of the balance box. Do check for chemicals under the balance pan by lifting it vertically off the pedestal. Brush the chemicals out and carefully replace the pan upon the pedestal.

Check that the air bubble is in the center of the level and,if necessary,correct this by turning the leveling feet.

Make sure the balance is plugged in.

Close all balance doors. Lightly press the control button down and then release. Immediately the digital mass display will show the following for a few seconds.

$$\boxed{8.8.8.8.8.8.8.8. \text{ g}}$$

This display will then be automatically followed by

$$\boxed{0.0000 \qquad\qquad \text{g}}$$

This cycle will normally take place only when turning on the balance. If 0.0000g is not displayed or is slow in its appearance on the digital mass display,it should be confirmed whether the balance is in a shock－proof and air－proof environment to ensure a stable zero point.

Before using,leave the balance connected to the power supply and switched on for some time, so that a thermal equilibrium can be established.

3.5　Taring and taking readings

Choose the right range,place weighing vessel on balance pan. Close all balance doors.

Push on the large,red square labeled "Tare",if re-zeroing is necessary. Repeat until only zeros are on the display.

Place the sample in the center of the pan or in the container.

It can be read when the display reading is stable and shows the weight unit g (mg). Read (record)the mass,remove the sample from the pan.

3.6　Cleaning up and shutting down the balance

Before leaving the balance,use a brush to clean up all solids from the balance pan,and wipe up any liquids.

When you have finished cleaning the area,it is courteous to close the balance doors and re-zero the display so that the balance is ready for the next person to use.

3.7　Notes

The extra material in the weighing process should be recycled to a waste liquid tank and can not be returned to the original container to avoid contamination of the entire bottle of reagents.

Close the balance door while weighing an object in order to prevent air currents from disturbing the reading. When finished, the operator should close the balance door to prevent dust and dirt from entering the balance.

Do not handle objects to be weighed with bare hands. Moisture, grease and dirt on your fingers will affect the weight of the objects.

To be weighed accurately, all objects must be at room temperature. A warm object sets up convection currents inside the balance enclosure, which will make an object appear lighter than it really is. Also, warm air inside the enclosure is less dense than the air that it displaces, which also leads to a negative determinate error.

Never weigh chemicals directly in contact with the balance pan. Use containers, such as beakers, flasks or weighing bottles.

All objects and materials that have recently been removed from a desiccator will absorb moisture and thereby gain weight. It is therefore good practice to record weights after identical time intervals. For example, if you are taking crucibles to constant weight, always record the weight of the crucible exactly 5 seconds after having placed it on the balance pan. In this way, it is possible to minimize the effect of moisture absorption.

Do not spill chemicals inside the balance enclosure. If a spill occurs, clean it up immediately.

第三节　有效数字的修约

一、有效数字

有效数字应反映结果的精确度，有效数字位数越多，精确度越高。有效数字表明数据中有意义的信息。

二、有效数字位数确定

如果数据中有欠准确的数值位数，那么该数据最好用科学计数法表示（例如，$x.xxx \times 10^y$）。

1. 示例

试说明下面的测定值有多少位有效数字：

（1）水中铜离子浓度是 0.00000572mol/L。

（2）血浆中葡萄糖的浓度是 5.0mmol/L。

（3）硝酸铵的质量是 5.20g。

2. 解决方案

（1）铜离子浓度，0.00000572mol/L，用科学计数法表示为 5.72×10^{-6} mol/L，共有 3 位有效数字。

（2）葡萄糖的浓度，5.0 mmol/L，用科学计数法表示为 5.0×10^{-3} mol/L，共有 2 位有效数字。

（3）硝酸铵的质量，5.20g 等同于 5200mg，用科学计数法表示为 5.20×10^3 mg，共有 3

位有效数字。

3. 注解

铜离子浓度 0.00000572mol/L 中"5"之前所有的"0"仅用于定位小数点位置，而不作为有效数字。可以通过改变单位来改变有效数字的数值。

在血糖样品中"0"作为原始数据给出，说明实验中已知葡萄糖的浓度数值为 5.0，而不是 5.1 或 4.9，但可能是 4.95 到 5.04 间的某个值。

对于硝酸铵的质量 5200mg，不知道其中的两个 0 是不是有效数字，因此假设不管是不是，都认为有效数字只有 2 位。质量表达为 5.20g，说明 5200mg 的第一个 0 是有效数字，而第二个 0 不是。单位的前缀带上 m 或 μ，是科学计数法的一种方式。

三、有效数字的位数

在现代仪器分析中，测定数值通常采用数字化方式输出。即使真正的有效位数不明确，也应全部采用，只在最后书写结果时才四舍五入到合适的有效数字位数。可以利用电子表格进行计算，而不管中间过程的有效数字，在最后结果表达时才进行有效数字的修约过程。为了正确表达数据，必须知道测定的不确定度。这可能取决于分析者的知识、经验、常识及重复测定的标准偏差。

例如，以毫米为刻度单位的 30cm 的尺测定 10cm 的长度，测定结果准确到毫米或半毫米是合理的（如 10.3cm 或 10.25cm）。如果结果的标准偏差已知，或按 95% 的置信区间计算，这对有效数字的位数保留有指导作用。

标准偏差和不确定度应表达为两位有效数字。

用相同的数量级表达结果（例如，10 的次幂，小数点的位置）。

因此，如果在滴定反应中的乙酸浓度测定结果是 0.1146mol/L，95% 的置信区间为 0.0096mol/L，那么乙酸的浓度可表达为（0.1146 ± 0.0096）mol/L（95% 置信区间），而如果不确定度为 0.011mol/L，那么乙酸的浓度表达为（0.115 ± 0.011）mol/L（95% 置信区间）。

Section 3　Rounding of Significant Figures

1. Significant figures

The significant figures should tell something about the precision of the result. The more figures quoted, the greater the implied precision.

Significant figures are those imparting useful information.

2. Counting significant figures

If there are inaccurate numerical digits in the data, then the number of significant figures is best determined by writing the result in scientific notation (i. e., $x.xxx \times 10^y$) and counting the digits.

2.1　Example

State how many significant figures are there in the following measured amounts:

The concentration of copperion in water is 0.00000572mol/L.

The concentration of glucose in blood is 5. 0mmol/L.

The mass of ammonium nitrate is 5. 20g.

2. 2　Solution

Expressing the concentration of copper ion in scientific notation, 0. 00000572mol/L becomes 5.72×10^{-6} mol/L. Hence there are three significant figures, the one digit before the decimal point and the two digits after the decimal point.

The 5. 0mmol/L concentration of glucose in blood can be revoiced as 5.0×10^{-3} mol/L and therefore the number of significant figures is two.

5. 20g of ammonium nitrate is equivalent to 5200mg. Expressed in scientific notation, the mass is 5.20×10^{3} mg with three significant figures.

2. 3　Annotation

In the copper ion concentration of 0. 00000572mol/L, the zeros before the 5 do not count as significant figures because the zeros are only being used to locate the decimal point. If this were not the case, we could simply alter the number of significant figures by changing our units.

In the blood glucose example, the zero is counted as it is listed in the original value, which suggests we know the glucose concentration is 5. 0, not 5. 1 or 4. 9. However, we do not know whether 5. 0 is really 5. 01 or somewhere between 4. 95 and 5. 04.

Note that with the mass of ammonium nitrate being 5200mg we have no idea whether either of the two zeros is significant or not, and therefore, we would make the assumption that neither is significant and we would conclude there are only two significant figures. The expression of the mass as 5. 20g, however, tells us that the first zero is significant as it is included in the scientific notation and that the second is not. The use of units with prefixes, such as m or μ is a way of applying scientific notation.

3. The number of significant figures of significant figures

For a measurement made by a modern instrument, the figures are usually put out digitally and should be used as given even if it is not clear that all are really significant. It is only when finally writing the result that the number should be rounded to an appropriate number of significant figures. Let the spreadsheet do all the calculations and leave any concerns about significant figures until the end when the final result is required.

To decide what the correct number is, it is necessary to know about the uncertainty of the measurement. This may be derived from the analyst's knowledge, experience or common sense, or may be determined from the standard deviation of repeated experiments.

For example, the use of a 30cm ruler, graduated in millimeters, to measure a length of about 10cm, will be reasonably given to the nearest millimeter or half millimeter (e. g. , 10. 3cm or 10. 25cm). If the standard deviation of a result is known, or if a 95% confidence interval has been calculated, this is a guide to the number of significant figures.

Write the standard deviation or uncertainty to two significant figures.

Then write the result to the same order of magnitude(i. e. , powers of 10, or decimal places).

Therefore, if the concentration of acetic acid in the titration competition was determined as 0. 1146mol/L with a 95% confidence interval of 0. 0096mol/L, then we could state the value of the concentration of acetic acid as (0.1146 ± 0.0096) mol/L (95% confidence interval). If the uncertainty was 0.011mol/L, then the concentration would be expressed as(0.115 ± 0.011) mol/L (95% confidence interval).

第四节　一般性规定

一、药品的外观、臭、味以及溶解度等

1. 外观性状是对药品的色泽和外表感观的规定。

2. 溶解度是药品的一种物理性质。各品种项下选用的部分溶剂及其在该溶剂中的溶解性能可供精制或制备溶液时参考；对在特定溶剂中的溶解性能需做质量控制时，在该品种检查项下另作具体规定。药品的近似溶解度表示为以下几种。

极易溶解	系指溶质 1g（ml）能在溶剂不到 1ml 中溶解；
易溶	系指溶质 1g（ml）能在溶剂 1 ~ 不到 10ml 中溶解；
溶解	系指溶质 1g（ml）能在溶剂 10 ~ 不到 30ml 中溶解；
略溶	系指溶质 1g（ml）能在溶剂 30 ~ 不到 100ml 中溶解；
微溶	系指溶质 1g（ml）能在溶剂 100 ~ 不到 1000ml 中溶解；
极微溶解	系指溶质 1g（ml）能在溶剂 1000 ~ 不到 10000ml 中溶解；
几乎不溶或不溶	系指溶质 1g（ml）在溶剂 10000ml 中不能完全溶解。

试验法：除另有规定外，称取研成细粉的供试品或量取液体供试品，置于 25℃ ±2℃ 一定容量的溶剂中，每隔 5min 强力振摇 30s；观察 30min 内的溶解情况，如无目视可见的溶质颗粒或液滴时，即视为完全溶解。

二、纯度和限度数值

包括上限和下限两个数值本身及中间数值。规定的这些数值不论是百分数，还是绝对数字，其最后一位数字都是有效位。

在运算过程中，可比规定的有效数字多保留一位数，然后根据有效数字的修约规则进舍至规定有效位。计算所得的最后数值或测定读数值均可按修约规则进舍至规定的有效位，取此数值与标准中规定的限度数值比较，以判断是否符合规定的限度。

除另有注明外，均按质量计。如规定上限为 100% 以上时，系指用规定的分析方法测定时可能达到的数值，它为规定的限度或允许偏差，并非真实含有量；如未规定上限时，系指不超过 101.0%。

制剂的含量限度范围系根据主药含量的多少、测定方法误差、生产过程不可避免的偏差和贮存期间可能产生降解的可接受程度而制定，生产中应按标示量 100% 投料。如已知某一成分在生产或贮存期间含量会降低，生产时可适当增加投料量，以保证在有效期内含量能符合规定。

三、计量单位

1. 法定计量单位名称和单位符号如下。

长度　　　　米（m）　分米（dm）　厘米（cm）　毫米（mm）　微米（μm）

　　　　　　　纳米（nm）

体积　　　升（L）　毫升（ml）　微升（μl）

质量　　　千克（kg）　克（g）　毫克（mg）　微克（μg）　纳克（ng）　皮克（pg）

物质的量　摩尔（mol）　毫摩尔（mmol）

压力　　　兆帕（MPa）　千帕（kPa）　帕（Pa）

温度　　　摄氏度（℃）

动力黏度　帕秒（Pa·s）　毫帕秒（mPa·s）

运动黏度　平方米每秒（m^2/s）　平方毫米每秒（mm^2/s）

波数　　　厘米的倒数（cm^{-1}）

密度　　　千克每立方米（kg/m^3）　克每立方厘米（g/cm^3）

放射性活度　吉贝可（GBq）　兆贝可（MBq）　千贝可（kBq）　贝可（Bq）

　　2. 本书使用的滴定液和试液的浓度，以 mol/L（摩尔/升）表示者，其浓度要求精密标定的滴定液用"XXX 滴定液（YYYmol/L）"表示；作其他用途无需精密标定其浓度时，用"YYYmol/L XXX 溶液"表示，以示区别。

　　3. 有关温度的描述，一般以下列名词术语表示。

水浴温度　　　　　　除另有规定外，均指 98～100℃

热水　　　　　　　　系指 70～80℃

微温或温水　　　　　系指 40～50℃

室温（常温）　　　　系指 10～30℃

冷水　　　　　　　　系指 2～10℃

冰浴　　　　　　　　系指约 0℃

放冷　　　　　　　　系指放冷至室温

　　4. 百分比用 % 符号表示，系指质量的比例；溶液的百分比，除另有规定外，系指溶液 100ml 中含有溶质若干克；乙醇的百分比，系指在 20℃时容量的比例。此外，可根据需要采用下列符号。

%（g/g）　　　　　　表示溶液 100g 中含有溶质若干克

%（ml/ml）　　　　　表示溶液 100ml 中含有溶质若干毫升

%（ml/g）　　　　　 表示溶液 100g 中含有溶质若干毫升

%（g/ml）　　　　　 表示溶液 100ml 中含有溶质若干克

　　5. 缩写 ppm 表示百万分比，系指质量或体积的比例。

　　6. 缩写 ppb 表示十亿分比，系指质量或体积的比例。

　　7. 液体的滴，系指在 20℃时，以 1.0ml 水为 20 滴进行换算。

　　8. 溶液后记示的（1→10）等符号，系指固体溶质 1.0g 或液体溶质 1.0ml 加溶剂使成 10ml 的溶液；未指明用何种溶剂时，均系指水溶液；两种或两种以上液体的混合物，名称间用半字线（－）隔开，其后括号内所示的（:）符号系指各液体混合时的体积（质量）比例。

　　9.《中国药典》所用药筛，选用国家标准的 R40/3 系列，分等如下。

筛号	筛孔内径（平均值）	目号
一号筛	2000μm±70μm	10 目

二号筛	850μm ±29μm	24 目
三号筛	355μm ±13μm	50 目
四号筛	250μm ±9.9μm	65 目
五号筛	180μm ±7.6μm	80 目
六号筛	150μm ±6.6μm	100 目
七号筛	125μm ±5.8μm	120 目
八号筛	90μm ±4.6μm	150 目
九号筛	75μm ±4.1μm	200 目

粉末的分等如下。

最粗粉　　指能全部通过一号筛，但混有能通过三号筛不超过20%的粉末

粗　粉　　指能全部通过二号筛，但混有能通过四号筛不超过40%的粉末

中　粉　　指能全部通过四号筛，但混有能通过五号筛不超过60%的粉末

细　粉　　指能全部通过五号筛，并含能通过六号筛不少于95%的粉末

最细粉　　指能全部通过六号筛，并含能通过七号筛不少于95%的粉末

极细粉　　指能全部通过八号筛，并含能通过九号筛不少于95%的粉末

10. 乙醇未指明浓度时，均系指95%（ml/ml）的乙醇。

四、取样量的准确度和试验精度

1. 试验中供试品与试药等"称重"或"量取"的量，均以阿拉伯数字表示，其精确度可根据数值的有效数位来确定，如称取"0.1g"，系指称取质量可为 0.06 ~ 0.14g；称取"2g"，系指称取质量可为 1.5 ~ 2.5g；称取"2.0g"，系指称取质量可为 1.95 ~ 2.05g；称取"2.00g"，系指称取质量可为 1.995 ~ 2.005g。遵循"四舍六入五成双"的原则。

"精密称定"系指称取质量应准确至所取质量的千分之一；"称定"系指称取质量应准确至所取质量的百分之一；"精密量取"系指量取体积的准确度应符合国家标准中对该体积移液管的精确度要求；"量取"系指可用量筒或按照量取体积的有效数位选用量具。取用量为"约"若干时，系指取用量不得超过规定量的 ±10%。

2. 恒重，除另有规定外，系指供试品连续两次干燥或炽灼后称量的差异在 0.3mg 以下的质量；干燥至恒重的第二次及以后各次称重均应在规定条件下继续干燥 1h 后进行；炽灼至恒重的第二次称重应在继续炽灼 30min 后进行。

3. 试验中规定"按干燥品（或无水物，或无溶剂）计算"时，除另有规定外，应取未经干燥（或未去水，或未去溶剂）的供试品进行试验，并将计算中的取用量按检查项下测得的干燥失重（或水分，或溶剂）扣除。

4. 试验中的"空白试验"系指在不加供试品或以等量溶剂替代供试液的情况下按同法操作所得的结果；含量测定中的"并将滴定的结果用空白试验校正"系指按供试品所耗滴定液的量（ml）与空白试验中所耗滴定液量（ml）之差进行计算。

5. 试验时的温度，未注明者，系指在室温下进行；温度高低对试验结果有显著影响者，除另有规定外，应以 25℃ ±2℃ 为准。

五、试验用水

除另有规定外，试验用水均系指纯化水。酸碱度检查所用的水均系指新沸并放冷的水。

六、酸碱性试验

酸碱性试验，如未指明用何种指示剂，均系指石蕊试纸。

七、原子量

计算相对分子质量以及换算因子等使用的原子量均按最新国际原子量表推荐的原子量。

Section 4　General Notices

1. Appearance, odour, taste and solubility of the drug

1. 1　Appearance of a drug is the requirements of color and external appearance.

1. 2　Solubility refers to the physical property of a drug substance. Solvents described under the monograph and the relevant solubility behaviors are stated for reference for purification or preparation of solution of a drug substance. Requirement should be stated under the item of test of the drug, if specific quality control is needed for the solubility behavior of the solvent accordingly.

Approximate solubilities of drugs are indicated by the following descriptive phases：

Very soluble indicates that 1g(ml) of solute is soluble in less than 1ml of solvent.

Freely soluble indicates that 1g(ml) of solute is soluble in 1ml to less than 10ml of solvent.

Soluble indicates that 1g(ml) of solute is soluble in 10ml to less than 30ml of solvent.

Sparingly soluble indicates that 1g(ml) of solute is soluble in 30ml to less than 100ml of solvent.

Slightly soluble indicates that 1g(ml) of solute is soluble in 100ml to less than 1000ml of solvent.

Very slightly soluble indicates that 1g(ml) of solute is soluble in 1000ml to less than 10000ml of solvent.

Practical insoluble indicates that 1g(ml) of solute is not soluble completely in 10000ml of solvent.

Testing method：unless otherwise specified, weigh out finely powdered sample or measure an amount of liquid sample, place the sample in a certain volume of the solvent at a temperature of 25℃ ± 2℃, shake strongly for 30s at an interval of 5min. Observe the solubility behavior for 30min. It is considered to be completely soluble if none of the particles or droplets of the solute is observed.

2. Limits of purity and content

Purity requirements and limits of purity of a drug substance as well as the weight (or content) variation of a preparation or dosage form stated in the monograph concerned include the values of upper and lower limits and the medium value. Whether these values are expressed in percentage or in absolute numerical value, the last decimal is a significant value.

In calculating testing result, the last effective figure is measured in one decimal place more than the significant decimal place indicated in the requirement and round up or down to the specified decimal place by the rule of commensuration, the value obtained is compared with the limits of the standard to determine the conformity with the specified limits.

The percentage content of the drug substance is calculated by weight, unless otherwise specified. If an upper limit of the content of a drug is stated as over 100%, it refers to a value possibly obtained by the assigned assay method in the monograph, representing the limit or permissible deviation stated in this book. If no upper limit is stated, the upper limit is considered to be not more than the equivalent amount of 101.0%.

The limit range of content of a preparation or dosage form is assigned on the basis of contents of active ingredient(s), assay method being applied and possible change occurred in the process of manufacturing and/or storage. A 100% labeled amount of active ingredient(s) should be used in manufacturing process. If a certain active ingredient is known to be lowering its content in the manufacturing process or in the storage period, sufficient amount of active ingredient concerned may be used to ensure that the content of the drug produced or being used in its shelf life complies with the requirements of the Pharmacopoeia.

3. Units of measurement in this book

3.1   The official names and symbols of units of measurement are listed as follows.

Units of length: meter(m), decimeter(dm), millimeter(mm), micrometer(μm), nanometer(nm).

Units of volume: liter(L), milliliter(ml), microliter(μl).

Units of mass(weight): kilogram(kg), gram(g), milligram(mg), microgram(μg), nanogram(ng), picogram(pg).

Units of amount of substance: mole(mol), micromole(mmol).

Units of pressure: megapascal(MPa), kilopascal(kPa), pascal(Pa).

Units of temperature: degree Celsius(℃).

Units of kinetic viscosity: pascal second(Pa·s).

Units of kinematic viscosity: square meter per second(m^2/s), square millimeter per second(mm^2/s).

Units of wave number: reciprocal of centimeter(cm^{-1}).

Units of density: kilogram per cubic meter(kg/m^3), gram per cubic centimeter(g/cm^3).

Units of radioactivity: gigabecquerel(GBq), megabecquerel(MBq), kilobecquerel(kBq), becquerel(Bq).

3.2   Where the strengths or concentrations of the volumetric solutions and test solutions are expressed in terms of mol/L in this book, the expression of "XXX volumetric solution(YYYmol/L)" is adopted for the volumetric solution which should be accurately standardized. The expression of "YYYmol/L XXX solution" is adopted for the solution of other purpose without specific accuracy of their concentration.

3.3   Temperature is expressed in the following terms.

The temperature of a water bath is 98～100℃, unless otherwise specified.

Hot water refers to that at the temperature of 70～80℃.

Slightly warm or *Warm water* refers to that at the temperature of 40 ~ 50℃.

Room temperature refers to the temperature of 10 ~ 30℃.

Cold water refers to that at the temperature of 2 ~ 10℃.

Ice bath refers to bath temperature at about 0℃.

Allow to cool indicates that the object is cooled to room temperature.

3.4　The symbol used for the expression of percentage is %, usually by weight, but the percentage of solutions, unless otherwise specified, refers to the number of grams of solute in 100ml of the solution. The percentage of ethanol refers to the percentage by volume at 20℃.

The following symbols may be used when necessary.

%(g/g) expresses the number of grams of a solute in 100g of solution.

%(ml/ml) expresses the number of milliliters of a solute in 100ml of solution.

%(ml/g) expresses the number of milliliters of a solute in 100g of solution.

%(g/ml) expresses the number of grams of a solute in 100ml of solution.

3.5　The ppm refers to the abbreviation of part per million, the proportion of the weight or volume.

3.6　The ppb refers to the abbreviation of part per billion, the proportion of the weight or volume.

3.7　The drop of a liquid refers to 1.0ml of water being equivalent to 20 drops at the temperature of 20℃.

3.8　The expression (1→10) stated under the solution refers to the solution of 10ml produced by adding sufficient quantity of solvent to dissolve 1.0g or 1.0ml of a solute. It is understood to be aqueous solution, if the solvent is not specified. If two or more solvents are used as a mixture, a hyphen is inserted between different solvents indicated by names; the following parenthesis expresses the proportion of each solvent by volume(or weight) in the mixture.

3.9　Sieves of Chinese National Standard R40/3 series are adopted in the book and the numbers are assigned as follows.

Sieve No.	Average internal diameter of aperture(μm)	Mesh No.
1	2000 ± 70	10
2	850 ± 29	24
3	355 ± 13	50
4	250 ± 9.9	65
5	180 ± 7.6	80
6	150 ± 6.6	100
7	125 ± 5.8	120
8	90 ± 4.6	150
9	75 ± 4.1	200

Powders are graded as follows：

Very coarse　　All particles pass through sieve No.1, not more than 20% passing through sieve No.3.

Coarse	All particles pass through sieve No. 2, not more than 40% passing through sieve No. 4.
Medium	All particles pass through sieve No. 4, not more than 60% passing through sieve No. 5.
Fine	All particles pass through sieve No. 5, not less than 95% passing through sieve No. 6.
Very fine	All particles pass through sieve No. 6, not less than 95% passing through sieve No. 7.
Ultra fine	All particles pass through sieve No. 8, not less than 95% passing through sieve No. 9.

3.10　Ethanol refers to that of 95% (ml/ml) in strength, unless otherwise specified.

4. Accuracy of sampling quantity and precision of testing defined

4.1　The quantity obtained by weighing or measuring the substance being examined and reagent being used is expressed in Arabic figures. The required precision is expressed by the significant numerical place. For example, the measurement of 0.1g by weight, refers to that 0.06 ~ 0.14g of the substance being weighed; for 2g, 1.5 ~ 2.5g of the substance may be weighed; for 2.0g, it indicates 1.95 ~ 2.05g of the substance may be weighed; for 2.00g, it indicates that 1.995 ~ 2.005g of the substance may be weighed. That means banker's rounding.

"*Weigh accurately*" indicates that the precision of measurement should be made to an accuracy of 0.1%; "weigh" indicates an accuracy being made to 1%. "*Measure accurately*" indicates the accuracy of the volume being measured complies with the national standard of pipet being used for the measurement of required volume. "*Measure*" indicates that the measuring cylinder or other measuring apparatus being used complies with the requirements for the measurement of volume to the significant numerical place. The word about states that the measuring quantity should not exceed ±10% of the specified quantity.

4.2　Constant weight, unless otherwise specified, indicates that the drying or ignition of a substance or material in two consecutive weightings do not differ by more than 0.3mg. The second and subsequent weighing are made after an additional hour of drying each time under the similar conditions. The second weighing of the substance or material made to constant weight by ignition is made after 30min under similar conditions.

4.3　The expression of "calculated on the dried (anhydrous or solvent free) basis" indicates that, unless otherwise specified, the undried substance or solvent containing the substance is used for the required testing. The result of "loss on drying (moisture or solvent)" should be subtracted from the amount of substance.

4.4　Blank test refers to a test carried out in the similar manner without the substance being examined or using the same amount of solvent instead of the solution being tested. To make any necessary correction of the result with a blank test indicates that the result is calculated by subtracting the number of milliliters of titrant used in the blank test from that consumed in the assay of the substance being examined.

4.5　The temperature for a test is at room temperature whenever the temperature is not stated. In the case that the temperature variation significantly influences the testing result, the test should be carried out at a temperature of 25℃ ±2℃, unless otherwise specified.

5. Test water

Water being used in tests and assays refer to purified waters. Water being used for the test of acidity or alkalinity is of the water freshly boiled and cooled to room temperature.

6. Aicd base experiment

Test for acidity or alkalinity of a solution without the statement of indicator being used refers to that Litmus paper is used.

7. Atomic weights

The atomic weights adopted for calculating the molecular weights and the conversion factors are the values recently published by the International Union of Pure and Applied Chemistry.

第五节　实验记录及报告格式

一、实时、真实、完整的记录

1. 在实验本上实时记录实验过程、现象和数据。
2. 真实反映实验过程中的问题，包括出现的错误。
3. 完整记录实验过程，以便进行原因分析。
4. 认真总结实验中的经验，分析实验成败的原因。

二、报告格式

实 验 名 称

日期：　　　　　　　天气：　　　　　　　实验人：

一、目的

二、实验内容

三、试药与仪器

　　1. 试药（所用的试剂和药品，包括纯度和浓度）。

　　2. 仪器（真实记录所用仪器的品牌、型号）。

四、实验方法

　　可以用流程图表示实验过程。

五、结果与分析

　　1. 记录实验现象、数据及典型示意图等，注意及时记录原始数据，如称样量和滴定体积等。

　　2. 数据计算分析。

六、结论

七、讨论

分析本次实验的成败原因，注意事项等，如有后续实验，则展望改进方向。

Section 5　Experiment Record and Report Format

1. Record real-timely, actually, intactly

1.1　Record the process, phenomena, and data of the experiment on the lab notebook real-timely.

1.2　Record the problems truly, including possible mistakes.

1.3　Record the process intactly, to analysis possible reasons.

1.4　Summarize the experience carefully, and discuss the results.

2. Report format

Title

Date：　　　　　　　　**Weather：**　　　　　　　　**Operator：**

1. Aim

2. Contents

3. Reagents and equipments

3.1　Equipment(record all the equipment actually, including brand and type).

3.2　Reagents (all the reagents and drugs used, including purity and concentration).

4. Method

It can be described as flow diagram.

5. Result and data process

5.1　Record phenomena, data and typical diagram, and record the raw data promptly, such as weight and volume.

5.2　Data process.

6. Conclusion

7. Discuss

Discuss the results, key points, and prospect.

（宋　敏）

第二章 药物的性状、鉴别和检查

Chapter 2 Description，Identification and Tests of Drugs

实验一 葡萄糖的性状、鉴别和检查

一、目的

（1）了解药品鉴别、检查的目的和意义。

（2）掌握药品性状测定方法和性状的正确描述。

（3）掌握药品常用鉴别方法和原理。

（4）掌握药品中一般杂质检查的方法原理和限量计算方法。

二、仪器与试药

1. 仪器

100ml 容量瓶、10ml 离心管、旋光仪、纳氏比色管、试砷瓶。

2. 试药

葡萄糖、葡萄糖注射液。

三、实验方法

（一）葡萄糖

本品为 D－（＋）－吡喃葡萄糖一水合物。

1. 葡萄糖的结构式、分子式、相对分子质量

$$OH \quad O \quad OH \quad OH \quad OH \quad \cdot H_2O$$

（Glucose，$C_6H_{12}O_6 \cdot H_2O$，$M\mathrm{w} = 198.17$）

2. 性状

本品为无色结晶或白色结晶性或颗粒性粉末；无臭，味甜。本品在水中易溶，在乙醇中微溶。

比旋度　取本品约 10g，精密称定，置 100ml 量瓶中，加水适量与氨试液 0.2ml，溶解后用水稀释至刻度，摇匀，放置 10min，在 25℃时依法测定，比旋度为 ＋52.6°至 ＋53.2°。

19

3. 鉴别

（1）取本品约 0.2g，加水 5ml 溶解后，缓缓滴入温热的碱性酒石酸铜试液中，即生成氧化亚铜的红色沉淀。

（2）本品的红外光吸收图谱应与对照的图谱（图 2-1）一致。

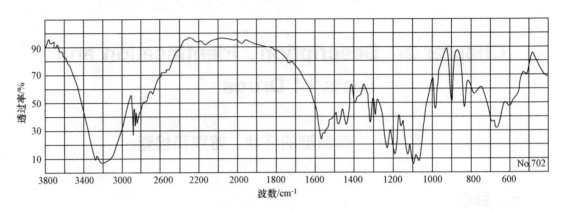

图 2-1 葡萄糖的红外对照图谱

4. 检查

（1）**酸度** 取本品 2.0g，加水 20ml 溶解后加酚酞指示液 3 滴与氢氧化钠滴定液（0.02mol/L）0.20ml，应显粉红色。

（2）**溶液的澄清度与颜色** 取本品 5.0g，加热水溶解后放冷，用水稀释至 10ml，溶液应澄清无色；如显浑浊，与 1 号浊度标准液比较，不得更浓；如显色，与对照液（取比色用氯化钴液 3.0ml、比色用重铬酸钾液 3.0ml 与比色用硫酸铜液 6.0ml，加水稀释成 50ml）1.0ml 加水稀释至 10ml 比较，不得更深。

（3）**乙醇溶液的澄清度** 取本品 1.0g，加乙醇 20ml，置水浴上加热回流约 40min，溶液应澄清。

（4）**氯化物** 取本品 0.6g，依法检查，与标准氯化钠溶液 6.0ml 制成的对照液比较，不得更浓（0.01%）。

（5）**硫酸盐** 取本品 2.0g，依法检查，与标准硫酸钾溶液 2.0ml 制成的对照液比较，不得更浓（0.01%）。

（6）**亚硫酸盐与可溶性淀粉** 取本品 1.0g，加水 10ml 溶解后加碘试液 1 滴，应即显黄色。

（7）**干燥失重** 取本品，在 105℃ 干燥至恒重，减失重量为 7.5%～9.5%。

（8）**炽灼残渣** 不得过 0.1%。

（9）**蛋白质** 取本品 1.0g，加水 10ml 溶解后加磺基水杨酸溶液（1→5）3ml，不得出现沉淀。

（10）**铁盐** 取本品 2.0g，加水 20ml 溶解后加硝酸 3 滴，缓缓煮沸 5min，放冷，加水稀释使成 45ml，加硫氰酸铵溶液（30→100）3ml，摇匀，如显色，与标准铁溶液 2.0ml 用同一方法制成的对照液比较，不得更深（0.001%）。

（11）**重金属** 取本品 4.0g，加水 23ml 溶解后，加乙酸盐缓冲液（pH 3.5）2ml，依法检查，含重金属不得过百万分之五。

（12）**砷盐** 取本品 2.0g，加水 5ml 溶解后加稀硫酸 5ml 与溴化钾溴试液 0.5ml，置水浴上加热约20min，使保持稍过量的溴存在，必要时，再补加溴化钾溴试液适量，并随时补充蒸散的水分，放冷，加盐酸5ml与水适量使成28ml，依法检查，应符合规定（0.0001%）。

（二）葡萄糖注射液

本品为葡萄糖或无水葡萄糖的灭菌水溶液。含葡萄糖（$C_6H_{12}O_6 \cdot H_2O$）应为标示量的95.0%～105.0%。

1. 性状

本品为无色或几乎无色的澄明液体，味甜。

2. 鉴别

取本品，缓缓滴入温热的碱性酒石酸铜试液中，即生成氧化亚铜的红色沉淀。

3. 检查

（1）pH值 取本品或本品适量，用水稀释制成含葡萄糖为5%的溶液，每100ml加饱和氯化钾溶液0.3ml，依法检查，pH值应为3.2～6.5。

（2）5-羟甲基糠醛 精密量取本品适量（约相当于葡萄糖1.0g），置100ml量瓶中，加水稀释至刻度，摇匀，照紫外-可见分光光度法，在284nm的波长处测定，吸收度不得大于0.32。

（3）重金属 取本品适量（约相当于葡萄糖3g），必要时，蒸发至约20ml，放冷，加乙酸盐缓冲液（pH 3.5）2ml与水适量使成25ml，依法检查，按葡萄糖含量计算，含重金属不得过百万分之五。

四、预习提要

（1）纳氏比色管的使用方法。
（2）一般杂质限量的计算方法。
（3）古蔡氏试砷法中使用各试剂的作用。

五、实验指导

（一）旋光度测定法

1. 原理及测定方法

平面偏振光通过含有某些光学活性化合物的液体或溶液时，能引起旋光现象，使偏振光的平面向左或向右旋转。旋转的角度称为旋光度。偏振光透过长1dm且每毫升中含有旋光物质1g的溶液，在一定波长与温度下测得的旋光度，称为比旋度。测定比旋度（或旋光度）可以区别或检查某些药品的纯杂程度，亦可用以测定含量。

除另有规定外，本法系采用钠光谱的D线（589.3nm）测定旋光度，测定管长度为1dm（如使用其他管长，应进行换算）。测定温度为20℃。使用读数至0.01°并检定旋光计。

测定旋光度时，将测定管用供试液体或溶液（取固定供试品，按该品种项下的方法制成）冲洗数次，缓缓注入供试液体或溶液适量（注意勿产生气泡），置于旋光计内检测读数，即得供试液的旋光度，使偏振光向右旋转者（顺时针方向）为右旋，以"＋"符号表示，使偏振光向左旋转者（反时针方向）为左旋，以"－"符号表示。用同法读取旋光度3次，取3次的平均数，照下列公示计算，即得供试品的比旋度。

对液体供试品：
$$[\alpha]_D^{20} = \frac{\alpha}{ld}$$

对固体供试品：
$$[\alpha]_D^{20} = \frac{100\alpha}{lC}$$

式中，$[\alpha]$ 为比旋度；D 为钠光谱的 D 线；α 为测得的旋光度；l 为光路长度（即测定管长度，dm），C 为溶液的浓度（g/100ml）；d 为液体的相对密度。

旋光度可用标准石英旋光管检定，读数误差应符合规定。

2. 注意事项

（1）每次测定前应以溶剂作空白校正，测定后，再校正 1 次，以确定在测定时零点有无变动；如第 2 次校正时发现零点有变动，则应重新测定旋光度。

（2）配制溶液及测定时，均应调节温度至 20℃ ±0.5℃（或各药品项下规定的温度）。

（3）配制溶液的浓度大都根据药品比旋度大小，使配成的测定液旋光度一般应在左旋或右旋 2°~8°范围，测定值太小，读取旋光度时容易造成误差。溶解度小的样品可以例外。用旋光法作含量测定时应称取 2 份做平行试验。

（4）钠光灯启动至少 20min 后发光才能稳定，测定或读数时应在钠光灯稳定后读取，测定时钠光灯尽量使用直流电路供电。测定间隔期间可置于交流供电，以延长钠灯寿命。

（5）测定零点或停点时，必须按动复测按钮数次，使检偏镜分别向左或向右偏离光学零位，以减少仪器的机械误差。同时通过观察左右复测数次的停点，检查仪器的重复性和稳定性，必要时也可用旋光标准石英管校正仪器的准确度。读取零点或停点应重复3次。

（6）供试的液体或固体物质的溶液应不显浑浊或含有混悬的小粒。如有上述情形时，应预先滤过，并弃去初滤液。

（7）往测试管加入供试品溶液时，应反复用供试品溶液冲洗测试管数次，以免供试液浓度改变。装入测定溶液时应避免产生气泡。

（8）有些化合物见光后旋光度变化很大，应绝对避光操作；有些化合物对放置时间有要求（如葡萄糖测定），必须完全按照规定的条件测定读数。

（9）仪器的各个光学镜片应保持干燥清洁，防止灰尘和油污污染，钠灯有一定的使用寿命，连续使用一般不超过 4h，亦不准瞬间内反复开关。

（10）测定结束后测试管必须洗净晾干，以备下次再用，不准许将盛有供试品的测试管长时间放置在仪器的样品室内。仪器不使用时样品室可放硅胶吸潮。

（11）物质的比旋度与测定光源、测定波长、溶剂、浓度和温度等因素有关。因此，表示物质的比旋度时应注明测定条件。

3. 葡萄糖的旋光性

葡萄糖分子结构中含有多个手性碳原子，具有旋光性。《中国药典》2015 年版采用旋光度法测定葡萄糖注射液的含量。本法简便、准确，亦可适用于测定葡萄糖注射液中葡萄糖。

该测定方法须提前加入氨试液，原理是葡萄糖有 α 及 β 两种互变异构体，在水溶液中存在如图 2 - 2 所示的变旋平衡。

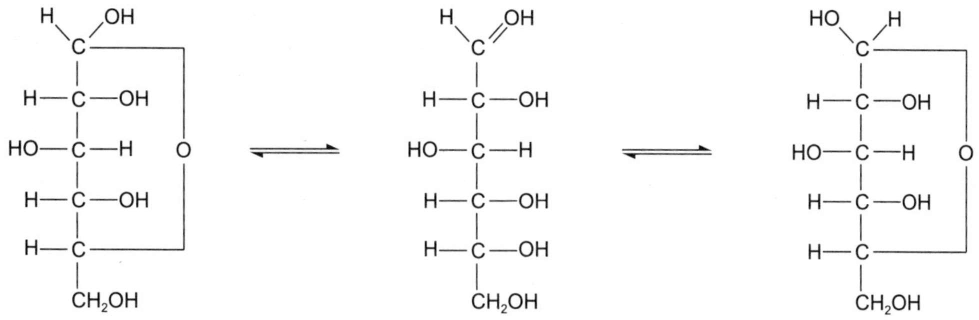

α-D-葡萄糖	醛式-D-葡萄糖	β-D-葡萄糖
$[\alpha]_D^{20}=+113.4^{\circ}$	$[\alpha]_D^{20}=+52.75^{\circ}$	$[\alpha]_D^{20}=+19.7^{\circ}$
（占36%）	（占0.024%）	（占64%）

图 2 - 2 葡萄糖在水溶液中的互变异构体

α 和 β 两种互变异构体的比旋度相差甚远，而在水溶液中两者互变，逐渐平衡，此时的比旋度也趋于恒定，为 + 52.5°～ + 53.0°，这种现象称为葡萄糖的变旋现象。因此，测定葡萄糖旋光度时，应首先使上述反应达到平衡状态，一般放置至少 6 小时。若加热、加酸或加弱碱，均可加速进入平衡状态。《中国药典》采用加氨试液的方法，加速反应变化到达平衡状态。

（二）pH 值测定法

除另有规定外，水溶液的 pH 值应以玻璃电极为指示电极、饱和甘汞电极为参比电极的酸度计进行测定。酸度计应定期进行计量检定，并符合国家有关规定。测定前，应采用标准缓冲液校正仪器，也可用国家标准物质管理部门发放的标示 pH 值准确至 0.01pH 单位的各种标准缓冲液校正仪器。

1. 仪器校正用的标准缓冲液

（1）草酸盐标准缓冲液 精密称取在 54℃ ±3℃ 干燥 4～5h 的草酸三氢钾 12.71g，加水使溶解并稀释至 1000ml。

（2）苯二甲酸盐标准缓冲液 精密称取在 115℃ ±5℃ 干燥 2～3h 的邻苯二甲酸氢钾 10.21g，加水使溶解并稀释至 1000ml。

（3）磷酸盐标准缓冲液 精密称取在 115℃ ±5℃ 干燥 2～3h 的无水磷酸氢二钠 3.55g 与磷酸二氢钾 3.40g，加水使溶解并稀释至 1000ml。

（4）硼砂标准缓冲液 精密称取硼砂 3.81g（注意避免风化），加水使溶解并稀释至 1000ml，置聚乙烯塑料瓶中，密塞，避免空气中二氧化碳进入。

（5）氢氧化钙标准缓冲液 于 25℃ 用无二氧化碳的水制备氢氧化钙的饱和溶液，取上清液使用。存放时应防止空气中二氧化碳进入。一旦出现浑浊，应弃去重配。

这些标准缓冲溶液必须用 pH 值基准试剂配制。不同温度时各种标准缓冲液的 pH 值如表 2 - 1 所示。

表 2-1　不同温度时各标准缓冲液的 pH 值

温度/℃	草酸盐 标准缓冲液	苯二甲酸盐 标准缓冲液	磷酸盐 标准缓冲液	硼砂 标准缓冲液	氢氧化钙 标准缓冲液（25℃）
0	1.67	4.01	6.98	9.64	13.43
5	1.67	4.00	6.95	9.40	13.21
10	1.67	4.00	6.92	9.33	13.00
15	1.67	4.00	6.90	9.28	12.81
20	1.68	4.00	6.88	9.23	12.63
25	1.68	4.01	6.86	9.18	12.45
30	1.68	4.02	6.85	9.14	12.29
35	1.69	4.02	6.84	9.10	12.13
40	1.69	4.04	6.84	9.07	11.98
45	1.70	4.05	6.83	9.04	11.84
50	1.71	4.06	6.83	9.01	11.71
55	1.72	4.08	6.83	8.99	11.57
60	1.72	4.09	6.84	8.96	11.45

2. 注意事项

测定 pH 值时，应严格按仪器的使用说明书操作，并注意下列事项。

（1）测定前，按各品种项下的规定，选择两种 pH 值约相差 3 个 pH 单位的标准缓冲液，并使供试液的 pH 值处于两者之间。

（2）取与供试液 pH 值较接近的第一种标准缓冲液对仪器进行校正（定位），使仪器示值与表列数值一致。

（3）仪器定位后，再用第二种标准缓冲液核对仪器示值，误差应不大于 ±0.02 pH 单位。若大于此偏差，则应小心调节斜率，使示值与第二种标准缓冲液的表列数值相符。重复上述定位与斜率调节操作，至仪器示值与标准缓冲液的规定数值相差不大于 0.02 pH 单位。否则，须检查仪器或更换电极后，再进行校正至符合要求。

（4）每次更换标准缓冲液或供试液前，应用纯化水充分洗涤电极，然后将水吸尽，也可用所换的标准缓冲液或供试液洗涤。

（5）在测定高 pH 值的供试品和标准缓冲液时，应注意碱误差的问题，必要时选用适当的玻璃电极测定。

（6）对弱缓冲液（如水）的 pH 值测定，先用苯二甲酸盐标准缓冲液校正仪器后测定供试液，并重取供试液再测，直至 pH 值的读数在 1min 内改变不超过 ±0.05 止；用硼砂标准缓冲液校正仪器，再如上法测定；二次 pH 值的读数相差不超过 0.1，取二次读数的平均值为其 pH 值。

（7）配制标准缓冲液与溶解供试品的水应是新沸过并放冷的纯化水，其 pH 值应为5.5～7.0。

（8）标准缓冲液一般可保存 2～3 个月，但发现有浑浊、发霉或沉淀等现象时，不能继续使用。

（三）溶液澄清度检查法

本法系在室温条件下，将用水稀释至一定浓度的供试品溶液与等量的浊度标准液分别置于配对的比浊用玻璃管（内径 15~16mm，平底，具塞，以无色、透明、中性硬质玻璃制成）中，在浊度标准液制备 5min 后，在暗室内垂直同置于伞棚灯下，照度为 1000lx，从水平方向观察、比较，用以检查溶液的澄清度或其浑浊程度。除另有规定外，供试品溶解后应立即检视。

品种项下规定的"澄清"系指供试品溶液的澄清度相同于所用溶剂，或未超过 0.5 号浊度标准液。

（1）浊度标准比色液的制备　称取于 105℃ 干燥至恒重的硫酸肼 1.00g，置 100ml 量瓶中，加水适量使溶解，必要时可在 40℃ 的水浴中温热溶解，并用水稀释至刻度，摇匀，放置 4~6h；取此溶液与等量的 10% 乌洛托品混合，摇匀，于 25℃ 避光静置 24h，即得。本液置冷处避光保存，可在两个月内使用，用前摇匀。

（2）浊度标准原液的制备　取浊度标准储备液 15.00ml，置 1000ml 量瓶中，加水稀释至刻度，摇匀，取适量，置 1cm 吸收池中，照紫外 - 可见分光光度法（《中国药典》四部通则 0401），在 550nm 的波长处测定，其吸光度应在 0.12~0.15 范围内。本液应在 48h 内使用，用前摇匀。

（3）浊度标准液的制备　取浊度标准原液与水，按表 2-2 配制，即得。本液应临用时制备，使用前充分摇匀。

表 2-2　浊度标准液的制备

级号	0.5	1	2	3	4
浊度标准原液/ml	2.50	5.0	10.0	30.0	50.0
水/ml	97.50	95.0	90.0	70.0	50.0

（四）溶液颜色检查法

药物溶液的颜色及其与规定颜色的差异能在一定程度上反应药物的纯度。本法将药物溶液的颜色与规定的标准比色液相比较，或规定的波长处测定其吸光度，以检查其颜色。

品种项下规定的"无色或几乎无色"，其"无色"系指供试品溶液的颜色相同于所用溶剂，"几乎无色"系指浅于用水稀释 1 倍后的相应色调 1 号标准比色液。

1. 第一法

除另有规定外，取各品种项下规定量的供试品，加水溶解，置于 25ml 的纳氏比色管中，加水稀释至 10ml。另取规定色调和色号的标准比色液 10ml，置于另一 25ml 的纳氏比色管中，两管同置白色背景上，自上向下透视，或同置白色背景前，平视观察；供试品呈现的颜色与对照管比较，不得更深。如供试品管呈现的颜色与对照管的颜色深浅非常接近或色调不尽一致，使目视观察无法辨别两者的深浅时，应改用第三法（色差计法）测定，并将其测定结果作为判定依据。

（1）比色用重铬酸钾液　精密称取在 120℃ 干燥至恒重的基准重铬酸钾 0.4000g，置 500ml 量瓶中，加适量水溶液并稀释至刻度，摇匀，即得。每毫升溶液中含 0.8000mg 的重铬酸钾（$K_2Cr_2O_7$）。

（2）比色用硫酸铜液　取硫酸铜约 32.5g，加适量的盐酸溶液（1→40）使溶解成 500ml，精密量取 10ml，置碘量瓶中，加水 50ml、乙酸 4ml 与碘化钾 2g，用硫代硫酸钠滴定液（0.1mol/L）滴定，至近终点时，加淀粉指示液 2ml，继续滴定至蓝色消失。每毫升硫代硫酸钠滴定液（0.1mol/L）相当于24.97mg的$CuSO_4 \cdot 5H_2O$。根据上述测定结果，在剩余的原溶液中加适量的盐酸溶液（1→40），使每毫升溶液中含62.4mg的$CuSO_4 \cdot 5H_2O$，即得。

（3）比色用氯化钴液　取氯化钴约32.5g，加适量的盐酸溶液（1→40）使溶解成500ml，精密量取2ml，置锥形瓶中，加水200ml，摇匀，加氨试液至溶液由浅红色转变至绿色后，加乙酸-乙酸钠缓冲液（pH 6.0）10ml，加热至60℃，再加二甲酚橙指示液5滴，用乙二胺四乙酸钠滴定液（0.05mol/L）滴定至溶液成黄色，每毫升乙二胺四乙酸钠滴定液（0.05mol/L）相当于11.90mg的$CoCl_2 \cdot 6H_2O$。根据上述测定结果，在剩余的原溶液中加适量的盐酸溶液（1→40），使每毫升溶液中含59.5mg的$CoCl_2 \cdot 6H_2O$，即得。

（4）各种色调标准储备液的制备　按表2-3量取比色用氯化钴液、比色用重铬酸钾液、比色用硫酸铜液与水，摇匀，即得。

表2-3　各种色调标准储备液的配制表

色调	比色用氯化钴溶液/ml	比色用重铬酸钾溶液/ml	比色用硫酸铜溶液/ml	水/ml
黄绿色	1.2	22.8	7.2	68.8
黄色	4.0	23.3	0	72.7
橙黄色	10.6	19.0	4.0	66.4
橙红色	12.0	20.0	0	68.0
棕红色	22.5	12.5	20.0	45.0

（5）各种色调色号标准比色液的制备　按表2-4量取各色调标准储备液与水，摇匀，即得。

表2-4　各种色号调标准比色液的配制表

色号	1	2	3	4	5	6	7	8	9	10
贮备液/ml	0.5	1.0	1.5	2.0	2.5	3.0	4.5	6.0	7.5	10.0
加水量/ml	9.5	9.0	8.5	8.0	7.5	7.0	5.5	4.0	2.5	0

2. 第二法

除另有规定外，取各品种项下规定量的供试品，加水溶解成10ml，必要时滤过，滤液照分光光度法与规定波长处测定，吸光度不得超过规定值。

3. 第三法（色差法）

本法是通过色差计直接测定溶液的透射值，对其颜色进行定量表述和分析的方法。当目视比色法较难于判定供试品与标准比色液之间的差异时，应考虑采用本法进行测定与判断。

供试品与标准比色液之间的颜色差异可以通过分别比较它们与水之间的色差值来得到，也可以通过直接比较它们之间的色差值来得到。

（五）氯化物检查法

除另有规定外，取各品种项下规定量的供试品，加水溶解成25ml（溶液如显碱性，可滴加硝酸，使之呈中性），再加稀硝酸10ml；溶液如不澄清，应滤过；置50ml纳氏比色管中，加水成约40ml，摇匀，即得供试溶液。另取该品种向下规定量的标准氯化钠溶液，置

50ml 纳氏比色管中，加稀硝酸10ml，加水成40ml，摇匀，即得对照溶液。于供试品溶液与对照溶液中，分别加入硝酸银溶液1.0ml，用水稀释成50ml，摇匀，在暗处放置5min，同置黑色背景上，从比色管上方向下观察、比较，即得。

供试溶液如带颜色，除另有规定外，可取供试溶液两份，分置50ml 纳氏比色管中，一份中加硝酸银试液1.0ml，摇匀，放置10min，如显浑浊，可反复滤过，至滤液完全澄清，再加规定量的标准氯化钠溶液与水适量成50ml，摇匀，在暗处放置5min，作为对照溶液；另一份中加硝酸银试液1.0ml 与水适量成50ml，摇匀，在暗处放置5min，按上述方法与对照溶液比较，即得。

标准氯化钠溶液的制备　称取氯化钠0.165g，置1000ml 量瓶中，加水适量，使溶解并稀释至刻度，摇匀，作为储备液。

临用前，精密量取储备液10ml，置100ml 量瓶中，加水稀释至刻度，摇匀，即得（每毫升相当于10μg 的 Cl）。

用滤纸滤过时，滤纸中如含有氯化物，可预先用含有硝酸的水溶液洗净后使用。

（六）炽灼残渣检查法

取供试品1.0～2.0g 或各品种项下规定的质量，置已炽灼至恒重的坩埚（如供试品分子中含有碱金属元素或氟元素，则应使用铂坩埚）中，精密称定，缓缓炽灼至完全炭化，放冷；除另有规定外，加硫酸0.5～1ml 使湿润，低温加热至硫酸蒸气除尽后在700～800℃炽灼至完全灰化，移至干燥器内，放冷，精密称定后在700～800℃炽灼至恒重，即得。

如须将残渣留作重金属检查，则炽灼温度必须控制在500～600℃。

（七）重金属检查法

重金属系指在规定条件下能与硫代乙酰胺或硫化钠作用显色的金属杂质。

标准铅溶液的制备　称取硝酸铅0.160g，置1000ml 量瓶中，加硝酸5ml 与水50ml 溶解后，用水稀释至刻度，摇匀，作为储备液。

临用前，精密量取储备液10ml，置100ml 量瓶中，加水稀释至刻度，摇匀，即得（每毫升相当于10μg 的 Pb）。

配置与储存的用的玻璃容器不得含铅。

1. 第一法

除另有规定外，取25ml 纳氏比色管两支，甲管中加一定量标准铅溶液与乙酸盐缓冲液（pH 3.5）2ml 后，加水或各品种项下规定的溶剂稀释成25ml，乙管中加入按该品种项下规定的方法制成的供试品溶液25ml。若供试品带颜色，可在甲管中滴加少量的稀焦糖溶液或其他无干扰的有色溶液，使之与乙管一致；在甲乙两管中分别加硫代乙酰胺试液各2ml，摇匀，放置2min，同置白纸上，自上向下透视，乙管中显示的颜色与甲管比较，不得更深。

如在甲管中滴加稀焦糖溶液仍不能使颜色一致时，可取该品种项下规定的两倍量的供试品和试液，加水或该品种项下规定的溶剂成30ml，将溶液分成甲乙两等份，乙管中加水或该品种项下规定的溶剂稀释成25ml；甲管中加入硫代乙酰胺试液2ml，摇匀，放置2min，经滤膜（孔径3μm）滤过，然后甲管中加入标准铅溶液一定量，加水或该品种项下规定的溶剂成25ml；分别在乙管中加硫代乙酰胺试液2ml，甲管中加水2ml，照上述方法比较，即得。供试品如含高铁盐影响重金属检查时，可取该品种项下规定方法制成的供试品溶液，加抗坏血酸0.5～1.0g，并在对照溶液中加入相同量的抗坏血酸，再照上述方法检查。

配制供试品溶液时，如使用的盐酸超过 1.0ml（或与盐酸 1.0ml 相当的稀盐酸），氨试液超过 2ml，或加入其他试剂进行处理者，除另有规定外，对照溶液中应取同样同量的试剂置瓷皿中蒸干，加乙酸盐缓冲液（pH 3.5）2ml 与水 15ml，微热溶解后，移至纳氏比色管中，加标准铅溶液一定量，再用水稀释成 25ml。

2. 第二法

除另有规定外，取该品种炽灼残渣项下遗留的残渣，加硝酸 0.5ml，蒸干，至氧化氮蒸气除尽后（或取供试品一定量，缓缓炽灼至完全炭化，放冷，加硫酸 0.5～1.0ml 使恰湿润，用低温加热使硫酸除尽后，加硝酸 0.5ml，蒸干，至氧化氮蒸气除尽，放冷，在 500～600℃炽灼使完全灰化），放冷，加盐酸 2ml，置水浴上蒸干后加水 15ml，滴加氨试液至对酚酞指示液显中性，再加乙酸盐缓冲液（pH 3.5）2ml，微热溶解后移置纳氏比色管中，加水稀释成 25ml；取配制供试溶液的试剂，置瓷皿中蒸干，加乙酸盐缓冲液（pH 3.5）2ml 与水 15ml，微热溶解后移置纳氏比色管中；加标准铅溶液一定量，再用水稀释成 25ml。照上述第一法检查，即得。

3. 第三法

除另有规定外，取供试品适量，加氢氧化钠试液 5ml，与水 20ml 溶解后置纳氏比色管中，加硫化钠试液 5 滴，摇匀，与一定量的标准铅溶液同样处理后的颜色比较，不得更深。

4. 第四法

仪器装置　滤器由具有螺纹丝扣并能密封的上下两部，以及垫圈、滤膜和尼龙垫网所组成，如图 2-3 所示。

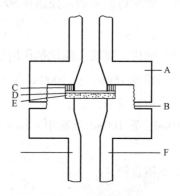

图 2-3　滤器示意图

A. 滤器上盖部分，入口处应能与 50ml 注射器紧密连接；

B. 连接头；C. 垫圈（外径 10mm，内经 6mm）；

D. 滤膜，直径 10mm，孔径 3.0μm，用前在水中浸泡 24h 以上；

E. 尼龙垫网（孔径不限），直径 10mm；F. 滤器下部，出口处套上一合适橡皮管

标准铅斑的制备　精密量取标准铅溶液一定量，置小烧杯中，用水或各品种项下规定的溶剂稀释成 10ml，加入乙酸盐缓冲液（pH 3.5）2ml 与硫代乙酰胺试液 1ml，摇匀，放置 10min，用 50ml 注射器转移至上述滤器中进行压滤（滤速约为每分钟 1ml），滤毕，取下滤膜，放在滤纸上干燥，即得。

检查法　取按各品种项下规定方法制成的供试品溶液 10ml，照标准铅斑的制备，自"加入乙酸盐缓冲液（pH 3.5）2ml"起依法操作，将生成的斑点与标准铅斑比较，不得更深。

若供试溶液有颜色或浑浊，应用滤膜进行预滤，如滤膜上有污染，应换滤膜再滤，直

至滤膜不再染色；取滤液 10ml，照标准铅斑的制备法，自"加入乙酸盐缓冲液（pH 3.5）2ml"起依法操作，并照上述检查法中所述比较，即得。

（八）砷盐检查法

标准砷溶液的制备　称取三氧化二砷 0.132g，置 1000ml 量瓶中，加 20% 氢氧化钠溶液 5ml 溶解后用适量的稀硫酸中和，再加稀硫酸 10ml，用水稀释至刻度，摇匀，作为储备液。

临用前，精密量取储备液 10ml，置 1000ml 量瓶中，加稀硫酸 10ml，用水稀释至刻度，摇匀，即得（每毫升相当于 10μg 的砷）。

1. 第一法（古蔡法）

仪器装置　如图 2-4 所示：A 为 100ml 标准磨口锥形瓶；B 为中空的磨口塞，上连导气管 C（外径 8.0mm，内径 6.0mm），全长约 180mm；D 为具孔的有机玻璃旋塞，其上部为圆形平面，中央有一圆孔，孔径与导气管 C 的内径一致，其下部孔径与导气管 C 的外径相适应，将导气管 C 的顶端套入旋塞下部孔内，并使管壁与旋塞的圆孔相吻合，黏合固定；E 为中央具应有圆孔径（孔径 6.0mm）的有机玻璃旋塞盖，与 D 紧密吻合。

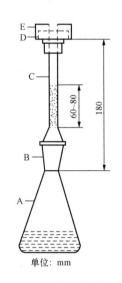

单位：mm

图 2-4　古蔡氏仪器装置图

测试时，于导气管 C 中装入乙酸铅棉花 60mg（装管高度为 60~80mm），再于旋塞 D 的顶端平面上放一片溴化汞试纸（试纸大小以能覆盖孔径而不露出平面外为宜），盖上旋塞盖 E 并旋紧，即得。

标准砷斑的制备　精密量取标准砷溶液 2ml，置 A 瓶中，加盐酸 5ml 与水 21ml，再加碘化钾试液 5ml 与酸性氯化亚锡试液 5 滴，在室温放置 10min 后加锌粒 2g，立即将照上法装妥的导气管 C。密塞于 A 瓶上，并将 A 瓶置 25~40℃ 水浴中，反应 45min，取出溴化汞试纸，即得。

若供试品须经有机破坏后再检砷，则应取标准砷溶液代替供试品，照该品种项下规定的方法同法处理后依法制备标准砷斑。

检查法　取按各品种项下规定方法制成的供试品溶液，置 A 瓶中，照标准铅斑的制备法，自"再加碘化钾试液 5ml"起依法操作。

将生成的砷斑与标准砷斑比较，不得更深。

2. 第二法（二乙基二硫代氨基甲酸银法）

仪器装置　如图 2-5 所示：A 为 100ml 标准磨口锥形瓶；B 为中空的标准磨口塞，上连导气管 C（一端的外径为 8mm，内径为 6mm；另一端长 140mm，外径 4mm，内径 1.6mm，尖端内径为 1mm）；D 为平底玻璃管（长 180mm，内径 10mm，于 5.0ml 处有一刻度）。

测试时，于导气管 C 中装入乙酸铅棉花 60mg（装管高度为 60~80mm），并于 D 管中精密加入二乙基二硫代氨基甲酸银试液 5ml。

标准砷对照液的制备　精密量取标准砷溶液 5ml，置 A 瓶中，加盐酸 5ml 与水 21ml，再加碘化钾试液 5ml 与酸性氯化亚锡试液 5 滴，在室温放置 10min 后加锌粒 2g，立即将导气管 C 与 A 瓶密塞，使生成的砷化氢气体导入 D 管中，并将 A 瓶置 25~40℃ 水浴中反应 45min，取出 D 管，添加三氯甲烷至刻度，混匀，即得。

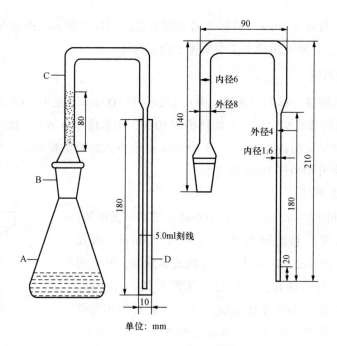

单位：mm

图2-5 二乙基二硫代氨基甲酸银法仪器图

若供试品须经有机破坏后再检砷，则应取标准砷溶液代替供试品，照各品种项下规定的方法同法处理后依法制备标准砷对照液。

检查法 取照各品种项下规定制成的方法供试品溶液，置 A 瓶中，照标准砷对照液的制备法，自"再加碘化钾试液 5ml"起依法操作。将所得溶液与标准砷对照液同置白色背景上，从 D 管上方向下观察、比较，所得溶液的颜色不得比标准砷对照液更深。必要时，可将所得溶液转移至 1cm 吸收池中，照紫外－可见分光光度法在 510nm 波长处以二乙基二硫代氨基甲酸银试液做空白，测定吸光度，与标准砷对照液按同法测得的吸光度比较，即得。

注意

（1）所用仪器和试液等照本法检查，均不应生成砷斑，或至多生成仅可辨认的砷斑痕。

（2）制备标准砷斑或标准砷对照液，应与供试品检查同时进行。

（3）本法所用锌粒应无砷，以能通过一号筛的细粒为宜；如使用的锌粒较大，用量应酌情增加，反应时间亦应延长为 1h。

（4）乙酸铅棉花系取脱脂棉 1.0g，浸入 12ml 乙酸铅试液与水的等容混合液中，湿透后挤压除去过多的溶液，并使之疏松，在 100℃ 以下干燥后，贮于玻璃塞瓶中备用。

（九）干燥失重测定法

取供试品，混合均匀（如为较大的结晶，应先迅速捣碎，使成 2mm 以下的小粒），取约 1g 或各品种项下规定的质量，置与供试品相同条件下干燥至恒重的扁形称量瓶中，精密称定，除另有规定外，在 105℃ 干燥至恒重。由减失的质量和取样量计算供试品的干燥失重。

供试品干燥时，应平铺在扁形称量瓶中，厚度不可超过 5mm，如为疏松物质，厚度不可超过 10mm。放入烘箱或干燥器进行干燥时，应将瓶盖取下，置称量瓶旁，或将瓶盖半开进行干燥；取出时，须将称量瓶盖好。置烘箱内干燥的供试品应在干燥后取出置干燥器中放冷，然后称定质量。

供试品如未达到规定的干燥温度即融化，应先将供试品于较低的温度下干燥至大部分水除去后再按规定条件干燥。

用减压干燥器或恒温减压干燥器时，除另有规定外，压力应在 2.67kPa（20mmHg）以下；干燥器中常用的干燥剂为五氧化二磷，除另有规定外，温度为 60℃。干燥剂应保持在有效状态。

六、讨论

（1）鉴别检查在药品质量控制中的意义及一般杂质检查的主要项目是什么？

（1）比色比浊操作应遵循的原则是什么？

（3）试计算葡萄糖重金属检查中标准铅溶液的取用量。

（4）古蔡试砷法中所加各试剂的作用与操作注意点是什么？

（5）根据样品取用量、杂质限量及标准砷溶液的浓度，计算标准砷溶液的取用量。

（6）炽灼残渣测定的成败关键是什么？什么是恒重？

Experiment 1   Description，Identification and Tests of Glucose

1. Purposes

1.1   To understand the aims and purposes of the drug quality control.

1.2   To learn about the methods for the determination and the special words for the description of the characteristics of drugs.

1.3   To grasp the common methods and principles of drug identification.

1.4   To grasp the priciple and method on purity test and know how to caculate the limits.

2. Instruments and chemical reagents

2.1   Instruments

100ml volumetric flask，10ml centrifuge tube，polarimeter，color comparison tube，arsenic test bottle.

2.2   Chemical reagents

Glucose，glucose injection.

3. Procedures and methods

3.1   Glucose

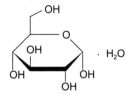

$(C_6H_{12}O_6 \cdot H_2O, M_W = 198.17)$

扫码"学一学"

Glucose is D – (+) – glucopyranose monohydrate.

3. 1. 1　Description　Colorless crystals or a white crystalline or granular powder; odourless; taste, sweet. Freely soluble in water; slightly soluble in ethanol.

3. 1. 2　Specific optical rotation　Dissolve, about 10g, weighed accurately, with a quantity of water and 0. 2ml of ammonia TS in a 100ml volumetric flask and dilute with water to volume. Mix well and allow to stand for 10 minutes. The specific optical rotation of the resulting solution is + 52. 6° ~ + 53. 2° at 25℃.

3. 1. 3　Identification

a. Dissolve about 0. 2g in 5ml of water, add dropwise hot alkaline cupric tartrate TS; a red precipitate of cuprous oxide is produced.

b. The infrared absorption spectrum is concordant with the reference spectrum of glucose (Figure 2 – 1).

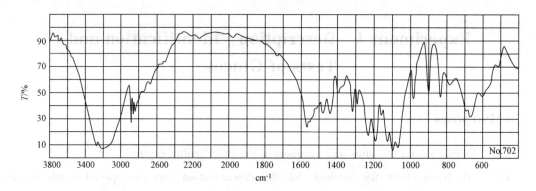

Figure 2 – 1　Reference IR spectrum of glucose

3. 1. 4　Test

Acidity　Dissolve 2. 0g in 20ml of water, add 3 drops of phenolphthalein IS and 0. 20ml of sodium hydroxide(0. 02mol/L)VS; a pink color is produced.

Clarity and color of solution　Dissolve 5. 0g in hot water, cool, dilute to 10ml with water; the solution is clear and colorless. Any opalescence produced is not more pronounced than that of reference suspension 1. Any color produced is not more intense than that of a solution prepared by diluting 1. 0ml of a reference solution(mix 3. 0ml of standard cobaltous chloride CS and 3. 0ml of standard potassium dichromate CS with 6. 0ml of standard copper sulfate CS and add sufficient water to produce 50ml)with water to 10ml.

Clarity of ethanolic solution　To 1. 0g add 20ml of ethanol and reflux on a water bath for about 40 minutes; the solution is clear.

Chloride　Carry out the limit test for chlorides, using 0. 60g. Any opalescence produced is not more pronounced than that of a reference using 6. 0ml of sodium chloride standard solution (0. 01%).

Sulfate　Carry out the limit test for sulfates, using 2. 0g. Any opalescence produced is not more pronounced than that of a reference using 2. 0ml of potassium sulfate standard solution(0. 01%).

Sulfites and soluble starch　Dissolve 1. 0g in 10ml of water, add 1 drop of iodine TS; a yellow color is produced.

Loss on drying　When dried to constant weight at 105℃, it loses between 7.5% ~9.5% of its weight.

Residue on ignition　Not more than 0.1%.

Protein　Dissolve 1.0g in 10ml of water, add 3ml of sulfosalicylic acid solution, no precipitate is produced.

Iron　Dissolve 2.0g in 20ml of water, add 3 drops of nitric acid, boil gently for 5 minutes. Allow to cool, dilute to 45ml with water, add 3ml of ammonium thiocyanate solution(30→100) and mix well. Any color produced is not more intense than that of a reference solution prepared in the same manner using 2.0ml of iron standard solution(0.001%).

Heavy metals　Dissolve 4.0g in 23ml of water, add 2ml of sodium acetate BS(pH 3.5), carry out the limit test for heavy metals: not more than 0.0005%.

Arsenic　Dissolve 2.0g in 5ml of water, add 5ml of dilute sulfuric acid and 0.5ml of potassium bromide-bromine TS. Heat on a water bath for about 20 minutes and maintain the presence of excess of bromine. Add a quantity of potassium bromide-bromine TS, if necessary. Replace the evaporated water constantly and cool, then add 5ml of hydrochloric acid and dilute with water to 28ml. The solution complies with the limit test for arsenic(0.0001%).

3.2　Glucose injection

Glucose injection is a sterile solution of glucose in water for injection. It contains not less than 95.0% and not more than 105.0% of the labeled amount of glucose($C_6H_{12}O_6 \cdot H_2O$).

3.2.1　Description　A clear, colorless or almost colorless liquid; taste, sweet.

3.2.2　Identification　Add a few drops of the injection to hot alkaline cupric tartrate TS; a red precipitate of cuprous oxide is produced.

3.2.3　Test

pH　3.2 ~6.5.

5-Hydroxymethylfurfural　Transfer an accurately measured volume equivalent to 1.0 g of glucose to a 100ml volumetric flask, dilute with water to volume and mix well. Measure the absorbance at 284nm; the absorbance is not greater than 0.32.

Heavy metals　Measure a volume equivalent to 3g of glucose, evaporate to about 20ml and cool. Add 2ml of acetate BS(pH 3.5) and sufficient water to produce 25ml. Carry out the limit test for heavy metals: not more than 0.0005%, calculated with reference to the content of glucose.

4. Prepare lessons before class

4.1　How to use and clear the color comparison tube?

4.2　How to figure out the limit of arsenic or heavy metals?

4.3　What is the effect for the reagents used in the Gutzeit method in detection of the limit of arsenic?

5. Guide for experiment

5.1　Optical rotation

5.1.1　Principle and procedures

When rotate light transmit through solutions of optically active substances, the transmitted light emerges at a measurable angle to the plane of the incident light. Those that rotate light in a clockwise direction as viewed towards the light source are dextrorotatory, or (+) optical isomers. Those that rotate light in the opposite direction are called levorotatory or (−) optical isomers. Substances that show optical rotatory power are chiral. Specific rotation is the measured angle of optical light, while transmitting through the solution in a 1dm cell and 1ml contain 1g optical substance, under specific temperature and light source. Specific rotation is an important physical constant and useful for distinguishing from each other, purity test and determination of chiral substances.

Rotation of substance is correlated with its chemical structure, concentration, pathlength of solution, temperature and wavelength of rotate light. Unless otherwise specified in monograph, measurements of optical rotation are made at 589nm at 20℃ with 1dm polarimeter tube, and the measured rotation is expressed as $[\alpha]_D^{20}$ under this condition.

For liquid sample:
$$[\alpha]_D^{20} = \frac{\alpha}{ld}$$

For solid sample:
$$[\alpha]_D^{20} = \frac{100\alpha}{lC}$$

Where is the specific rotation with D line of sodium source lamp, 20 is the temperature, l is the pathlength in decimeters, C is the concentration of the analyte in g per 100ml, d is relative density of liquid sample.

5.1.2　Cautions

a. Blank correction with solvent should be done before and after zero checking. Appropriate cell check should be conducted when required.

b. Experimental temperature should be kept around 20℃ ±0.5℃ (unless otherwise specified in individual monograph) during the preparation of test solution and determination of rotation.

c. Appropriate concentration of the test solution is decided to yield a rotation between(±)2° ~ 8°, except for slightly soluble substances, for very small rotation value may probably lead to a big error, and at least 2 tests should be conducted concomitantly.

d. Sodium source lamp would take 20min to get stable after irradiation, and the user has to wait patiently for the instrumental initialization and being ready for measurement. Direct current is preferred for light source to alternating current which can be employed during break of assay to prolong the life-span time of light.

e. Zero check should be conducted by push retesting button repeatedly to minimize instrumental error. If necessary, standard quartz tube can be employed for the validation of polarimeter. Zero or stopping point should be recorded for three times.

f. Test solution should be clear, if necessary, filter and take successive solution for test.

g. Polarimeter tube should be rinsed thoroughly and filled carefully to make sure it is free of bubble.

h. Rotation of some compounds change with light, where preparation of solution and determination should be protected from direct sunlight. Allow the test solution to stand for some time if it is required in the monograph.

i. All optical glasses of polarimeter must be kept in clean and dry conditions and keep away from dust and stain. Source lamp has limited working hours and do not keep it working for more than 4h at one time.

j. Tube must be washed thoroughly and dried for storage after determination. Polarimeter must be stored with drying agent.

k. Specific rotation is affected by light source, detecting wavelength, solvent, concentration and temperature, so experimental conditions need to be specified where necessary.

5.1.3　Optical rotation of glucose

Glucose is an optical rotation substance, for there are several chiral carbons in its structure. Glucose is analyzed by optical rotation in many dosage forms which contain glucose in Ch. P. Determination of optical rotation is simple and convenient and can be applied for assay of chiral substances.

Ammonia TS is needed because there are α and β enantiomers, which make a balance in the solution(Figure 2 – 2).

α –D–glucose
$[\alpha]_D^{20} = +113.4°$
（36%）

Aldehyde–D–glucose
$[\alpha]_D^{20} = +52.75°$
（0.024%）

β –D–glucose
$[\alpha]_D^{20} = +19.7°$
（64%）

Figure 2 – 2　Multirotation of glucose in water

The equation shows that different enantiomers have different specific rotations, and they reach a balance gradually with specific rotation between + 52.5° ~ + 53.0°, which is called multirotation. Warming, adding of acid or base can help to accelerate the making up of balance. Ammonia TS is employed in Ch. P.

5.2　Determination of pH value

The pH value of an aqueous solution is determined by a pH meter using a glass electrode as the indicator electrode, and a saturated calomel electrode as the reference electrode. Metrological verification of the pH meter should be carried out at regular intervals to meet the related motional requirements. Before each measurement, the pH meter should be calibrate with the standard buffer solutions prepared as follows, or those of a declared pH valve accurate to 0.01pH unit distributed by national administrative department of certified reference material(CRM).

5.2.1　Standard buffer solution used for the calibration of pH meters

a. Standard tetraacetate BS　Dissolve 12.71g of potassium tetraacetate, previously dried at

54℃ ±3℃ for 4 ~ 5 hours and accurately weighted, in water to produce 1000ml.

b. Standard biphthalate BS　Dissolve 10. 21g of potassium biphthalate, previously dried at 115℃ ±5℃ for 2 ~ 3 hours and accurately weighted, in water to produce 1000ml.

c. Standard phosphate BS　Dissolve 3. 55g of anhydrous disodium hydrogen phosphate and 3. 40g of potassium dihydrogen phosphate, previously dried at 115℃ ± 5℃ for 2 ~ 3 hours and accurately weighted, in water to produce 1000ml.

d. Standard sodium tetraborate BS　Dissolve 3. 81g of sodium tetraborate, accurately weighted (avoid efflorescence), in water to produce 1000ml. Preserve the solution in well closed polyethylene contained from carbon dioxide in the air.

e. Standard calcium hydroxide BS　Use the supernatant of a saturated solution of calcium hydroxide, saturated with carbon dioxide-free water at 25℃. Store protected from carbon dioxide in the air. Discard and repeat the preparation if the solution becomes turbid.

Standard buffer solutions mentioned above must be prepared from the certified reagents for pH determination. The exact pH values of the saturated buffer solutions at different temperatures mentioned above are given in the following table.

The standard buffer solutions are numbered here in the same sequence as above in the Table 2 – 1.

Table 2 – 1　pH values of standard buffer solutions at different temperature

Temp/℃	Oxalate standard buffer	Phthalate standard buffer	Phosphate standard buffer	Sodium borate standard buffer	Calcium hydroxide standard buffer (25℃)
0	1. 67	4. 01	6. 98	9. 64	13. 43
5	1. 67	4. 00	6. 95	9. 40	13. 21
10	1. 67	4. 00	6. 92	9. 33	13. 00
15	1. 67	4. 00	6. 90	9. 28	12. 81
20	1. 68	4. 00	6. 88	9. 23	12. 63
25	1. 68	4. 01	6. 86	9. 18	12. 45
30	1. 68	4. 02	6. 85	9. 14	12. 29
35	1. 69	4. 02	6. 84	9. 10	12. 13
40	1. 69	4. 04	6. 84	9. 07	11. 98
45	1. 70	4. 05	6. 83	9. 04	11. 84
50	1. 71	4. 06	6. 83	9. 01	11. 71
55	1. 72	4. 08	6. 83	8. 99	11. 57
60	1. 72	4. 09	6. 84	8. 96	11. 45

5. 2. 2　Notices

Announcements operate the pH meter according to the manufacturer's instructions and pay attention to the following precautions when pH value is determined.

a. Select two standard buffer solutions with difference in pH value 3 units before determining test solution, and the pH value of the test solution is between that of two standard buffer solutions.

b. Calibrate the apparatus using the primary standard buffer solution where pH value is closer to test solution, adjusting the meter(fixed position) to read the appropriate pH value given in the table mentioned above.

c. Calibrate the apparatus using the second standard buffer solution. The deviation should not be more than ± 0.02 pH units, adjusting the slope carefully to make the observed pH value meet the value in the table mentioned above if it is not. Repeat the adjusting procedure for fixed position and slope until the difference between the observed value on the apparatus and the value of standard buffer solution is not more than 0.02 pH units. Otherwise the apparatus should be examined or the electrode should be exchanged till comply with the requirement.

d. The electrode should be rinsed with water and dried (or rinsed with the solution being examined) before each measurement.

e. A highly alkaline glass electrode should be used if the pH value of solution being examined is high. The error caused by alkalinity should be corrected if the electrode used is apt to produce such an error.

f. The determination of the pH value of a liquid with weak buffering capacity (e.g. water) should be conducted after the pH meter is calibrated with standard potassium biphthalate BS and repeated after the pH meter is calibrated with standard sodium tetraborate BS. The reading should not be recorded until the shift in 1 minute is within 0.05 unit. The pH value of the liquid being examined is the mean value of the two readings provided that they do not differ by more than 0.1 unit.

g. Freshly boiled and cooled distilled water with a pH value 5.5—7.0 should be used for preparing standard buffer solution and dissolving the substance to be examined in pH determinations.

h. Usually, the standard buffer solutions can be kept for 2—3 months, but should not be used if any turbidity, mould or precipitate is discovered.

5.3 Clarity of solution

Clarity of Solution is a method for testing of clarity or opalescence of a solution. Place the solution of the substance being examined and reference suspension of appropriate concentration into separate method, flat-bottomed test tubes, 15 ~ 16 mm in diameter, of colorless, transparent, neutral hard glass, accurately measured. Compare the contents of the test tubes after 5 minutes in preparation of the reference suspension against a blank background by viewing under diffused light down the vertical axes of the tubes. Or place the tubes under the light source of the illuminating shade chamber of 1000lx, view horizontally through the tubes.

A solution which is termed "clear" means that the clarity of solution of the substance being used for the preparation of the solution, or its opalescence is not more pronounced than that of reference suspension No 0.5.

Preparation of opalescence reference standard stock solution　Dissolve 1.00g of hydrazine sulfate, previously dried to constant weight at 105℃, in 100ml volumetric flask with water, warm in a water both at 40℃ if necessary, and dilute with water to volume, shake thoroughly and allow to stand for 4 ~ 6 hours. Mix the solution with equal volume of 10% urotropine solution, shake thoroughly and to stand for 24 hours at 25℃, protected from light. The suspension is stable for 2 months in a cool place, protected from light. Shake thoroughly before using.

Preparation of opalescence reference standard solution   Dilute 15. 0ml of opalescence reference standard stock solution with water in 1000ml volumetric flask and make up to volume, shake thoroughly. Transfer a quantity to a 1 cm cell, measure absorbance at 550nm, the absorbance is 0. 12 – 0. 15. The solution should be used within 48 hours of preparation. Shake thoroughly before using.

Preparation of reference suspension   Prepare the following reference suspensions (Table 2 – 2) using the opalescence reference standard solution and water. This solution should be freshly prepared. Shake thoroughly before using.

Table 2 – 2   Preparation of reference suspension

Reference suspension No.	0. 5	1	2	3	4
Opalescence reference standard solution /ml	2. 50	5. 0	10. 0	30. 0	50. 0
Water /ml	97. 50	95. 0	90. 0	70. 0	50. 0

5. 4   Color of solution

The color of solution and its difference from the specified color can, to some extent, demonstrate the purity of drug. Color of solution is a method for testing the color of a solution, by comparing the color of solution of drug with that of the reference solutions specified, or, measuring the absorbance at the specified wavelength.

A solution which is termed "colorless" specified in an individual monograph means that the color of solution of drug is the same as that of the solvent being used for the preparation of the solution, and a solution which is termed "almost colorless" means that the color of solution of drug is less intense than that of a reference solution, prepared by diluting reference solution No. 1 with same volume of water.

5. 4. 1   Method 1

Unless otherwise specified, dissolve a quantity of the substance being remained specified in an individual monograph with water in a 25ml Nessler cylinder, dilute with water to 10ml. Place in another Nessler cylinder 10ml of reference solution of specified tins and color. View down vertically the cylinders against a white background, or view horizontally against a white background in diffused light. The color in the cylinder containing the test solution is not more intense than that in the cylinder containing the reference solution. If the color in the cylinder containing the test solution is, or is almost, the same as that in the cylinder containing the reference solution, or the tint between cylinders not consistent, so that it is unable to estimate the result by naked eye. Method 3 (Color Difference Meter Method) should be used, and the result should be accorded for justifying.

Potassium dichromate standard solution for color comparison   Dissolve 0. 4000g of reference potassium dichromate ($K_2Cr_2O_7$), previously dried to constant weight at 120℃ and accurately weighed, in water in a 500ml volumetric flask and dilute with water to volume, shake thoroughly. Each 1ml of the solution contains 0. 8000mg of $K_2Cr_2O_7$.

Cupric sulfate standard solution for color comparison   Dissolve about 32. 5g of cupric sulfate in a quantity of hydrochloric acid solution (1→40) to produce 500ml. Transfer 10ml of the solution, accurately measured, to an iodine flask, add 50ml of water, 4ml of acetic acid and 2g of potassium iodide. Titrate with sodium thiosulfate(0.1mol/L)VS, add 2ml of starch IS toward the end point of the titration and continue to titrate until the blue color disappears. Each 1ml of sodium thiosulfate (0.1mol/L)VS is equivalent to 24.97mg of $CuSO_4 \cdot 5H_2O$. Dilute the rest of cupric sulfate solution with hydrochloric acid solution(1→40) to contain 62.4mg of $CuSO_4 \cdot 5H_2O$ per milliliter, based on the above assay result.

Cobaltous chloride standard solution for color comparison　Dissolve about 32.5g of cobaltous chloride in a quantity of hydrochloric acid solution(1→40) to produce 500ml. Transfer 2ml of the solution, accurately measured, to a flask, add 200ml of water, mix well. Add ammonia TS until the solution turns from pink to green color, add 10ml of acetic acid-sodium acetate BS(pH 6.0), heat to 60℃ and then add 5 drops of xylenol orange IS. Titrate with disodium edetate(0.05mol/L)VS until the solution turns to yellow. Each 1ml of disodium(0.05mol/L)VS is equivalent to 11.90mg of $CoCl_2 \cdot 6H_2O$. Dilute the rest of cobaltous chloride solution with hydrochloric acid solution(1→40) to contain 59.5mg of $CoCl_2 \cdot 6H_2O$, based on the above assay result.

Preparation of stock reference solutions　Prepare the following stock reference solutions, using the 3 standard solutions, dipited in Table 2-3.

Table 2-3　Preparation of stock reference solutions(expressed in 1ml)

Color	Cobaltous chloride standard solution/ml	Potassium dichromate standard solution/ml	Cupric sulfate standard solution/ml	Water/ml
yellowish green(YG)	1.2	22.8	7.2	68.8
yellow(Y)	4.0	23.3	0	72.7
orange yellow(Y)	10.6	19.0	4.0	66.4
orange red(OY)	12.0	20.0	0	68.0
brownish red(BR)	22.5	12.5	20.0	45.0

Preparation of reference solutions　Prepare the following reference solutions, using the stock reference solutions, shown in Table 2-4.

Table 2-4　Preparation of reference solutions(expressed in1ml)

Number of reference solutions	1	2	3	4	5	6	7	8	9	10
Stock Reference Solutions/ml	0.5	1.0	1.5	2.0	2.5	3.0	4.5	6.0	7.5	10.0
Water/ml	9.5	9.0	8.5	8.0	7.5	7.0	5.5	4.0	2.5	0

5.4.2　Method 2

Unless otherwise specified, dissolve quantity of the substance being examined specified in an individual monograph with water to produce a solution of 10ml, filter if necessary. Measure the absorbance at the wavelength specified, it gives not more than required value.

5.4.3　Method 3(Color Different Meter Method)

This is a method describing and analyzing the color of a solution quantitatively by direct measurement of its tristimulus value of transmittance using color difference meter. Using this method for determination recognition when it is difficult to identify the color difference between a test specimen and a reference solution visually.

Color difference between a test specimen and a reference solution is achieved by comparing their tristimulus value directly or by comparing them with those of water respectively.

5.5　Limit test for chlorides

Test preparation　Unless otherwise specified, weigh a quantity of the substance being examined as under individual monographs, dissolve it in about 25ml of water (if the solution is alkaline, neutralize with nitric acid dropwise). Add 10ml of dilute nitric acid and filter if necessary, transfer the solution to a 50ml Nessler cylinder, add water to produce 40ml and mix well.

Reference preparation　Transfer a volume of sodium chloride standard solution as prescribed under individual monographs to a 50ml Nessler cylinder, add 10ml of dilute nitric acid and sufficient water to produce 40ml, mix well.

Procedure　To each of the Nessler cylinders described above add 1.0ml of silver nitrate TS, dilute with water to 50ml and mix well. Allow to stand in the dark for 5 minutes, compare the opalescence produced by viewing down the vertical axis of the cylinders against a black background.

If the test preparation is colored, unless otherwise specified, place two aliquots of the test preparation in Nessler cylinders separately, to one cylinder add 1.0ml of silver nitrate TS, mix and allow to stand for 10 minutes, filter the content of the cylinder repeatedly until the filtrate is perfectly clear, then add the prescribed volume of standard sodium chloride solution to the filtrate, use it as the reference preparation. To the other cylinder add 1.0ml of silver nitrate TS, use it as the test preparation. Dilute the test preparation and the reference preparation with water to 50ml, mix well and allow to stand in the dark for 5 minutes, compare the opalescence as described above.

Sodium chloride standard solution　Dissolve 0.165g of sodium chloride in water in a 1000ml volumetric flask, and dilute to the volume, mix well (stock solution). Transfer 10ml of the stock solution, accurately measured, into a 100ml volumetric flask immediately before use, dilute with water to the volume and mix well (each 1ml is equivalent to 10μg of Cl).

The filter paper used in this test, if necessary, should be previously washed with water containing nitric acid until the washing is free from chlorides.

5.6　Determination of residue on ignition

Place 1.0 ~ 2.0g or the quantity specified under individual monographs of the substance being examined, accurately weighed, in a suitable crucible (if the substance being examined contains alkali metals or fluorine element, the platinum crucible should be used). Previously ignited to constant weight. Heat gently until it is thoroughly charred, cool and moisten the residue with 0.5 ~ 1ml of sulfuric acid, unless otherwise directed. Heat gently until white fumes are no longer evolved and then ignite at 700 ~ 800℃ until the incineration is complete. Cool in a desiccator and weight accurately. Ignite against at 700 ~ 800℃ to constant weight.

If the residue is to be used in the limit test for heavy metals, the ignition temperature should be controlled at 500 ~ 600℃.

5.7　Limit test for heavy metals

The term "heavy metals" refers to those metals that react with thioacetamide or sodium sulfide under the specified condition to produce a colored compound.

Lead standard solution   Dissolve 0. 160g of lead nitrate in 5ml of nitric acid and 50ml of water in a 1000ml volumetric flask, dilute to volume with water, mix well(stock solution) .

Transfer 10ml of the stock solution, accurately measured, to a 100ml volumetric flask, dilute with water to volume and mix well(each 1ml is equivalent to 10μg of Pb). This solution should be prepared immediately before using.

All glassware used for the preparation and preparation of standard lead solution should be free from lead.

5. 7. 1   Method 1

Unless otherwise specified, use two 25ml Nessler cylinders. To cylinder A add the specified volume of lead standard solution and 2ml of acetate BS(pH 3. 5) , dilute with water or other solvent as specified under individual monographs to 25ml. To cylinder B add 25ml of the test preparation containing a quantity of the substance being examined as specified under individual monographs.

If the original test preparation is colored, it may be matched by the addition of a few drops of dilute caramel solution or other suitable solution to cylinder A.

To each cylinder add 2ml of thioacetamide TS and mix well, allow to stand for 2 minutes, compare the color produced by viewing down the vertical axis of the cylinders against a white background. The color produced in cylinder B is not more intense than that produced in cylinder A.

If the color cannot be matched by the addition of caramel solution, dissolve the double amount of the substance being examined and the reagent, in water or other solvent as specified under individual monographs to produce 30ml of test preparation. Divide the test preparation into two equal portions and transfer to Nessler cylinders A and B. To cylinder B add sufficient water or other solvent as specified under individual monographs to produce 25ml. To cylinder A add 2ml of thioacetamide TS, mix well and allow to stand for 2 minutes, filter through filter membrane of 3μm in porosity. To cylinder A add the prescribed volume of lead standard solution and dilute with water of other solvent as specified under individual monographs to produce 25ml. Then add 2ml of thioacetamide TS to cylinder A and compare the color as described above.

If substance being examined contains a ferric salt which interferes with the test, 0. 5 ~ 1. 0g of ascorbic acid should be added to each cylinder.

Unless otherwise specified, evaporate the same quantity of the same reagents to dryness in a porcelain dish. Dissolve the residue in 2ml of acetate buffer(pH 3. 5) and 15ml of water. Transfer the solution to a Nessler cylinder, add the specified quantity of lead standard solution and water to 25ml. The solution is used as reference solution for the test solution which is prepared by using more than 1. 0ml of hydrochloric acid or equivalent amount of dilute hydrochloric acid, 2ml of ammonia TS or by treating with other reagents.

5. 7. 2   Method 2

Unless otherwise specified, use the residue obtained from the Determination of residue on ignition, add 0. 5ml of nitric acid, evaporate to dryness, heat until nitrous oxide fumes are no longer evolved(or alternatively, ignite a quantity of the substance being examined in a crucible until sulfurous acid fumes are no longer evolved, add 0. 5ml of nitric acid, evaporate to dryness, heat until nitrous oxide fumes are no longer evolved and ignite at 500 ~ 600℃ until the incineration is complete). Cool, add 2ml of hydrochloric acid, evaporate to dryness on a water bath, add 15ml of water, followed by ammonia TS dropwise until the solution is neutral to phenolphthalcin IS, then add 2ml of acetate BS(pH 3.5) and warm to effect dissolution. Transfer the resulting solution to Nessler cylinders B, dilute with water to 25ml and proceed as described under method 1. The reference preparation of test solution in a porcelain dish and evaporate to dryness, heat gently to dissolve in 2ml of acetate BS(pH 3.5) and 15ml of water, transfer to the Nessler cylinders A and add the specified volume of standard lead solution, dilute with water to 25ml.

5.7.3 Method 3

Unless otherwise specified, dissolve a quantity of the substance being examined in 5ml of sodium hydroxide TS and 20ml of water. Transfer the solution to a Nessler cylinder, add 5 drops of sodium sulfide TS and mix well, the color produced is not more intense than that of a reference preparation containing the specified volume of lead standard solution and treated in the same manner.

5.7.4 Method 4

Apparatus　The filter bolder is composted of tightly scaled upper and lower parts with screw thread, washer, filter membrane and nylon pad web, shown in Figure 2－3.

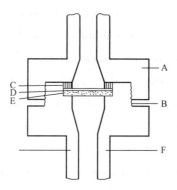

Figure 2－3　The schematic diagram of filter bolder

A. the top part of the filter bolder, the entrance may be fitted with a 50ml syringe; B. The joint; C. The washer (external diameter is 10mm, internal diameter is 6mm); D. The filter membrane with 10mm in diameter and 3.0μm of porosity diameter, soaked in water for more than 24 hours before use; E. The nylon pad web (porosity diameter is not required) with 10mm in diameter; F. The lower part of the filter bolder, the exit is fitted with a suitable rubber tube.

A is the top part of the filter bolder, the entrance may be fitted with a 50ml syringe; B is joint; C is washer(external diameter is 10mm, internal diameter is 6mm); D is filter membrane with 10mm in diameter and 3.0μm in of porosity, soaked in water for more than 24 hours before using; E is nylon pad web(porosity diameter is not required) with 10mm in diameter; F is the lower part of the filter bolder, the exit is fitted with a suitable rubber tube.

Lead standard stain　Measure accurately a quantity of lead standard solution to a small beaker, dilute to 10ml with water or other solvent as specified under individual monographs, add 2ml of acetate BS (pH 3.5) and 1.0ml of thioacetamide TS, mix well, allow to stand for 10 minutes. Transfer to the above filter holder with a 50ml syringe and filter it on applying an even pressure(filter rate is about 1ml per minute), then place the filter membrane on a piece of filter paper and dry it.

Procedure   Transfer 10ml of the test preparation prepared as described under individual monographs and proceed as described under lead standard stain, beginning with the words "add 2ml of acetate BS(pH 3. 5)". Any stain produced is not more intense than the standard stain.

If the test preparation is colored or turbid, filter it previously with filter membrane and repeat the filtration until the filter membrane remains uncontaminated. Proceed as described under lead standard stain, beginning with the words "add 2ml of acetate BS(pH 3. 5)", using 10ml of filter, and compare the stain as described above.

5. 8   Limit test for arsenic

Arsenic standard solution   Dissolved 0. 132g of arsenic trioxide in 5ml of 20% sodium hydroxide solution in a 1000ml volumetric flask, neutralize with dilute sulfuric acid and add 10ml in excess, dilute with water to volume and mix well, as a stock solution.

Transfer 10ml of the stock solution, accurately measured, to a 1000ml volumetric flask immediately before using, add 10ml of dilute sulfuric acid, dilute with water to volume and mix well (each 1ml is equivalent to 1μg of As).

5. 8. 1   Method 1(Gutzeit's method)

Apparatus   As shown in Figure 2 −4, A is a 100ml conical flask with standard ground joint; B is a standard bellow ground glass stepper connected to glass conduit C(external diameter 8. 0mm, internal diameter 6. 0mm), the total length of B and C is about 180mm; D is a place screw, the upper part of which has an aperture 6. 0mm in diameter; E is a plastic screw can which has an aperture 5. 0mm in diameter. A wad of lead acetate cotton wool weighting about 60mg is packed into tube C to a depth of about 50—80mm. A disc of mercuric bromide test paper is placed between the contesting surfaces of D and E.

Arsenic standard stain   Place 2ml of standard arsenic solution, accurately measured, in flask A, add 5ml of hydrochloric acid and 21ml of water. Then add 5ml of potassium iodide TS and 5 drops of acid stannous chloride TS, allow to stand at room temperature for 10 minutes and add 2g of zinc granules. Insert the stopper B and conduit C into the mouse of flask A and immerse the flask in a water both at 25—40℃ for 45 minutes. Remove the mercuric bromide test paper.

Use arsenic standard solution instead of the substance being examined and treat it in the same manner described under the individual monographs, prepared arsenic standard stain as described above, if the substance needs to be destroyed originally before carrying out the limit test for arsenic.

Procedure   Transfer the test preparation prepared as described under individual monographs to flask A and proceed as described under arsenic standard stain, beginning with the words "Then add 5ml of potassium iodide TS". Any stain produced is not more intense than the standard stain.

5. 8. 2   Method 2(Silver diethyldithiocarbamate method)

Apparatus   As shown in Figure 2 −5, A is a 100ml conical flask with standard ground joint; B is a standard hollow ground glass stopper connected to glass conduct C(at one end, the external diameter is 8. 0mm; the internal diameter is 1. 6mm; the other end is in length of 140 mm, in external diameter of 1 mm and in internal diameter of 1. 6mm, the internal diameter of sharp end is 1mm). D is a glass tube with flat bottom (length 180mm, internal diameter 10mm, and with a graduation at 5.0ml). A wad of cotton wool previously moistened with lead acetate TS and dried weighting about 60mg is packed into conduit C to a depth of about 80mm, and measure accurately 5ml of silver diethyldithiocarbamate TS in tube D.

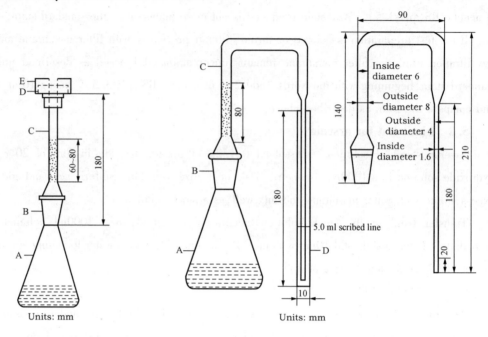

Figure 2 – 4   The equipment of Gutzert's method

Figure 2 – 5   The equipment of Silver diethyldithiocarbamate method

Standard arsenic reference solution   Transfer 5ml of arsenic standard solution as described under Method 1 to flask A, accurately measured, add 5ml of hydrochloric acid and 21ml of water. Then add 5ml of potassium iodide TS and 5 drops of acid stannous chloride TS, allow to stand at room temperature for 10 minutes and add 2g of zinc granules. Connect conduit C into flask A immediately, and allow the evolved arsine to enter tube D. Immerse the flask A in a water bath at 25 – 40℃ for 45 minutes. Remove tube D, add chloroform to the graduation, mix well.

Use arsenic standard solution instead of substance being examined and treat in the same manner described under the individual monographs, prepare arsenic standard stain as described above, if the substance being examined needs to be destroyed organically before carrying out the test for arsenic.

Procedure   Transfer the test preparation prepared as described under individual monographs to flask A and proceed as described under standard arsenic reference solution, beginning with the words "Then add 5ml of potassium iodide TS".

Compare the above two solutions against a white background. Any color produced by the test preparation is not more intense than that produced by the standard arsenic reference solution. If necessary, determine the absorbance at the wavelength of 510nm, using silver diethyldithiocarbamate TS as the blank.

Notes

a. Make sure that a blank test produces no arsenic stain or only a barely visible stain.

b. The preparation of standard stain and test stain must be carried out concomitantly.

c. The zinc granules should be arsenic free and the size is small such that they will pass through a No. 1 sieve. The quantity used should be increased and the reaction time should be extended up to 1 hour, if the granules are of large size.

d. Lead acetate cotton wool is prepared by immersing 1. 0g of absorbent cotton in 12ml of a mixture of equal volumes of lead acetate TS and water. Drain out excess liquid and make the cotton wool fluffy, allow it to dry at a temperature below 100℃ and preserve in a well closed glass container.

5. 9 Determination of loss on drying

Mix the substance being examined thoroughly, if it is in the form of large crystals, reduce them to a size of about 2mm by crushing. Place about 1g or the amount specified under individual monographs of the substance being examined in a trace, shallow weighting bottle, previously dried to constant weight at 105℃, unless otherwise directed.

The substance being examined should be evenly distributed to form a layer of not more than 5mm in thickness, or not more than 10mm in the case of bulky material. When the loaded bottle is placed in the drying chamber of desiccator, remove the stopper and put it beside the bottle, or leave it on the bottle in half open position. Upon the opening of the drying chamber or desiccator, the bottle should be closed promptly. If the substance is dried by heating, allow it to cool to room temperature in a desiccator before weighting. If the substance melts at a lower temperature until most of the water is removed, then dry it under the specified condition. If a vacuum desiccator or constant temperature vacuum desiccator is to be used, a pressure of 2. 67kPa (20mmHg) or less should be maintained unless otherwise directed. The desiccants used in a desiccator are usually anhydrous calcium chloride, sillies gel or phosphorus pentoxide. Phosphorus pentoxide is used in a constant temperature vacuum desiccator at 60℃, unless otherwise directed. The desiccants should be kept fully effective.

6. Discussion

6. 1   What are the purposes of drug identification and test? What are the usual items of drug tests?

6. 2   What are the standard operation procedures for the clarity test?

6. 3   How much of the lead standard solution should be taken for the limit test for heavy metals in this experiment?

6. 4   What precautions should be taken for the limit test for arsenic (method 1)?

And what is the function for each of the test solutions added?

6. 5   Figure out the amount of the arsenic standard solution that should be taken for the limit test for arsenic(0. 0001%) in this experiment with the specified quantity of 2. 0g of sample.

6. 6   What is the key step during the determination of residue on ignition? What does "ignite or dry to constant weight" mean?

（徐新军）

实验二 醋酸氢化可的松或醋酸氢化可的松片的鉴别和检查

一、目的

（1）了解甾体激素类药物中有关物质的来源和检查的意义。

（2）掌握醋酸氢化可的松的鉴别和有关物质检查方法。

二、仪器与试药

1. 仪器

试管、研钵、电子天平、100ml 量瓶、50ml 量瓶、紫外分光光度仪、比色皿、水浴锅、薄层板、点样毛细管、喷瓶。

2. 试药

醋酸氢化可的松、醋酸氢化可的松片。

三、实验方法

（一）醋酸氢化可的松的鉴别检查

本品为 11β，17α，21 - 三羟基孕甾 - 4 - 烯 - 3，20 - 三酮 - 21 - 乙酸酯。按干燥品计算，含 $C_{23}H_{32}O_6$ 应为 $97.0\% \sim 102.0\%$。

1. 醋酸氢化可的松的结构、分子式、相对分子质量

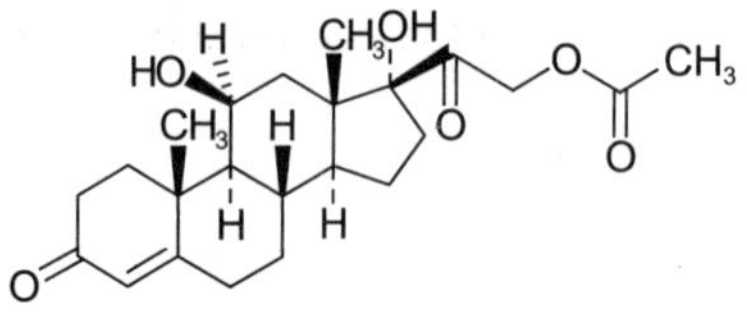

（$C_{23}H_{32}O_6$，$Mw = 404.50$）

2. 性状

本品为白色或几乎白色的结晶性粉末，无臭。

本品在乙醇或三氯甲烷中微溶，在水中不溶。

比旋度 取本品，精密称定，加二氧六环溶解并定量稀释制成每毫升中含 10mg 的溶液，依法测定，比旋度为 +158° 至 +165°。

3. 鉴别

（1）取本品约 0.1mg，加乙醇 1ml 溶解后，加新制的硫酸苯肼试液 8ml，在 70℃ 加热 15min，即显黄色。

（2）取本品约 2mg，加硫酸 2ml 使溶解，即显黄至棕黄色，并带绿色荧光。

（3）在含量测定项下记录的色谱图中，供试品溶液主峰的保留时间应与对照品溶液主峰的保留时间一致。

（4）本品的红外光吸收图谱应与对照的图谱（光谱集 552 图）一致。

（5）取本品，精密称定，加无水乙醇溶解并定量稀释制成每毫升中约含 10μg 的溶液，

照紫外－可见分光光度法在241nm的波长处测定吸光度，吸收系数（$E_{1cm}^{1\%}$）为383～407。

4. 检查

（1）其他甾体　取本品，加三氯甲烷：甲醇（9:1）制成每毫升中含3.0mg的溶液，作为供试品溶液；精密量取适量，加三氯甲烷：甲醇（9:1）稀释成每毫升中含60μg的溶液，作为对照溶液。照薄层色谱法试验，吸取上述两种溶液各10μl，分别点于同一硅胶G薄层板上，以1，2－二氯乙烷：甲醇：水（95:5:0.3）为展开剂，展开后，晾干，在105℃干燥10min，放冷，喷以碱性四氮唑蓝试液，立即检视。供试品溶液如显杂质斑点，其颜色与对照溶液的主斑点比较，不得更深。

（2）干燥失重　取本品，在105℃干燥至恒重，减失重量不得过0.5%。

（二）乙酸氢化可的松片

本品含醋酸氢化可的松（$C_{23}H_{32}O_6$）应为标示量的90.0%～110.0%。

1. 性状

本品为白色片。

2. 鉴别

取本品的细粉适量（约相当于乙酸氢化可的松60mg），用三氯甲烷提取2次，每次10ml，合并三氯甲烷液，滤过，滤液置水浴上蒸干，残渣照乙酸氢化可的松项下的鉴别（1）、鉴别（2）项试验，显相同的反应。

3. 检查

含量均匀度　取本品1片，置乳钵中研磨，加无水乙醇适量，分次将乙酸氢化可的松移入200ml量瓶中，振摇使乙酸氢化可的松溶解，用无水乙醇稀释至刻度，摇匀，滤过，取续滤液为供试品溶液；精密称取乙酸氢化可的松对照品20mg，置200ml量瓶中，加无水乙醇溶解并稀释至刻度，摇匀，作为对照品溶液。精密量取供试品溶液与对照品溶液各1ml，分别置干燥具塞试管中，各精密加无水乙醇9ml与氯化三苯四氮唑试液1ml，摇匀，再各精密加氢氧化四甲基铵试液1ml，摇匀，在25℃的暗处放置40～45min，照紫外－可见分光光度法在485nm的波长处分别测定吸光度，计算含量，应符合规定。

四、预习提要

（一）分光光度法测定原理

分光光度法是通过测定物质在特定波长处或一定波长范围内的吸光度或发光强度，对该物质进行定性和定量分析的方法。

常用的波长范围：①200～400nm的紫外光区；②400～760nm的可见光区；③2.5～25μm（按波数记为4000～400cm⁻¹）的红外光区。所用仪器为紫外－分光光度计、可见－分光光度计（或比色计）、红外－分光光度计或原子吸收－分光光度计。为保证测量的精密度和准确度，所用仪器应按照国家计量检定规程或药典附录规定，定期进行校正检定。

单色光辐射穿过被测物质溶液时，在一定的浓度范围内被该物质吸收的量与该物质的浓度和液层的厚度（光路长度）成正比，其关系式为

$$A = -\lg T = ECL$$

式中，A为吸光度；T为透光率；E为吸收系数，采用的表示方法是$E_{1cm}^{1\%}$，其物理意义为当溶液浓度为1%（g/ml），液层厚度为1cm时的吸光度值；C为100ml溶液中所含被测物质

的质量（按干燥品或无水物计算），g；L 为液层厚度，cm。

物质对光的选择性吸收波长，以及相应的吸收系数是该物质的物理常数。已知某纯物质在一定条件下的吸收系数后，可用同样条件将该供试品配成溶液，测定其吸光度，即可由上式计算出供试品中该物质的含量。在可见光区，除某些物质对光有吸收外，很多物质本身并没有吸收，但可在一定条件下加入显色试剂或经过处理使其显色后再测定，故又称为比色分析。

（二）TLC 基本原理和操作方法

薄层色谱法系指将供试品溶液点样于薄层板上，经展开、检视所得的色谱图，与适宜的对照物按同法所得的色谱图进行对比，用于药品鉴别或杂质检查。

1. 仪器与材料

（1）薄层板

自制薄层板　除另有规定外，玻板要求光滑，平整，洗净后不附水珠，晾干。最常用的固定相有硅胶 G、硅胶 GF$_{254}$、硅胶 H 和硅胶 HF$_{254}$，其次有硅藻土、硅藻土 G、氧化铝、氧化铝 G、微晶纤维素、微晶纤维素 F$_{254}$ 等。一般要求其颗粒粒径为 5 ~ 40μm。

薄层涂布　一般可分为无黏合剂和含黏合剂两种。前者系将固定相直接涂布于薄板上，后者系在固定相中加入一定量的黏合剂，一般常用 10% ~ 15% 煅石膏（CaSO$_4$·2H$_2$O 在 140℃ 加热 4h），混匀后加水适量使用，或用羧甲基纤维素钠水溶液（0.2% ~ 0.5%）适量调成糊状，均匀涂布于玻板上。使用涂布器涂布应能使固定相在玻板上涂成一层符合厚度要求的均匀薄层。

市售薄层板　分普通薄层板和高效薄层板，如硅胶薄层板、硅胶 GF$_{254}$ 薄层板、聚酰胺薄膜和铝基片薄层板等。

（2）点样器　同纸色谱项。

（3）展开缸　应使用同适合薄层板大小的玻璃质薄层色谱展开缸，并有严密的盖子，底部应平整光滑，或有双槽。

（4）显色剂　见各品种项的规定。可采用喷雾显色、浸渍显色或置碘蒸气中显色，用以检出斑点。

（5）显色装置　喷雾显色要求用压缩气体使显色剂呈均匀细雾状喷出；浸渍显色可用专用玻璃器皿或用适宜的玻璃缸代替；蒸气熏蒸显色可用双槽玻璃缸或适宜大小的干燥器代替。

（6）检视装置　为装有可见光、短波紫外光（254nm）、长波紫外光（365nm）光源及相应滤片的暗箱，可附加摄像设备供拍摄色谱用，暗箱内光源应有足够的光照度。

2. 操作方法

（1）薄层板制备

自制薄层板　除另有规定外，将 1 份固定相和 3 份 CMC - Na 水溶液在研钵中按同一方向研磨混合，去除表面的气泡后倒入涂布器中，在玻板上平稳地移动涂布器进行涂布（厚度为 0.2 ~ 0.3mm），取下涂好薄层的玻板，置水平台上于室温下晾干后在 110℃ 活化 30min，即置有干燥剂的干燥箱中备用。使用前检查其均匀度（可通过透射光和反射光检视）。

市售薄层板　临用前一般应在 110℃ 活化 30min。聚酰胺薄膜无须活化。铝基片薄层板可根据需要剪裁，但须注意剪裁后的薄层板底部的硅胶层不得破损。如在储放期间被空气中杂质污染，使用前可用适宜的溶剂在展开容器中上行展开预洗，110℃活化后放干燥器中备用。

（2）点样器　除另有规定外，用点样器点样于薄层板上，一般为圆点，点样基线距底边2.0cm，样点直径为2～4mm，点间距离可视斑点扩散情况以下不影响检出为宜，一般为1.0～2.0cm。点样时必须注意勿损伤薄层板表面。

（3）展开缸　展开缸如需预先用展开剂饱和，可在缸中加入足够量的展开剂，并在壁上贴两条与缸一样高、宽的滤纸条，一端浸入展开剂中，密封顶盖，使系统平衡或按各品种项的规定操作。

将点好供试品的薄层板放入展开缸中，浸入展开剂的深度为距薄层板底边0.5～1.0cm（切勿将样点浸入展开剂中），密封顶盖，待展开至规定距离（一般为10～15cm），取出薄层板，晾干，按各品种项的规定检测。

展开剂可以单向展开，即向一个方向进行；可以进行双向展开，即先向一个方向展开，取出，待展开剂完全挥发后，将薄层板转动90°，再用原展开剂或另一种展开剂进行展开，亦可多次展开。

（4）显色与检视　荧光薄层板可用荧光淬灭法；普通薄层板、有色物质可直接检视，无色物质可直接用物理或化学方法检视。物理方法可检出荧光斑点的荧光颜色及强度；化学方法一般用化学试剂显色后立即覆盖同样大小的玻板，并检视。

（三）含量均匀度检查

含量均匀度系指小剂量或单剂量的固体制剂、半固体制剂和非均相液体制剂的每片（个）含量符合标示量的程度。

除另有规定外，片剂、硬胶囊剂或注射用无菌粉末，每片（个）标示量不大于25mg或主药含量不大于每片（个）重量25%者；内容物非均一溶液的软胶囊、单剂量包装的口服混悬液、透皮贴剂、吸入剂和栓剂，均应检查含量均匀度。复方制剂仅检查符合上述条件的组分。

凡检查含量均匀度的制剂一般不再检查重（装）量差异。

五、实验指导

（一）紫外－可见分光光度法测定注意事项

1. 对溶剂的要求

含有杂原子的有机溶剂通常均具有很强的末端吸收。因此，作溶剂使用时，它们的使用范围均不能小于截止使用波长，如甲醇、乙醇的截止使用波长为205nm。另外，当溶剂不纯时，也可能增加干扰吸收。因此，在测定供试品前，应先检查所用的溶剂在供试品所用的波长附近是否符合要求，即将溶剂置1cm石英吸收池中以空气为空白（即空白光路中不置任何物质）测定其吸光度。溶剂和吸收池的吸光度在220～240nm范围内不得超过0.40，在241～250nm范围内不得超过0.20，在251～300nm范围内不得超过0.10，在300nm以上时不得超过0.05。

2. 测定法

测定时，除另有规定外，应以配置供试品溶液的同批溶剂为空白对照，采用1cm石英吸收池，在规定的吸收峰波长±2nm以内测试几个点的吸光度，或由仪器在规定波长附近自动扫描测定，以核对供试品的吸收峰波长位置是否正确。除另有规定外，吸收峰波长应在该品种项规定的 ±2nm 以内，并以吸光度最大的波长作为测定波长。一般供试品溶液的吸光度读数，以在 0.3～0.7 之间的误差较小。仪器的狭缝波带宽度应小于供试品吸收带的半宽度的十分之一，否则测得的吸光度会偏低；狭缝宽度应以减小狭缝宽度时供试品的吸光度不再增大为准。由于吸收池和溶剂本身可能有空白吸收，因此测定供试品的吸光度后应减去空白读数，或由仪器自动扣除空白读数后再计算含量。当溶液的 pH 值对测定结果有影响时，应将供试品溶液和对照品溶液的 pH 值调成一致。

（二）TLC 法系统适用性试验

按各品种项要求对检测方法进行系统适用性试验，使斑点的检测灵敏度、比移值（R_f）和分离效能符合规定。

1. 检测灵敏度

系指杂质检查时，采用对照溶液稀释若干倍的溶液与供试品溶液和对照溶液在规定的色谱条件下，在同一块薄层板上点样、展开、检视，前者应显示清晰的斑点。

2. 比移值

系指从基线至展开斑点中心的距离与从基线至展开剂前沿的距离的比值：

$$R_f = \frac{\text{从基线至展开斑点中心的距离}}{\text{从基线至展开剂前沿的距离}}$$

可用供试品溶液主斑点与对照品溶液主斑点的比移值进行比较，或用比移值来说明主斑点或杂质斑点的位置。

3. 分离效能

鉴别时，在对照品与结构相似的药物的对照品制成混合对照溶液的色谱图中，应显示两个清晰分离的斑点。杂质检查时，在杂质对照品用供试品自身对照溶液或同品种对照品溶液溶解制成混合对照溶液的色谱图中，应显示两个清晰分离的斑点，或待测成分与相邻的杂质斑点应清晰分离。

（三）含量均匀度的计算方法

除另有规定外，取供试品 10 片（个），照各品种规定的方法，分别测定每片（个）以标示量为 100 的相对含量 X，求其均值 $\overline{X}$ 和标准差 S $\left[S = \sqrt{\dfrac{\sum (X - \overline{X})^2}{n-1}} \right]$ 以及标示量与均值之差的绝对值 A（$A_i = |100 - \overline{X}|$）：若 $A + 1.80S \leqslant 15.0$，则供试品的含量均匀度符合规定；若 $A + S > 15.0$，则不符合规定；若 $A + 1.80S > 15.0$，且 $A + S \leqslant 15.0$，则应另取 20 片（个）复试。根据初试、复试结果，计算 30 片（个）的均值、标准差 S 和标示量与均值之差的绝对值 A：如 $A + 1.45S \leqslant 15.0$，则供试品的含量均匀度符合规定；$A + 1.45S > 15.0$，则不符合规定。

六、讨论

（1）醋酸氢化可的松的鉴别原理是什么？

（2）甾体激素中"其他甾体"检查的意义和常用方法是什么？

（3）哪类甾体激素可与四氮唑蓝产生反应，是结构中的何种基团参与反应，反应式是什么？ 反应式是什么？反应式是什么？反应式是什么？

Experiment 2 Description，Identification and Tests of Hydrocortisone Acetate or Hydrocortisone Acetate Tablets

1. Purposes

1. 1   To study the origins of the related compounds of steroidal drugs and the significance of the limit tests for them.

1. 2   To grasp the identification and the limit test for the related compounds of hydrocortisone acetate.

2. Instruments and chemical reagents

2. 1   Instruments

Test tube, mortar, electronic balance, 100ml volumetric flask, 50ml volumetric flask, UV spectrometer, 1cm cell, thermostat-controlled water-bath, thin layer plate, spotting capillary, spraying bottle.

2. 2   Chemical reagents

Hydrocortisone acetate, hydrocortisone acetate tablets.

3. Procedures and methods

3. 1   Hydrocortisone Acetate

Hydrocortisone acetate is $11\beta, 17\alpha, 21$ – trihydroxypregn – 4 – ene – 3, 20 – dione – 21 – acetate. It contains not less than 97. 0% and not more than 102. 0% of $C_{23}H_{32}O_6$, calculated on the dried basis.

3. 1. 1   Structure, molecular formula and molecular weight of hydrocortisone acetate

$$(C_{23}H_{32}O_6, M_w = 404. 50)$$

3. 1. 2   Description

A white or almost white crystalline powder, odourless. Slightly soluble in ethanol or chloroform, insoluble in water.

Specific optical rotation   + 158° to + 165°, in a solution of 10mg/ml in dioxane.

3. 1. 3   Identification

a. Dissolve about 0. 1mg in 1ml of ethanol, add 8ml of freshly prepared phenylhydrazine sulfate TS, heat at 70℃ for 15minutes, a yellow color is produced.

b. Dissolve about 2mg in 2ml of sulfuric acid, a yellow or brownish-yellow colour is produced with green fluorescence.

c. The retention time of the principal peak in the chromatogram of the test solution obtained in the assay is identical with that of hydrocortisone acetate CRS peak in the chromatogram of the reference solution.

d. The infrared absorption spectrum is concordant with the reference spectrum.

e. Measure the absorbance of a solution of 10μg/ml in dehydrated ethanol at 241nm, the value of $E_{1cm}^{1\%}$ is 383 ~ 407.

3.1.4 Test

a. Other steroids   Carry out the method for thin-layer chromatography, using silica gel G as the coating substance and a mixture of dichloromethane : methanol : water (95 : 5 : 0.3) as the mobile phase. Apply separately to the plate 10μl each of two solutions in chloroform-methanol (9 : 1) containing (1) 3.0mg/ml and (2) 60μg /ml of the substance being examined. After developing and removal of the plate, dry it in air and then at 105℃ for 10 minutes, cool and spray with alkaline tetrazolium blue TS. Examine immediately. Any spot in the chromatogram obtained with solution(1) other than the principal spot is not more intense than the principal spot obtained with solution(2).

b. Loss on drying   When dried to constant weight at 105℃, loses not more than 0.5% of its weight.

3.2 Hydrocortisone Acetate Tablets

Hydrocortisone acetate tablets contain not less than 90.0% and not more than 110.0% of the labeled amount of hydrocortisone acetate($C_{23}H_{32}O_6$).

3.2.1 Description

White tablets.

3.2.2 Identification

Powder a quantity of tablets equivalent to 60mg of hydrocortisone acetate, extract with two quantities of 10ml each of chloroform, combine the chloroform solutions, filter and evaporate to dryness on a water bath. The residue complies with the tests (a.) and (b.) for Identification described under hydrocortisone acetate.

3.2.3 Test

Content uniformity   Comply with the requirements for content uniformity. Triturate 1 tablet with dehydrated ethanol and transfer completely into a 200ml volumetric flask, dilute with dehydrated ethanol to volume, shake thoroughly and filter, and use successive filtrate as the test solution. Dissolve 20mg of hydrocortisone acetate CRS in a 200ml volumetric flask in dehydrated ethanol, dilute with dehydrated ethanol to volume, shake thoroughly, used as the reference solution. To 1ml each of two solutions, accurately measured, in separate stoppered test tubes, add accurately 9ml of dehydrated ethanol and 1ml of triphenyltetrazolium chloride TS and mix well; then add accurately 1ml of tetramethylammonium hydroxide TS and mix well. Allow to stand in dark at 25℃ for 40 ~ 50 minutes and measure the absorbance at 485nm. Calculate the content of $C_{23}H_{32}O_6$.

4. Prepare lessons before class

4.1 Theory of Spectrophotometry

Spectrophotometry is method used in qualitative and quantitative analysis in which the light absorbance or the intensity of light emission of the substance being examined is measured at a definite wavelength or within a definite range of wavelength.

The spectral ranges involved in pharmaceutical analysis mainly consist of 3 regions: ① the ultraviolet region(200 ~ 400nm); ②the visible region(400 ~ 760nm); ③the infrared region(2.5 – 25μm or 4000 ~ 400cm^{-1}). The instructions used are the ultraviolet-visible spectrophotometer, visible spectrophotometer (or colorimeter), infrared spectrophotometer or atomic absorbance spectrophotometer. All instruments should be calibrated regularly to insure the precision and the accuracy.

When monochromatic radiation passes through an absorbing medium, the absorbance of the radiation is proportional to the concentration of the absorbing substance and the thickness following the absorbing medium, this relation is expressed by the following equation.

$$A = -\lg T = ECL$$

Where A is the absorbance, T is the transmittance, E is the absorption coefficients, C is the concentration of the substance expressed in g/ml, calculated on the dried or dehydrated basis and L is the absorption path length expressed in cm. The term is used in this pharmacopoeia to denote the absorbance of a 1% solution in a 1cm cell.

The wavelength of the selective absorption and the corresponding absorption coefficient are physical constants of the substance being examined. When the absorption coefficient of a substance is known, its content can be calculated from the above equation. In the visible region, the content of a colorless substance can be determined colorimetrically after the addition of a color developing agent or any other treatment.

4.2 Procedure of TLC

Thin-layer chromatography is a separation technique in which the test solutions are deposited on the thin layer plate. The chromatogram obtained after on the thin layer plate and visualization can be compared with that of appropriate reference substance under the same condition. The result can be used for drug identification and impurity testing.

4.2.1 Apparatus and materials

a. Thin layer plate

Home made plate   Unless otherwise specified, the glass plate should be smooth, flat and dry, no bead on it after being washed.

Silica gel G   Silica gel GF$_{254}$, silica gel H, silica gel H$_{254}$, diatomaceous earth, diatomaceous earth G, aluminum oxide, aluminum oxide G, microcrystalline cellulose, microcrystalline cellulose G, etc, are commonly used as stationary phases. Their particle size is usually 5 ~ 40μm in diameter.

Coating the plate   The absorbent or support can be applied to the glass plate with or without a binder. When the binder is needed, mix the absorbent or support with 10% ~ 15% of gypsum (CaSO$_4$ · 2H$_2$O, dried at 140℃ for 4 hours) and sufficient water, or with a 0.2% ~ 0.5% solution of carboxymethy-celluose sodium as binder. Triturate the mixture to a homogeneous paste and spraid the slurry on the glass plate. Spreader is used to spread the slurry on the glass plate to form a uniform layer of definite thickness.

Precoated plates　It contains normal thin-layer plates and high-performance thin-layer plates, such as silica gel thin-layer plates, silica gel GF$_{254}$ thin-layer plates polyamide thin-layer plates, aluminum thin-layer plates etc.

b. Sample applicator　Same as described under Paper Chromatography.

c. Developing chamber　Glass chamber of suitable size with tight lid and a flat bottom or twin trough may be used.

d. Visualization reagent　As specified in the monograph. The spots can be visualized by spraying, exposure to vapour of I$_2$ or immersion.

e. Visualization device　The spray visualization requires that the visualizing reagent should be ejected by the compressed gas as fine and even fogdrops. Special glass apparent or suitable glass tank can be used for the immersion visualization. The twin trough chamber or dessicator with suitable size can be used for vapour method.

f. Detection device　It consists of a dark chamber with filter, a light source with visible light, short (254nm) and long (360nm) UV wavelengths light, and photographic equipment. The light source should have enough illumination.

4.2.2　Procedure

a. Preparation of thin-layer plate

Home made plates　Unless otherwise specified, one part of station phase and three parts of CMC − Na solution are triturated in one direction to a homogeneous paste, remove gas bubbles on the surface, put the paste in the spreader, spread on glass plates. The thickness of the layer is generally 0.2 ~ 0.3mm. Allow the plate to dry on a horizontal plane, activate at 110°C for 30 min and store in a dessicator with silica gel.

Commercial precoated plates　The plates should be usually activated in an over at 110℃ and stored in a dessicator.

b. Sample application　Unless otherwise specified, apply the sample to the plate using a sample applicator, circular sports are spread 2.0cm from the end of the plate. The distance between the adjacent spots is usually 1.0 ~ 2.0cm, which can be adjusted according to the diffusion of the spot in order not to interface with the detection. It is essential not to damage the thin layer in applicating the sample.

c. Developing　If the developing should be equilibrated previously with the vapor of the developer, add sufficient developer into the chamber and line the inner walls of the developing chamber with two filter paper strips of the same dimension of the wall, seal the cover of the chamber and allow the system to equilibrate or by the method specified in the monograph.

Place the plate into the developing chamber with the test spots toward the bottom and into the develop about 5 ~ 10mm in depth, seal the cover until the solvent frontal, air-dry the plates, and observe the spots by the method specified in the monograph.

One dimensional chromatography is that the developing proceeds along one direction, sometimes two-dimensional chromatography may be performed by turning the plate at right angle and developing with the original developer or a different solvent system. Multiple dimensional developing may also be used.

d. Visualization and diction   The fluorescence quenching method can be used for the fluorescence thin-layer plate. For the culinary thin-layer plate, the color substance could be detected visually, the colorless substance could be detected by physical or chemical method. The color and the intensity of the fluorescence spot can be detected by physical method. The plate may be visualized by chemical method with chemical reagent. A glass plate of the same size is immediately covered on the visualized plate for inspection.

4.3   Test of content uniformity

Test for content uniformity is expressed as the contents of single ingredient of solid preparations, semi-solid preparations, and unhomogeneous liquid preparations small dosage or comply with the labelled amount.

Unless otherwise specified, the labelled amount of each tablet, capsule or sterile powder for injection is not more than 25mg or the content of the active ingredient is not more than 25% of each weight; the soft capsule filled with inhomogeneous solution, the single-dose oral suspension, transdermal patches, aerosol for inhalant and suppositories, are all carried on the test for content uniformity. The component which complies with the above requirement is tested for compound preparations.

When the test for content uniformity is specified in the monograph, it is understood that the test for weight variation(and of content) can be exempted.

5. Guide for experiment

5.1   Ultraviolet-visible spectrophotometry

5.1.1   Requirements for the solvents

The organic solvents containing heteroatoms usually have strong absorption at the lower wavelength. Thus, their ranges of use should be less than the cut off wavelength. For example, the cut off wavelength of methanol and ethanol is 205nm. Otherwise, impurity of solvents would enhance the interference of absorption. The solvent used in spectrophotometric determination should be checked for any interfering absorption peak around the selected wavelength for the measurement of the absorbance being examined. The absorbance of a solvent should not exceed 0.40 in the range of 220nm to 240nm, 0.20 in the range of 241nm to 250nm, 0.10 in the range of 251nm to 300nm and 0.05 at wavelength above 300nm, where measured in a 1cm quartz cell against air.

5.1.2   Procedure

Unless otherwise specified, the same batch of solvent used to prepare the solution of the substance being examined should be employed as the blank in matched 1cm quartz cell. The wavelength of maximum absorption should be checked by measuring the absorbance of the substance being examined in the vicinity of the specified wavelength, within a range of ±2nm, to check the wavelength of absorption maximum is correct or not. Unless otherwise specified, the absorption maximum must be within ±2nm as specified in the monograph, otherwise, the identity, purity of the substance or the correctness of the wavelength of the spectrophotometer should be considered. The assay should be carried out at the wavelength of maximum absorption. The concentration of the solution should be adjusted to give an absorbance reading of 0.3 to 0.7 where the experimental error is the smallest. The width of the specified slit must be smaller than the tenth of half-width of the absorption bend, otherwise low absorbance will be resulted. The slit width is appropriate if further reduction does not result in an increase of the absorbance reading. The absorbance of as unmatched cell with the solvent concerned as a blank must be subtracted from the absorbance of the substance being examined or be automatically deducted by the spectrophotometer. When the pH affects the results determined, the pH of the test preparation should be adjusted equal to that of the reference preparation.

5.2 Thin-layer Chromatography system suitability test

The system suitability test should be carried out according to the testing method specified under monograph, the detection sensitivity of the spots. Rf value and separating power should be in conformity with the requirements.

5.2.1 Detection sensitivity

For the testing of impurity, a spot is clearly visible in the chromatogram obtained with the most dilute reference solution. The test solution and the series dilute reference solution are spotted, developed and visualized at the same thin layer and under the prescribed chromatographic system.

5.2.2 Retention factor

It is defined as the ratio of the distance from the point of application to the center of the spot and the distance traveled by the solvent from the point of application.

$$R_f = \frac{\text{the dictance from baseline to the spot center}}{\text{the dictance from baseline to the solvent front}}$$

The principle spot in the chromatogram obtained with test solution is compared visually with the corresponding spot in the chromatogram obtained with the reference solution by comparing the retention factor, or the position of the principal spot and the impurity spot is expressed by the retention factor.

5.2.3 Separating power

Where identification testing is carried out, two well separated clean spots should be detected in the chromatogram of a mixed solution prepared with the reference substance of the substance being examined and the reference substance of the substance with the similar structure. Where impurity testing is conducted, two well separated clear spots should be detected in the chromatogram of a reference solution prepared with the impurity reference substance and the substance being examined or the reference substance of the substance being examined. The spots of the substance being examined and the adjacent impurity should be clearly separated.

5.3 The calculation of content uniformity

Unless otherwise specified, take 10 tablets (unit) of the substance being examined, as specified in the individual monograph, determine separately the relative content X of each tablet which express 100 as the labelled amount, caculate its mean value $\overline{X}$, the standard deviation S $\left[S = \sqrt{\dfrac{(X - \overline{X})^2}{n - 1}}\right]$ and the absolute value A ($A_i = |100 - \overline{X}|$) which is the difference between the labelled amount and the mean value: if $A + 1.80S \leq 15.0$, the substance being examined complies with the test for content uniformity; if $A + S > 15.0$, the substance being examined fails to comply with the test for content uniformity; if $A + 1.80S > 15.0$ and $A + S \leq 15.0$, then repeat the determination using another 20 tablets. According to the results of first and second test, calculate the mean value A, the difference between the labeled amount and the mean value: if $A + 1.45S \leq 15.0$, the substance being examined complies with the test for content uniformity; if $A + 1.45S > 15.0$, the substance being examined fails to comply with the test for content uniformity.

6. Discussion

6.1 What are the principles of the identification of hydrocortisone acetate?

6.2 What are the commonly used method for and the significance of the limit test for other steroids for the steroidal drugs?

6.3 What kind of steroidal drugs can react with the alkaline tetrazolium blue TS? What is the chemical reaction equation?

（徐新军）

实验三 甲苯咪唑的性状、鉴别和检查

一、目的

（1）了解药物晶型对药效的影响。

（2）熟悉药物晶型检查的方法及原理。

（3）熟悉药物吸收系数测定方法。

二、仪器与试药

1. 仪器

分析天平，紫外－可见分光光度计，红外光谱仪，玛瑙研钵，量瓶（5ml、10ml、100ml、200ml），10ml量筒，0.5移液管和1ml移液管，滴管，50ml烧杯，硅胶GF_{254}薄层板，紫外光灯，干燥箱，称量瓶，坩埚，电炉，马弗炉，纳氏比色管。

2. 试药

甲苯咪唑原料、10% A晶型甲苯咪唑、甲酸、异丙醇、液状石蜡、丙酮、三氯甲烷、甲醇、硝酸、硫酸、盐酸、氨试液、酚酞指示液、乙酸盐缓冲液（pH 3.5）、标准铅溶液、水。

三、实验方法

1. 甲苯咪唑的结构、分子式、相对分子质量

（$C_{16}H_{13}N_3O_3$，$Mw = 295.30$）

本品为 5 - 苯甲酰基 - 2 - 苯并咪唑氨基甲酸甲酯，按干燥品计算，含 $C_{16}H_{13}N_3O_3$ 应为 98.0% ~ 102.0%。

2. 性状

本品为白色、类白色或微黄色结晶性粉末，无臭。

本品在甲酸中易溶，在冰乙酸中略溶，在丙酮或三氯甲烷中极微溶解，在水中不溶。

吸收系数 取本品约 50mg，精密称定，加甲酸 5ml 溶解，用异丙醇定量稀释制成每毫升中约含 10μg 的溶液，照紫外 - 可见分光光度法，在 312nm 的波长处测定吸光度，按干燥品计算吸收系数（$E_{1cm}^{1\%}$）为 485 ~ 505。

3. 鉴别

（1）取本品约 50mg，加甲酸 5ml 溶解，用异丙醇稀释制成每毫升中约含 10μg 的溶液，照紫外 - 可见分光光度法测定，在 312nm 的波长处有最大吸收。

（2）本品的红外光吸收图谱应与对照的图谱一致。

4. 检查

（1）A 晶型 取本品与含 A 晶型为 10% 的甲苯咪唑对照品各约 25mg，分别加液体石蜡 0.3ml，研磨均匀，制成厚度约 0.15mm 的石蜡糊片，同时制作厚度相同的空白液体石蜡糊片作参比，照红外分光光度法测定，并调节供试品与对照品在 803cm^{-1} 波数处的透光率为 90% ~ 95%，分别记录 620 ~ 803cm^{-1} 波数处的红外光吸收图谱。在约 620cm^{-1} 和 803cm^{-1} 波数处的最小吸收峰间连接一基线，再在约 640cm^{-1} 和 662cm^{-1} 波数处的最大吸收峰之顶处作垂线与基线相交，用基线吸光度法求出相应吸收峰的吸光度值。供试品在约 640cm^{-1} 与 662cm^{-1} 波数处吸光度之比，不得大于含 A 晶型为 10% 的甲苯咪唑对照品在该波数处的吸光度之比。

（2）有关物质 取本品 50mg，置 10ml 量瓶中，加甲酸 2ml 溶解后，用丙酮稀释至刻度，摇匀，作为供试品溶液；精密量取 1ml 和 0.5ml，分别置 200ml 量瓶中，用丙酮稀释至刻度，作为对照溶液①和②。照薄层色谱法试验，吸取上述两种溶液各 10μl，分别点于同一硅胶 GF$_{254}$ 薄层板上，以三氯甲烷:甲醇:甲酸（90:5:5）为展开剂，展开，晾干，置紫外光灯（254nm）下检视。对照溶液②应显一个明显斑点，供试品溶液如显杂质斑点，与对照溶液①的主斑点比较，不得更深。

（3）干燥失重 取本品，在 105℃ 干燥至恒重，减失重量不得过 0.5%。

（4）炽灼残渣 取本品 1.0g，依法检查，遗留残渣不得过 0.1%。

（5）重金属 取炽灼残渣项下遗留的残渣，依法检查，含重金属不得过百万分之二十。

四、预习提要

（1）甲苯咪唑是世界卫生组织推荐的首选广谱驱虫药。该药存在 3 种结晶变体（A、B、C），不同的晶型可以转化，C 晶型为有效晶型，A 晶型为无效晶型，B 晶型疗效有待证明，药物中存在的混晶主要是 A 晶型。《中国药典》规定用红外分光光度法检查 A 晶型杂质，不得过 10%。A 晶型在 640cm^{-1} 的波数处有强吸收，C 晶型有弱吸收；A 晶型在 662cm^{-1} 的波数处有弱吸收，C 晶型有强吸收。当供试品中有 A 晶型时，在上述二波数处吸光度比值变化。

（2）物质在结晶时由于受各种因素影响，使分子内或分子间键合方式发生变化，致使分子或原子在晶格空间排列不同，形成不同的晶体结构。同一物质具有两种或两种以上的空间排列和晶胞参数，形成多种晶型的现象称为多晶现象。虽然在一定的温度和压力下，只有一种晶型在热力学上是稳定的，但由于从亚稳态转变为稳态的过程通常非常缓慢，因此许多结晶药物都存在多晶现象。固体多晶型包括构象型多晶型、构型型多晶型、色多晶型和假多晶型。同一药物的不同晶型在外观、溶解度、熔点、溶出度、生物有效性等方面可能显著不同，从而影响药物的稳定性、生物利用度及疗效，该种现象在口服固体制剂方面表现得尤为明显。药物多晶型现象是影响药品质量与临床疗效的重要因素之一，因此对存在多晶型的药物进行研发及审评时，应对其晶型分析予以特别关注。目前，鉴别晶型主要是针对不同的晶型具有不同的理化特性及光谱学特征来进行的：X 射线衍射法、红外吸收光谱法、熔点法和热台显微镜法、热分析法、偏光显微镜法、核磁共振法、溶解度方法、扫描隧道显微镜法、药物多晶型计算机辅助预测。

（3）结晶固体的多晶现象是由于相同化学组成的物质具有不同的晶格结构或不同的分子构象。红外光谱和拉曼光谱是用于晶型鉴定的有效的振动光谱方法。红外光谱和拉曼光谱可用于药物多晶型研究是由于不同晶型药物分子中的某些化学键键长、键角有所不同，致使其振动—转动跃迁能级不同，与其相应的红外光谱的某些主要特征，如吸收带频率、峰形、峰位、峰强度等也会出现差异。

五、实验指导

（一）红外分光光度法

1. 仪器及校正

可使用傅里叶红外变换光谱仪或色散型红外分光光度计。用聚乙烯薄膜（厚度约为 0.04mm）校正仪器，绘制其光谱图，用 3027cm^{-1}、2851cm^{-1}、1601cm^{-1}、1028cm^{-1}、907cm^{-1} 处的吸收峰对仪器的波数进行校正。傅里叶红外变换光谱仪在 3000cm^{-1} 附近的波数误差应不大于 ±5cm^{-1}，在 1000cm^{-1} 附近的波数误差应不大于 ±1cm^{-1}。

用聚乙烯薄膜校正时，仪器的分辨率要求在 3110~2850cm^{-1} 范围内应能清晰地分辨出 7 个峰，峰 2851cm^{-1} 与谷 2870cm^{-1} 之间的分辨深度不小于 18% 透光率，峰 1583cm^{-1} 与谷 1589cm^{-1} 之间的分辨深度不小于 12% 透光率。仪器的标称分辨率，除另有规定外，应不低于 2cm^{-1}。

2. 供试品的制备及测定

（1）原料药鉴别 除另有规定外，应按照国家药典委员会编订的《药品红外光谱集》

各卷收载的各光谱图所规定的方法制备样品，具体操作技术参见《药品红外光谱集》的说明。

采用固体制样技术时，最常碰到的问题是多晶现象，固体样品的晶型不同，其红外光谱往往也会产生差异。当供试品的实测光谱与《药品红外光谱集》所收载的标准光谱不一致时，当排除各种可能影响光谱的外在或人为因素后，应按该药品光谱图中备注的方法或各品种项规定的方法进行预处理，再绘制光谱，并比对。如未规定该品种供药用的晶型或预处理方法，则可使用对照品，并采用适当的溶剂对供试品与对照品在相同的条件下同时进行重结晶，然后依法绘制光谱，并比对。如已规定特定的药用晶型，则应采用相应的晶型对照品依法对比。

制样技术不能满足鉴别需要时，可改用溶液法绘制光谱后比对。

（2）制剂鉴别　品种鉴别项应明确规定制剂的前处理方法，通常采用溶剂提取法。提取时应选择适宜的溶剂，以尽可能减少辅料的干扰，并力求避免导致可能的晶型转变。提取的样品再经适当干燥后依法进行红外光谱鉴别。

（3）多组分原料药鉴别　不能采用全光谱比对，可借鉴以下"3. 注意事项（2）③"的方法，选择主要成分的若干个特征谱带，用于组成相对稳定的多组分原料药鉴别。

（4）晶型、异构体限度检查或含量测定　供试品制备和具体测定方法均按各品种项有关规定操作。

3. 注意事项

（1）各品种项规定"应与对照的图谱（光谱集××图）一致"系指《药品红外光谱集》各卷所载的图谱。同一化合物的图谱若在不同卷上均有收载时，则以后卷所载的图谱为准。

（2）药物制剂经提取处理并依法绘制光谱，比对时应注意以下四种情况：

①辅料无干扰，待测成分的晶型无变化，此时可直接与原料药的标准光谱进行比对；

②辅料无干扰，但待测成分的晶型有变化，此种情况可用对照品经同法处理后的光谱比对；

③待测成分的晶型不变化，而辅料存在不同程度的干扰，此时可参照原料药的标准光谱，在指纹区内选择 3～5 个不受辅料干扰的待测成分的特征谱带作为鉴别的依据，鉴别时，实测谱带的波数误差应小于规定值的 0.5%；

④待测成分的晶型有变化，辅料也存在干扰，此种情况一般不宜采用红外光谱鉴别。

（3）由于各种型号的仪器性能不同，供试品制备时研磨程度的差异或吸水程度不同等原因，均会影响光谱的形状。因此，进行光谱比对时，应考虑各种因素可能造成的影响。

（二）红外分光光度法试样的制备方法

1. 压片法

取供试品约 1mg，置玛瑙研钵中，加入干燥的溴化钾或氯化钾细粉约 200mg，充分研磨混匀，移置于直径为 13mm 的压模中，使铺布均匀，抽真空约 2min 后，加压至 0.8～1GPa，保持 2～5min，除去真空，取出制成的供试片，目视检查应均匀透明，无明显颗粒（也可采用其他直径的压模制片，样品与分散剂的用量可相应调整以制得浓度合适的片子）。将供试片置于仪器的样品光路中，并扣除用同法制成的空白溴化钾或氯化钾片的背景，录制光谱图。

对溴化钾或氯化钾的质量要求 用溴化钾或氯化钾制成空白片，录制光谱图，基线应大于75%透光率；除在3440cm^{-1}及1630cm^{-1}附近因残留或附着水而呈现一定的吸收峰外，其他区域不应出现大于基线3%透光率的吸收谱带。

2. 糊法

取供试品约5mg，置玛瑙研钵中，滴加少量液状石蜡或其他适宜的液体，制成均匀的糊状物，取适量夹于两个溴化钾片（每片重约150mg）之间，作为供试片；以溴化钾约300mg制成空白片作为背景补偿，录制光谱图。可用其他适宜的盐片夹持糊状物。

3. 膜法

参照上述糊法所述的方法，将液体供试品铺展于溴化钾片或其他适宜的盐片中录制，或将供试品置于适宜的液体池内录制光谱图。若供试品为高分子聚合物，可先制成适宜厚度的薄膜，然后置样品光路中测定。

4. 溶液法

将供试品溶于适宜的溶剂内，制成1%～10%浓度的溶液，置于0.1～0.5mm厚度的液体池中录制光谱图，并以相同厚度装有同一溶剂的液体池作为背景补偿。

5. 衰减全反射法

将供试品均匀地铺展在衰减全反射棱镜的底面上，并紧密接触，依法录制反射光谱图。

6. 气体法

采用光路长度约为10cm的气体池，首先将气体池抽真空，然后充以适当压力（例如30～50mmHg）的供试气体，录制光谱图。

（三）甲苯咪唑的红外光谱图

见图2-6。

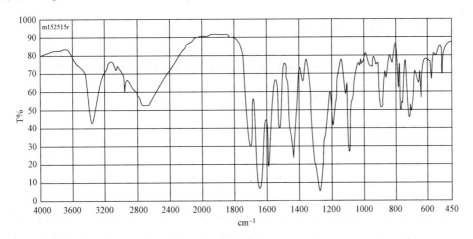

图2-6 甲苯咪唑的红外光谱图

仪器：傅里叶变换红外光谱仪；状态：溴化钾压片；四氢呋喃重结晶甲苯咪唑

六、讨论

（1）药物晶型测定的常用方法有哪些，各有什么特点？

（2）如何保证红外光谱测定数据结果真实可靠？

（3）红外分光光度法试样的制备方法有哪几种？

Experiment 3 Description, Identification and Tests of Mebendazole

1. Purposes

1.1 To learn about the influence of polymorphism of some drugs on their pharmacological effects.

1.2 To study the principle and methods for the test of polymorphism.

1.3 To grasp the measurement of specific absorbance.

2. Instruments and chemical reagents

2.1 Instruments

Analytic balance, UV spectrophotometer, infrared spectrometer, agate mortar, volumetric flask (5ml, 10ml, 100ml, 200ml), 10ml volumetric cylinder, pipette(0.5ml, 1ml), dropper, 50ml beaker, silica gel thin layer plate (GF$_{254}$), ultraviolet lamp, drying oven, weight flask, crucible, electric heater, Muffle furnace, Nessler's cylinder.

2.2 Chemical reagents

Mebendazole material, polymorph A (10%) mebendazole, formic acid, isopropyl alcohol, liquid paraffin, acetone, chloroform, methanol, nitric acid, sulfuric acid, hydrochloric acid, ammonia solution, phenolphthalein indicating liquid, acetate buffer(pH 3.5), standardization plumb solution, water.

3. Procedures and methods

3.1 Structure, molecular formula and molecular weight of mebendazole

(C$_{16}$H$_{13}$N$_3$O$_3$, Mw = 295.30)

Mebendazole is (5 – benzoyl – 1H – benzimidazol – 2 – yl) – carbamic acid methyl ester. It contains not less than 98.0% and not more than 102.0% of C$_{16}$H$_{13}$N$_3$O$_3$, calculated on the dried basis.

3.2 Description

A white, almost white or faintly yellow crystalline powder, odourless.

Freely soluble in formic acid; sparingly soluble in glacial acetic acid; very slightly soluble in acetone or chloroform; insoluble in water.

Specific absorbance　Dissolve about 50mg, accurately weighed, in 5ml of formic acid. Dilute with isopropanol to produce a solution of 10μg/ml. Measure the absorbance at 312nm, the value of A (1%, 1 cm) is 485 ~ 505.

3.3　Identification

3.3.1　Dissolve about 50mg, accurately weighed, in 5ml of formic acid, dilute with isopropanol to produce a solution of 10μg/ml. The light absorption exhibits a maximum at 312nm.

3.3.2　The infrared absorption spectrum is concordant with the reference spectrum(IR Album No. 101).

3.4　Test

Polymorph A　Weigh accurately about 25mg each of the substance being examined and mebendazole CRS which contains about 10% of polymorph A. Triturate with 0.3ml of liquid paraffin separately to form smooth creamy pastes. Mount the mull of about 0.15mm in thickness between rock salt plates, using a blank liquid paraffin mull as reference. Carry out the method for infrared spectrophotometry. Record the infrared spectra over the range $620 \sim 803cm^{-1}$ under the condition that the transmission of the substance being examined and mebendazole CRS at $803cm^{-1}$ is 90% ~ 95%. Draw a baseline between the minimum absorption occurring at $620cm^{-1}$ and $803cm^{-1}$ and lines from peaks at $640cm^{-1}$ and $662cm^{-1}$ perpendicular to the baseline. Calculate the absorbance of the corresponding absorption peak by the baseline absorption method. Calculate the ratio of the peak heights of the maximum at about $640cm^{-1}$ to that of the maximum at about $662cm^{-1}$. The peak height ratio of the substance being examined is not greater than that of mebendazole CRS containing 10% of polymorph A.

Related substances　Dissolve about 50mg, accurately weighed, in 2ml of formic acid in a 10ml volumetric flask, dilute with acetone to volume and mix well, as the test solution. Measure accurately a quantity of the test solution, dilute with acetone to produce two reference solutions containing 25μg/ml（Ⅰ）and 12.5μg/ml（Ⅱ）. Carry out the method for thin-layer chromatography, using silica gel GF_{254} as the coating substances and a mixture of chloroform：methanol：formic acid(90：5：5)as the mobile phase. Apply separately to the plate 10μl each of the three solutions. After developing and removing of the plate, dry it in air and examine under ultraviolet light at 254nm. The test is not valid unless the chromatogram obtained with the reference solution Ⅱ shows one clear spot. Any spot other than the principal spot in the chromatogram obtained with the test solution is not more intense than the principal spot obtained with the reference solution Ⅰ.

Loss on drying　When dried to constant weight at 105℃, loses not more than 0.5% of its weight.

Residue on ignition　Not more than 0.1%, using 1.00g.

Heavy metals　Carry out the limit test for heavy metals using the residue obtained in the test for residue on ignition：not more than 0.002%.

4. Prepare lessons before class

4.1　Mebendazole is a broad spectrum anthelminthic drug recommended by WHO, which is widely used in large scale deworming programmes. This active pharmaceutical ingredient exhibits three crystal forms, namely, polymorphs A, B, and C. Among the three crystal forms which could transform into each other, polymorph C is therapeutically favored, polymorph A is the inactive crystal form, while the effects of polymorphs B is still under estimation. Polymorph A is the main inactive crystal impurities in mebendazole. In Ch. P (2015), polymorph A is examined by infrared spectrophotometry, not greater than 10%. The principle of this test is as follows: in $640cm^{-1}$, polymorph A has strong absorption while polymorph C has weak absorption; in $662cm^{-1}$, polymorphs A has weak absorption while polymorphs C has strong absorption. If polymorph A exists in test samples, the ratio of absorbance under the two wave numbers will change.

4.2　Various factors in the process of drug preparation or refining may influence its crystal form. Polymorphism often exists in solid drugs, which is a very important factor affecting the quality and validity of drugs. A few methods for the analysis of drug crystal form were involved, such as X ray diffraction, infrared spectrometry, melting point method and heating stage microscopy, thermal analysis, polarization microscopy, nuclear magnetic resonance spectroscopy, dissolubility analysis, scanning tunnel microscopy, drug pleiomorphism computer-assisted calculation.

4.3　Polymorphism in crystalline solids is defined as materials with the same chemical composition, different lattice structures and/or different molecular conformations. Most prominent among the vibrational spectroscopic methods for polymorph identification are infrared and Raman spectroscopy. Both techniques offer information on structure and molecular conformation in the solid state by probing vibrations of atoms. These methods are especially important for the characterization of polymorphs because hydrogen-bonding patterns often differ among forms and the functional groups affected will display shifts of varying degrees. Other information gained from vibrational spectroscopies, which can be helpful in the distinction of polymorphs, includes low energy lattice vibrations caused by differences in crystal packing. Infrared spectroscopy observes vibrational modes associated with the absorption of a compound in the infrared region of the spectrum.

5. Guide for experiment

5.1　Infrared Spectrophotometry

5.1.1　Equipment and Calibration

Fourier-transform infrared spectrophotometer or dispersive infrared spectrophotometer are often used for pharmaceutical analysis. The wave-number scale of an infrared spectrophotometer may be calibrated by use of a polystyrene film of 0.04 mm thickness. The absorption peaks at $3027cm^{-1}$, $2851cm^{-1}$, $1601cm^{-1}$, $1028cm^{-1}$ and $907cm^{-1}$ are used for the calibration. Tolerance should be not more than $\pm 5cm^{-1}$ in the vicinity of $3000cm^{-1}$ and not more than $\pm 1cm^{-1}$ in the vicinity of $1000cm^{-1}$ for the Fourier-transform infrared spectrophotometer.

When a polystyrene film is used for calibration, the resolution factor of the instrument between $3110 \sim 2850cm^{-1}$ requires that seven peaks should be clearly isolated, the depth of the trough from the maximum absorption at about $1583cm^{-1}$ to the minimum at about $1589cm^{-1}$ should be not less than 12% transmittance and that from the maximum at about $2851cm^{-1}$ to the minimum at about $2870cm^{-1}$ should be not less than 18% transmittance. Unless otherwise specified, the nominal resolution factor of the instrument should not be less than $2cm^{-1}$.

5.1.2　Preparation and Determination

a. Identification for drug substances　Unless otherwise specified, for the identification test the substance being examined must be prepared according to the method described in each volume of "Atlas of Infrared Spectra of Drugs", edited by Chinese Pharmacopoeia Commission. Detailed procedures see also the Introduction of the Atlas.

If the spectrum obtained in the solid state with the substance being examined and the reference substance show differences due to polymorphism of solid specimen, in this case, after excluding the possibility of external or human factors, the substance being examined should be pre-treated according to the method for specified substance described in *Atlas of the Infrared Spectra of Drugs* or individual monograph, and then record the spectrum again. If the crystalline form and suitable pre-treatment method are not specified, the reference substance may be used, the substance being examined and the reference substance are re-crystallized using suitable solvent under the same condition and then be determined and compared. If the crystalline form is specified, the reference substance with corresponding crystalline form should be used.

When the solid sample preparation technique is not satisfactory for identification, Prepare a solution in a suitable solvent may be an alternative method used for comparison of spectrum.

b. Identification for preparations　The specimen should be prepared as described in the individual monograph, and solvent extraction method is often used. In order to minimize the interference of excipients and avoid the potential change of crystalline form as far as possible, suitable solvent should be chose for the extraction procedure, carry out the test for identification after the extract specimen has been dried by a suitable method.

c. Identification for multi-component drug substances　If it is not applicable to compare the spectrum in the region of $4000 \sim 400 cm^{-1}$, the method described in the "5. 1. 3 notes b(iii)" may be used, i. e. , carry out the identification test by comparison of main bands of major constituent provided that the substance being examined has a fixed composition.

d. Polymorphism inspection, limit test of the isomers and assay　The method of sample preparation and determination is performed according to the procedure described in the individual monograph.

5. 1. 3　Notes

a. In the monograph where infrared absorption spectrum is concordant with the reference spectrum refers to the spectrum specified in the above "*Atlas of Infrared Spectra of Drugs*". If the spectra for the same compound are described in different volume, the latter one should be taken as the reference.

b. Following are 4 approaches during the spectrum comparison for formulated preparations by extraction method.

i. The excipients in a formulated preparation do not interfere with the spectrum comparison and there is no change in the crystalline form of the substance being examined after the extraction, compare the recorded spectrum with the reference spectrum of its drug substance.

ii. The excipients in a formulated preparation do not interfere with the spectrum comparison, however, there is difference in the crystalline form of the substance being examined after the extraction, the reference substance may be used. The extracted sample and the reference substance should be treated under the same condition and then be determined and compared.

iii. There is no change in the crystalline form for substance being examined after the extraction, however, the excipients have somewhat interference with the spectrum comparison, based on the reference spectrum of its drug substances, select 3 ~ 5 specific bands of absorption in the fingerprint region, where excipients have no interference for the comparison, and perform the spectrum comparison refer to the above criteria for identification. In the identification, the deviation between the specified wave number and that of measured should be not more than 0.5%.

iv. There is difference in the crystalline form of the substance being examined after the extraction, and excipients also interfere with the comparison after treatment, infrared spectrophotometry is not recommended for the identification test due to the complicated conditions.

c. Several factors such as difference in instrument performance of various models, inadequate or successive grinding in preparation of the disc, or water sucking etc, may give rise to unsatisfactory spectrum in shape. It should be kept in mind during the comparison with the reference spectrum.

5.2　Procedures for preparation of samples in infrared spectrophotometry

5.2.1　Disc Method

Triturate about 1mg of the substance being examined with approximate 200mg of dried, finely powdered potassium bromide or potassium chloride in an agate mortar. Grind the mixture thoroughly and spread it uniformly in a die of 13mm in diameter. Compress the mixture under vacuum with a pressure applied to the die of 0.8 ~ 1Gpa from 2 to 5 minutes. Take out the die assembly has been evacuated about 2 minutes. Remove the vacuum and take off the disc. The resultant disc should be uniform transparent and free from any obvious particles by visual inspection. When and if the die of other diameters is used, the dosages of sample and dispersive reagent should be adjusted accordingly to prepare the disc with suitable concentration. Mount the disc in a suitable holder and place it into the sample beam of the spectrophotometer. Place a similarly prepared blank disc of potassium bromide or potassium chloride into the sample beam for background compensation. Record the spectrum with background deducted.

Quality requirement for potassium bromide or potassium chloride record the spectrum of a blank disc of potassium bromide or potassium chloride prepared as described above. The spectrum has a substantially flat baseline exhibiting no maxima with an absorbance greater than 3% of transmittance above the baseline, with the exception of maxima due to residual or absorbed water at about $3440cm^{-1}$ and $1630cm^{-1}$. The baseline should be more than 75% of transmittance.

5.2.2　Mull method

Triturate about 5mg of the substance being examined with a little amount of liquid paraffin or other suitable liquid to give a homogeneous creamy paste in an agate mortar. Compress and hold a portion of the mull between two flat potassium bromide plates (about 150mg each). Record the spectrum by using a blank disc of potassium bromide with about 300mg in weight for background compensation. Other suitable salt plates may be used instead of potassium bromide plates.

5.2.3　Film method

Use a capillary film of the liquid substance being examined held between two potassium bromide plates or other suitable salt plates with the method as described in the mull method. A filled cell of suitable thickness may be also used. For high polymer, prepare a film with suitable thickness. Mount the film in a suitable holder and place it into the sample beam. Record the spectrum.

5.2.4 Solution method

Prepare a solution of the substance being examined in a suitable solvent to the concentrations of 1% ~ 10% . Place the solution in a filled cell with a thickness of 0.1 to 0.5 mm. Record the spectrum when a matched cell filled with the same solvent as background.

5.2.5 ATR method

Place the substance being examined in a manner of homogeneous and close contact with an ATR(Attenuated Total Reflectance) prism, and record its reflectance spectrum.

5.2.6 Gas method

Examine gases in a cell with optical path length of about 10cm. Evacuate the cell and fill the gas being examined to a suitable pressure(for example, 30 ~ 50mmHg). Record the spectrum.

5.3 Infrared spectra of mebendazole

See Figure 2 – 6.

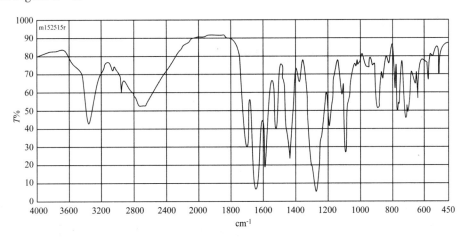

Figure 2 – 6   Infrared spectra of mebendazole

Instrument: Fourier Transform Infrared Spectrophotometer;

Phase: potassium bromide disc; Re-crystallized mebendazole(tetrahydrofuran).

6. Discussion

6.1   What are the commonly used methods for the test of polymorphism? And what are the characteristics of each of them?

6.2   What are the factors that influence the accuracy and reliability of infrared spectrophotometry?

6.3   What are the commonly used methods for preparation of samples in infrared spectrophotometry?

(徐新军)

实验四　维生素 B₁ 的性状、鉴别和检查

一、目的

（1）掌握维生素 B₁ 专属鉴别反应的原理和方法。

（2）掌握维生素 B₁ 有关物质检查方法。

（3）熟悉维生素 B₁ 一般杂质检查的原理和方法。

二、仪器与试药

1. 仪器

分析天平，荧光计或荧光分光光度计，高效液相色谱仪。

2. 试药

维生素 B₁ 对照品，铁氰化钾，氢氧化钠，盐酸，异丁醇，无水乙醇，甲醇，乙腈，庚烷磺酸钠，磷酸。

三、实验方法

1. 维生素 B₁ 的结构式、分子式和分子量

$$(C_{12}H_{17}ClN_4OS \cdot HCl \quad Mw = 337.27)$$

本品为氯化甲基 – 3 – ［（2 – 甲基 – 4 – 氨基 – 5 – 嘧啶基）甲基］ – 5 – （2 – 羟基乙基）噻唑鎓盐酸盐。按干燥品计算，含 $C_{12}H_{17}ClN_4OS \cdot HCl$ 不得少于 99.0%。

2. 性状

本品为白色结晶或结晶性粉末；有微弱的特臭，味苦；干燥品在空气中迅即吸收约 4% 的水分。

本品在水中易溶，在乙醇中微溶，在乙醚中不溶。

吸收系数　取本品，精密称定，加盐酸溶液（9→1000）溶解并定量稀释制成每 1ml 约含 12.5μg 的溶液，照紫外 – 可见分光光度法（《中国药典》四部通则 0401），在 246nm 的波长处测定吸光度，吸收系数（$E_{1cm}^{1\%}$）为 406 ~ 436。

3. 鉴别

（1）维生素 B₁ 的荧光鉴别　取 50ml 量瓶，精密加入对照品溶液 5ml，迅速加入（1 ~ 2s 内）氧化试剂 3.0ml，在 30s 内再加入异丁醇 20.0ml，密塞，剧烈振摇 90s；再加入无水乙醇 2ml，旋摇数秒，带分层后，取上层澄清的异丁醇液约 10ml，置荧光计测定池内，进行荧光扫描，确定维生素 B₁ 的最大激发波长（excitation wavelength）和发射波长（emission wavelength）。

对照品溶液的制备：取维生素 B₁ 对照品约 20mg，精密称定，溶于 300ml 的稀醇溶液

（1→5），用 3mol/L 盐酸溶液调节至 pH4.0，加稀醇稀释成 1000ml，作为储备液，避光冷藏，储存期 1 个月。精密吸取对照品储备液 1.0ml，置 10ml 量瓶中，用 0.2mol/L 盐酸溶液稀释至刻度，摇匀，得 2μg/ml 的溶液，再精密吸取 2μg/ml 的溶液 1.0ml，置 10ml 量瓶中，用 0.2mol/L 盐酸溶液稀释至刻度，摇匀，得 0.2μg/ml 的溶液，即得。

氧化试剂的制备　取新鲜配制的 1.0% 铁氰化钾溶液 4.0ml，加 3.5mol/L 氢氧化钠溶液制成 100ml，于 4h 内使用。

（2）取本品适量，加水溶解，水浴蒸干，在 105℃ 干燥 2 小时测定。本品的红外光吸收图谱应与对照的图谱（光谱集 1205 图）一致。

（3）本品的水溶液显氯化物鉴别（1）的反应（《中国药典》四部通则 0301）。

4. 检查

酸度　取本品 0.50g，加水 20ml 溶解后，依法测定（通则 0631），pH 值应为 2.8~3.3。

溶液的澄清度与颜色取本品 1.0g，加水 10ml 溶解后，溶液应澄清无色；如显色，与对照液（取比色用重铬酸钾液 0.1ml，加水适量使成 10ml）比较，不得更深。

硫酸盐　取本品 2.0g，依法检查（通则 0802），与标准硫酸钾溶液 2.0ml 制成的对照液比较，不得更浓（0.01%）。

硝酸盐　取本品 1.0g，加水溶解并稀释至 100ml，取 1.0ml，加水 4.0ml 与 10% 氯化钠溶液 0.5ml，摇匀，精密加稀靛胭脂试液［取靛胭脂试液，加等量的水稀释。临用前，量取本液 1.0ml，用水稀释至 50ml，照紫外－可见分光光度法（《中国药典》四部通则 0401），在 610nm 的波长处测定，吸光度应为 0.3~0.4］1ml，摇匀，沿管壁缓缓加硫酸 5.0ml，立即缓缓振摇 1 分钟，放置 10 分钟，与标准硝酸钾溶液（精密称取在 105℃ 干燥至恒重的硝酸钾 81.5mg，置 50ml 量瓶中，加水溶解并稀释至刻度，摇匀，精密量取 5ml，置 100ml 量瓶中，用水稀释至刻度，摇匀。每 1ml 相当于 50μg 的 NO_3）0.50ml 用同法制成的对照液比较，不得更浅（0.25%）。

有关物质　取本品，精密称定，用流动相溶解并稀释制成每 1ml 中约含 1mg 的溶液，作为供试品溶液；精密量取 1ml，置 100ml 量瓶中，用流动相稀释至刻度，摇匀，作为对照溶液。照高效液相色谱法（《中国药典》四部通则 0512）试验，用十八烷基硅烷键合硅胶为填充剂，以甲醇－乙腈－0.02mol/L 庚烷磺酸钠溶液（含 1% 三乙胺，用磷酸调节 pH 值至 5.5）（9：9：82）为流动相，检测波长为 254nm，理论板数按维生素 B_1 峰计算不低于 2000，维生素 B_1 峰与相邻峰的分离度均应符合要求。精密量取供试品溶液与对照溶液各 20μl，分别注入液相色谱仪，记录色谱图至主峰保留时间的 3 倍。供试品溶液色谱图中如有杂质峰，各杂质峰面积的和不得大于对照溶液主峰面积的 0.5 倍（0.5%）。

干燥失重　取本品，在 105℃ 干燥至恒重，减失重量不得过 5.0%（《中国药典》四部通则 0831）。

炽灼残渣　不得过 0.1%（《中国药典》四部通则 0841）。

铁盐　取本品 1.0g，加水 25ml 溶解后，依法检查（《中国药典》四部通则 0807），与标准铁溶液 2.0ml 制成的对照液比较，不得更深（0.002%）。

重金属　取本品 1.0g，加水 25ml 溶解后，依法检查（《中国药典》四部通则 0821 第一法），含重金属不得过百万分之十。

总氯量　取本品约 0.2g，精密称定，加水 20ml 溶解后，加稀醋酸 2ml 与溴酚蓝指示液

8~10 滴，用硝酸银滴定液（0.1mol/L）滴定至显蓝紫色。每1ml 硝酸银滴定液（0.1mol/L）相当于3.54mg 的氯（Cl）。按干燥品计算，含总氯量应为20.6%~21.2%。

四、预习提要

1. 简述维生素 B_1 的结构特点与理化性质。

2. 硫色素荧光反应为维生素 B_1 的专属鉴别反应，其反应原理是什么？

3. HPLC 法应用于药物的有关物质检查有哪几种方法？本实验中有关物质的检查采用哪一种方法？

4. 应用反相键合相色谱法分析有机弱酸或弱碱和完全离子化的强酸或强碱时，其色谱条件有何特点？

五、实验指导

（一）荧光光谱分析

某些物质吸收光能量后，可发射波长与激发光波长相同或不同的光，当激发光源停止照射试样时，再发射过程立即停止，这种再发射的光称为荧光（fluorescence）。荧光包括分子荧光和原子荧光。荧光分析法是通过测定物质分子产生的荧光强度进行物质的定性与定量分析的方法。采用荧光分析法来测量的仪器称为荧光光谱分析仪。

任何发射荧光的物质都具有两个特征光谱，即激发光谱（excitation spectrum）和荧光光谱（fluorescence spectrum）。

激发光谱：连续改变激发光波长，固定荧光发射波长，测定不同波长的激发光照射下，物质溶液发射的荧光强度的变化。以激发光波长为横坐标，荧光强 ERWQ 度为纵坐标作图，即可得到荧光物质的激发光谱。从激发光谱图上可找到发生荧光强度最强的激发波长 λ_{ex}。

荧光光谱：用 λ_{ex} 作激发光源，并固定强度，测定不同波长的荧光强度。以荧光波长为横坐标，荧光强度为纵坐标作图，便得荧光光谱。荧光强度最强的波长为 λ_{em}。荧光物质的 λ_{ex} 和 λ_{em} 是鉴定物质的依据，也是定量测定中所选用的最灵敏的波长。

荧光光谱仪的工作原理：在激发光的频率、强度以及液层厚度不变的情况下，荧光物质所发射的荧光强度与溶液的浓度成正比。因此，可以通过测定荧光强度来求出该物质的含量。

荧光分析法所测量的是待测物质所发射的荧光强弱，属于发射光谱分析，荧光光度计和荧光分光光度计属于发射光谱仪器。荧光光度计（fluorophotometer）：采用滤光片做单色器，结构较简单，功能也较差。荧光分光光度计（fluorospectrophotometer）：采用棱镜或光栅为色散元件，结构较复杂，功能较强，但价格远远高于荧光光度计。

（二）高效液相色谱法

（1）加校正因子的主成分自身对照法测定杂质含量时，可采用加校正因子的主成分自身对照法。在建立方法时，按各品种项下的规定，精密称（量）取杂质对照品和主成分对照品各适量，配制测定杂质相对于主成分校正因子的溶液，进样，记录色谱图，按下式计算杂质的校正因子。

$$校正因子 = \frac{C_A / A_A}{C_B / A_B}$$

式中，C_A 为杂质的浓度；A_A 为杂质的峰面积或峰高；C_B 为主成分的浓度；A_B 为主成分的峰面积或峰高。

也可精密称（量）取主成分对照品和杂质对照品各适量，分别配制成不同浓度的溶液，进样，记录色谱图，绘制主成分浓度和杂质浓度对其峰面积的回归曲线，以主成分回归直线斜率与杂质回归直线斜率的比计算校正因子。

校正因子可直接载入各品种项下，用于校正杂质的实测峰面积。需作校正计算的杂质，通常以主成分为参比，采用相对保留时间定位，其数值一并载入各品种项下。测定杂质含量时，按各品种项下规定的杂质限度，将供试品溶液稀释成与杂质限度相当的溶液，作为对照溶液；进样，记录色谱图，必要时，调节纵坐标范围（以噪声水平可接受为限）使对照溶液的主成分色谱峰的峰高约达满量程的 10% ~ 25% 。除另有规定外，通常含量低于 0.5% 的杂质，峰面积的相对标准偏差（RSD）应小于 10%；含量在 0.5% ~ 2% 的杂质，峰面积的 RSD 应小于 5 %；含量大于 2% 的杂质，峰面积的 RSD 应小于 2%。然后，取供试品溶液和对照溶液适量，分别进样，除另有规定外，供试品溶液的记录时间，应为主成分色谱峰保留时间的 2 倍，测量供试品溶液色谱图上各杂质的峰面积，分别乘以相应的校正因子后与对照溶液主成分的峰面积比较，计算各杂质含量。

（2）不加校正因子的主成分自身对照法

测定杂质含量时，若无法获得待测杂质的校正因子，或校正因子可以忽略，也可采用不加校正因子的主成分自身对照法。同上述（3）法配制对照溶液、进样调节纵坐标范围和计算峰面积的相对标准偏差后，取供试品溶液和对照品溶液适量，分别进样。除另有规定外，供试品溶液的记录时间应为主成分色谱峰保留时间的 2 倍，测量供试品溶液色谱图上各杂质的峰面积并与对照溶液主成分的峰面积比较，依法计算杂质含量。

（3）面积归一化法

按各品种项下的规定，配制供试品溶液，取一定量进样，记录色谱图。测量各峰的面积和色谱图上除溶剂峰以外的总色谱峰面积，计算各峰面积占总峰面积的百分率。用于杂质检查时，由于仪器响应的线性限制，峰面积归一化法一般不宜用于微量杂质的检查。

六、讨论

1. 采用荧光分析法时，应注意避免哪些干扰因素？

2. 可用"加校正因子的主成分自身对照法"测定杂质含量，这里的校正因子指的是什么？为什么要测定校正因子？

3. 根据维生素 B_1 的结构特点，对其有关物质检查的 HPLC 色谱条件进行分析。

Experiment 4　Description，Identification and Tests of Vitamin B_1

1. Purposes

1.1　To study the principles and methods of Vitamin B_1 exclusive identification reaction.

1.2　To experiment on the limit test for the related compounds of Vitamin B_1.

1.3　To be familiar with the principles and methods of Vitamin B_1 general impurity inspection.

2. Instruments and chemical reagents

2.1 Instruments

Analytical balance, fluorometer or fluorescence spectrophotometer, high performance liquid chromatography.

2.2 Chemical reagets

Vitamin B_1 reference substance, potassium ferricyanide, sodium hydroxide, hydrochloric acid, isobutanol, absolute ethanol, methanol, acetonitrile, sodium heptane sulfonate, phosphoric acid.

3. Procedures and methods

3.1 Structure, molecular formula and molecular weight of Vitamin B_1

$$(C_{12}H_{17}ClN_4OS \cdot HCl \quad Mw = 337.27)$$

Thisproduct is methyl-3-[(2-methyl-4-amino-5-pyrimidinyl) methyl]-5-(2-hydroxyethyl) thiazo – lium hydrochloride. Calculated as dry product, containing $C_{12}H_{17}ClN_4OS \cdot HCl$ should not be less than 99.0%.

3.2 Description

White crystal or crystalline powder; odour, slightly characteristic; taste, bitter. When exposed to air, the driedsubstance rapidly absorbs about 4% of water.

Freely soluble in water; slightly soluble in ethanol; and insoluble in ether.

Specific absorbance   Measure the absorbance of a solution of 12.5 μg per ml in hydrochloric acid solution (9 →1000) at 246 nm(0401), the value of A (1%, 1cm) is 406 to 436.

3.3 Identification

3.3.1   Transfer 5.0 ml standard solution to 50 ml volumetric flask, add 3.0 ml oxidation reagent rapidly (within 1~2s), add 20.0 ml n – butanol in 30s, replace the stopper with airproof, shake 90s severely; add 2 ml absolute ethyl alcohol, shake some seconds, after layer separation, transfer 10 ml clear liquid in the upper layer to the cell of the FR instrument, scan the FR figure.

Preparation of standard solution   weigh accurately 20 mg vitamin B_1 CRS, dissolve in 300 ml diluent ethanol (1→5), adjust pH to 4.0 with 3mol/L hydrochloric acid, and then dilute with diluent ethanol to 1000 ml as the stock solution. The stock solution is valid for 1 month when stored under refrigeration and protected from light. Transfer 1.0 ml stock solution to 10 ml volumetric flask, dilute with 0.2mol/L hydrochloric acid to volume, mix well to produce 2μg/ml solution. Then transfer 2μg/ml solution 1.0 ml to 10 ml volumetric flask, dilute with 0.2mol/L hydrochloric acid to volume, mix well to produce the 0.2μg/ml solution.

Preparation of oxidation reagent   take freshly prepared 1.0% potassium ferricyanide solution

4. 0ml,add 3. 5mol/L sodium hydroxide solution to make 100ml,use within 4h.

3. 3. 2　Dissolve a quantity in water and evaporate to dryness on a water bath. The infrared absorption spectrum of the residue dried at 105℃ for 2 hours (0402) is concordant with the reference spectrum (IR Album No. 1205).

3. 3. 3　The aqueous solution yields the reactions (1) characteristic of chloride (0301).

3. 3. 4　Test

Acidity　Dissolve 0. 50 g in 20 ml of water, , pH 2. 8 ~ 3. 3(0631).

Clarity and color of the solution　A solution of 1. 0 g in 10 ml of water is clear and colorless. Any color produced is not more intense than that of a reference solution prepared by diluting 0. 1 ml of standard potassium dichromate CS with water to 10 ml.

Sulfate　Carry out the limit test for sulfates (0802),using 2. 0g. Any opalescence produced is not more pronounced than that of a reference using 2. 0 ml of potassium sulfate standard solution (0. 01%).

Nitrate　Dissolve 1. 0g in water and dilute to 100ml,measure 1. 0 ml,add 4. 0ml of water and 0. 5ml of 10% sodium chloride solution,mix well,add accurately 1. 0ml of dilute indigocarmine TS[①] and mix well. Then add slowly,along the wall of the tube,5. 0 ml of sulfuric acid,shake gently for 1 minute and allow to stand for 10 minutes. The colour of the solution is not lighter than that of a reference solution prepared by treating 0. 50 ml of standard potassium nitrate solution[②] in the same manner (0. 25%).

Preparation of dilute indigocarmine TS：Dilute indigocarmine TS with an equal volume of water. The absorbance of a dilution (1→50) measured at 610 nm (0401) immediately before use is 0. 3 - 0. 4.

Preparation of standard potassium nitrate solution：Weigh accurately 81. 5 mg of potassium nitrate CRS,previously dried to constant weight at 105℃,to a 50 ml volumetric flask,dissolve in water and dilute to volume,mix well. Measure 5 ml accurately to a 100 ml volumetric flask,dilute with water to volumn and mix well. Each ml of the solution is equivalent to 50 μg NO_3.

Related substance　Carry out the method for high performance liquid chromatography (0512), using a column packed with octadecylsilane bonded silica gel and a mixture of methanol – acetonitrile – 0. 02mol/L heptanesulfonate solution (containing 1% triethylamine and adjust to pH 5. 5 with phosphoric acid) (9 : 9 : 82) as the mobile phase. Detection wavelength is 254nm,and the number of theoretical plates of the column is not less than 2000,calculated with reference to the peak of vitamin B_1. The resolution factor between the principal peak and its adjacent impurity peak complies with the related requirements.

Prepare asolution of 1. 0 mg per ml in mobile phase as test solution；Transfer accurately 1 ml of the test solution into 100 ml volumetric flask,dilute to volume with mobile phase,mix well and use as reference solution. Inject separately 20μl each of the test solution and the reference solution into the column and record the chromatogram for 3 times the retention time of the principal peak,the sum of the areas of all peaks other than the principal peak in the chromatogram obtained with the test solution is not more than 0. 5 time the area of the principal peak in the chromatogram obtained with the reference solution (0. 5%).

Loss on drying　When dried to constant weight at 105℃,loses not more than 5. 0% of its weight (0831).

Residue on ignition   Not more than 0.1% (0841)

Iron   Dissolve 1.0g in 25 ml of water, carry out the limit test for iron (0807). Any color produced is not more intense than that of a reference solution prepared by using 2.0ml of iron standard solution (0.002%).

Heavymetals   Dissolve 1.0g in 25 ml of water, carry out the limit test for heavy metals (0821, method 1): not more than 0.001%.

Total chlorine   Dissolve about 0.2 g, accurately weighed, in 20 ml of water, add 2 ml of dilute acetic acid and 8 ~ 10 drops of bromophenol blue IS, titrate with silver nitrate (0.1 mol/L) VS until the colour changes to bluish – violet. Each ml of silver nitrate (0.1 mol/L) VS is equivalent to 3.54 mg of Cl. It contains not less than 20.6% and not more than 21.2% of Cl, calculated on the dried basis.

4. Prepare lessons before class

4.1   Briefly describe the structural characteristics and physicochemical properties of Vitamin B_1.

4.2   The sulfur pigment fluorescence reaction is the exclusive identification reaction of Vitamin B_1.

What is thereaction principle?

4.3   What are the methods for the application of HPLC in the examination of related substances in drugs? Which method is used in this experiment?

4.4   What are the characteristics of chromatographic conditions when using reversed phase bonded phase chromatography to analyze organic weak or weak bases and fully ionized strong acids or bases?

5. Guide for experiment

5.1   Fluorescence spectroscopy

When some substances absorb light energy, they emit light of the same or different wavelength asthe wavelength of the excitation light. When the excitation source stops illuminating the sample, the re-emission process stops immediately. This re-emitted light is called fluorescence. Fluorescence includes molecular fluorescence and atomic fluorescence. Fluorescence analysis is a method of qualitative and quantitative analysis of a substance by measuring the intensity of fluorescence generated by a substance molecule. An instrument that uses fluorescence analysis to measure is called a fluorescence spectrum analyzer.

Any substance that emits fluorescence has two characteristic spectra, an excitation spectrum and a fluorescence spectrum.

Excitation spectrum   continuously change the wavelength of the excitation light, fix the fluorescence emission wavelength, and measure the change of the fluorescence intensity emitted by the substance solution under the excitation light of different wavelengths. The excitation spectrum of the fluorescent substance can be obtained by plotting the wavelength of the excitation light as the abscissa and the fluorescence intensity as the ordinate. The excitation wavelength λ_{ex} at which the fluorescence intensity is strongest can be found from the excitation spectrum.

Fluorescence spectrum　λ_{ex} was used as the excitation source, and the intensity was fixed to measure the fluorescence intensity at different wavelengths. The fluorescence spectrum is obtained by plotting the fluorescence wavelength as the abscissa and the fluorescence intensity as the ordinate. The wavelength with the strongest fluorescence intensity is λ_{em}. The λ_{ex} and λ_{em} of the fluorescent substance are the basis for identifying the substance and the most sensitive wavelength selected for the quantitative determination.

The working principle of the fluorescence spectrometer: under the condition that the frequency, intensity and thickness of the excitation light are constant, the fluorescence intensity emitted by the fluorescent substance is proportional to the concentration of the solution. Therefore, the content of the substance can be determined by measuring the fluorescence intensity.

The fluorescence analysis method measures the fluorescence intensity emitted by the substance to be tested, and belongs to the emission spectrum analysis. The fluorescence photometerand the fluorescence spectrophotometer belong to the emission spectrum instrument. Fluorescence photometer (fluorophotometer): The filter is used as a monochromator, which has a simple structure and poor function. Fluoroscopy spectrophotometer (fluorospectrophotometer): using prisms or gratings as dispersive components, the structure is more complicated, and the function is stronger, but the price is much higher than the fluorescence photometer.

5. 2　High performance liquid chromatography

5. 2. 1　When the impurity content is determined by the main component self – control method with the correction factor, the principal component self – control method with the correction factor can be used. When establishing the method, according to the provisions under each item, Precisely weigh the amount of the impurity reference substance and the main component reference substance, prepare a solution for measuring the impurity relative to the principal component correction factor, inject the sample, record the chromatogram, and calculate the correction factor of the impurity according to the following formula.

$$correction\ factor = \frac{C_A / A_A}{C_B / A_B}$$

Where C_A is the concentration of impurities, A_A is the peak area or peak height of impurities, C_B is the concentration of the main component, A_B is the peak area or peak height of the main component.

It can also be accurately weighed (quantity) the appropriate amount of the main component reference substance and the impurity reference substance, respectively, and prepare different concentrations of the solution, inject the sample, record the chromatogram, and draw a regression curve by taking the main component concentration (or impurity concentration) as the abscissa, and the correspondingpeak area as the ordinate. The correction factor is calculated by the ratio of the slope of the main component regression line to the slope of the impurity regression line.

The correction factor can be directly loaded under each category to correct the measured peak area of the impurity. Impurities that need to be corrected, usually based on the principal component, are positioned with relative retention time, and their values are included in each category. When measuring the impurity content, the test solution is diluted to a solution equivalent to the impurity limit according to the impurity limit specified in each item, as a control solution; inject, record the chromatogram, and if necessary, adjust the ordinate range (limit to acceptable noise levels) so that the peak height of the main component peak of the control solution is about 10% to 25% of full scale. Unless otherwise specified, the relative standard deviation (RSD) of the peak area should be less than 10% for impurities with a content of less than 0.5%; the RSD of the peak area should be less than 5% for impurities with a content between 0.5% and 2%. ; for impurities with a content greater than 2%, the RSD of the peak area should be less than 2%. Then, take the appropriate amount of the test solution and the control solution, and inject separately, unless otherwise specified, the recording time of the test solution shall be twice the retention time of the main component chromatographic peak. The peak area of each impurity on the chromatogram of the test solution shall be measured and multiplied by the corresponding correction factor. The corrected peak area of the impurity was compared with the peak area of the main component of the control solution, and the content of each impurity was calculated.

5.2.2　Main component self – control method without correction factor

When the impurity content is determined, if the correction factor of the impurity to be tested cannot be obtained, or the correction factor is negligible, the principal component self – control method without the correction factor may be used. With the above method (1), prepare the control solution, adjust the vertical coordinate range of the injection and calculate the relative standard deviation of the peak area, take the appropriate amount of the test solution and the reference solution, and inject respectively. Unless otherwise specified, the recording time of the test solution should be 2 times of the retention time of the main component chromatographic peak. The peak area of each impurity on the chromatogram of the test solution is measured and compared with the peak area of the main component of the control solution. Calculate the impurity content.

5.2.3　Area normalization method

According to the provisions under each item, prepare the test solution, take a certain amount of injection, and record the chromatogram. The area of each peak and the total chromatographic peak area on the chromatogram except the solvent peak were measured, and the percentage of each peak area to the total peak area was calculated. For impurity inspection, the peak area normalization method is generally not suitable for the inspection of trace impurities due to the linear limitation of the instrument response.

6. Discussion

6.1　What kinds of disturbances should be avoided when using fluorescence analysis?

6.2　The impurity content can be determined by the "Main component self – control method with correction factor". What is the correction factor here? Why measure the correction factor?

6.3　Please discuss the HPLC chromatographic conditions for the examination of related substances of Vitamin B$_1$ according to its structural characteristics.

（宋　瑞）

实验五 典型中药的鉴别

一、目的

（1）掌握薄层色谱法在中药化学成分鉴别中的应用。

（2）了解显微鉴别的方法与特点。

二、仪器与试药

1. 仪器

显微镜、加热回流装置、硅胶 G 薄层板（羧甲基纤维素钠为黏合剂）、紫外光灯、展开缸、点样器、喷雾显色装置、水浴锅、漏斗、滤纸、蒸发皿。

2. 试药

三黄片、吴茱萸、茯苓、人参、盐酸小檗碱对照品、黄芩苷对照品、大黄对照药材、大黄酚对照品、大黄素对照品、甲醇、乙酸乙酯、丁酮、甲酸、水、稀盐酸、三氯化铁乙醇溶液、乙醚、石油醚（30~60℃）、甲酸乙酯、浓氨水、槐花或槐米、芦丁对照品、乙醇、镁粉、盐酸。

三、实验方法

（一）药材的理化鉴别

1. 吴茱萸中生物碱及挥发油的鉴别

（1）取本品粉末 0.5g，置 10ml 带塞试管中，加盐酸溶液（1→100）8ml，用力振摇数分钟，滤过。取滤液 2ml，加碘化汞钾试液 1 滴，振摇后，发生黄白色沉淀；取滤液 1ml，缓缓加入对二甲氨基苯甲醛试液 2ml，置水浴上加热（勿振摇），两液接面出现红褐色环状带。

（2）取本品粉末适量，经微量升华得油状物，加硫酸 2 滴及香兰素结晶少量，观察颜色变化，另以乙醚溶液取适量升华所得油状物，点样于硅胶 G 薄层板上，以石油醚:乙酸乙酯（8:1）为展开剂展开，取出，晾干，喷以香兰素 – 浓硫酸试剂，观察挥发油斑点（可与水蒸气蒸馏所得挥发油对照）。

2. 茯苓中茯苓多糖的鉴别

取本品粉末 0.5g，置试管中加蒸馏水 10ml，以热水浴中振摇提取数分钟，过滤，取滤液 2ml，加新鲜配制 5% 的 α – 萘酚的乙醇液数滴，沿管缓缓加入硫酸 0.5ml，放置片刻，两液接界处显紫红色环，加热振摇后，管中液体呈紫色浑浊状，放置数小时后可见紫色沉淀。

3. 人参中人参皂苷的鉴别

（1）取人参粉末约 0.2g，加乙酐 2ml，在水浴上加温 2min，过滤。取滤液 1ml，缓缓加入浓硫酸 0.5ml，两液交界面红色变为红棕色，最后呈暗棕色。

（2）取人参粉末约 0.5g，加乙醇 5ml，振摇 5min，滤过，取滤液少量，置蒸发皿中蒸干，滴加三氯化锑的三氯甲烷饱和溶液，再蒸干，显紫色。

4. 槐花的鉴别

取本品粉末0.1g，加乙醇10ml，加热5min，滤过。取滤液1ml，加镁粉少量与盐酸2～3滴，即显樱红色。

（二）三黄片的鉴别

1. 处方

大黄300g，盐酸小檗碱5g，黄芩浸膏21g，制成1000片。

2. 性状

本品为糖衣片或薄膜衣片，除去包衣后显棕色；味苦、微涩。

3. 鉴别

（1）大黄显微鉴别　取本品2～3片，至乳钵中研成粉末，取适量置载玻片上，滴加甘油乙酸试液、水合氯醛试液或其他适当试液，盖上盖玻片，置显微镜下观察：草酸钙簇晶大，直径60～140μm。

（2）盐酸小檗碱和黄芩苷的鉴别　取本品5片，除去包衣，研细，取0.25g加甲醇5ml，超声处理5min，滤过，滤液作为供试品溶液。另取盐酸小檗碱对照品，加甲醇制成每毫升含0.2mg的溶液；取黄芩苷对照品，加甲醇制成每毫升含1mg的溶液，作为对照品溶液。照薄层色谱法试验，吸取上述三种溶液各3～5μl，分别点于同一硅胶G薄层板上，以乙酸乙酯：丁酮：甲酸：水（10:7:1:1）为展开剂，展开，取出，晾干，分别在紫外光灯（365nm）和紫外光灯（254nm）下检视。供试品色谱中，在与盐酸小檗碱对照品色谱相应的位置上，紫外光（365nm）下显相同颜色的荧光斑点；在与黄芩苷对照品色谱相应的位置上，紫外光（254nm）下显相同颜色的斑点。

（3）大黄对照药材的鉴别　取鉴别（2）项下的供试品溶液作为供试品溶液。另取大黄对照药材0.2g，加甲醇3ml，超声处理5min，取上清液作为对照药材溶液。照薄层色谱法试验，吸取上述两种溶液各5μl，分别点于同一硅胶G薄层板上，以环己烷：乙酸乙酯：甲酸（12:3:0.1）为展开剂，展开，取出，晾干，置紫外光灯（365nm）下检视。在供试品色谱中，在与对照药材色谱相应的位置上，显相同颜色荧光斑点。

四、预习提要

（1）显微法鉴别中药的操作方法和注意事项有哪些？

（2）中药鉴别的方法有哪些？

（3）如何铺制鉴别用薄层色谱板？进行展开时的注意事项有哪些？

五、实验指导

（一）中药制剂鉴别中检测药味的选择

对于中药制剂，原则上处方中的每一药味均应进行鉴别研究，并选择尽量多的药味制定在标准中。三黄片由大黄药材、盐酸小檗碱和黄芩提取物按一定制法制成，因此，在三黄片的质量标准中对这三种药味均进行鉴别。三黄片中含有大黄药材的粉末（见附：**三黄片的制法**），因此可以采用显微鉴别法鉴别大黄药材的特征。盐酸小檗碱、黄芩提取物中主要成分黄芩苷和大黄对照药材均采用薄层色谱法进行鉴别。本实验中的薄层色谱鉴别方法由《中国药典》收载。

附：三黄片的制法

黄芩浸膏系取黄芩，加水煎煮三次，第一次 1.5h，第二次 1h，第三次 40min，合并煎液，滤过，滤液加盐酸调节 pH 值至 1～2，静置 1h，取沉淀，用水洗涤使 pH 值至 5～7，烘干，粉碎成细粉。取大黄 150g，粉碎成细粉，过筛；取大黄 150g 粉碎成粗粉，加 30% 乙醇回流提取三次，滤过，合并滤液，回收乙醇并减压浓缩至稠膏状，加入大黄细粉、盐酸小檗碱细粉 5g、黄芩浸膏细粉 21g 及辅料适量，混匀，制成颗粒，干燥，压制成 1000 片，包糖衣，即得。

（二）显微鉴别法

显微鉴别法系指用显微镜对药材的切片、粉末、解离组织或表面制片及含药材粉末的制剂中药味的组织、细胞或内含物等特征进行鉴别的一种方法。鉴别时选择典型的供试品，根据各品种鉴别项的规定制片。在制片过程中，必要时滴加水合氯醛试液后在酒精灯上加热透化，并滴加甘油乙醇试液或稀甘油，再盖上盖玻片。

（三）TLC 鉴别

1. TLC 鉴别中对照物的选择

对照物分为对照品（主要为有效成分和特征成分的单体，也包括对照提取物）和对照药材两种。对照物的设置有以下四种方式。

（1）对照品对照　用已知中药制剂某一种有效成分或特征成分对照品制成对照液，与样品在同一条件下层析，比较相同位置有无同一颜色（或荧光）的斑点，来检测是否含有原料药材。可设置一种或数种对照品。

（2）对照药材对照　鉴于单一化学对照品不能反映药材的整体特征，并且多种药材共存时化学成分专属性较差，故采用对照药材对照，以对照药材的色谱整体性为特征进行鉴别。

（3）对照品和对照药材同时对照（双对照）　为了准确检验制剂投料的真实性，有时仅用对照品无法鉴别出来，这时可增加原药材作为对照药材。要求样品色谱图中的主要斑点应与对照品和对照药材色谱图中斑点相一致，从而大大提高方法的专属性和整体性。

（4）阴阳对照　由于中药制剂中许多化学成分和有效成分不明确，或有效成分虽已明确但又无对照品，此时可采用阴阳对照法进行鉴别。

2. 薄层色谱法的显色与检视

供试品含有可见光下有颜色的成分可直接在日光下检视，如没有颜色，可用喷雾法或浸渍法以适宜的显色剂显色或加热显色后在日光下检视。有荧光的物质或遇某些试剂可激发荧光的物质可在 365nm 紫外光灯下观察荧光色谱。对于在紫外光下有吸收的成分可用带有荧光剂的硅胶板，在 254nm 紫外光灯下观察荧光板面上的荧光猝灭物质形成的色谱。本实验中盐酸小檗碱、黄芩苷和大黄中蒽醌类化合物均有荧光，因此可在紫外光灯（365nm 和 254nm）下观察其荧光斑点。

六、讨论

（1）中药成分复杂，如何保证所建立的薄层色谱鉴别方法的专属性？

（2）显微鉴别法适用于什么特征的中药制剂鉴别？

（3）如何选择中药制剂鉴别的药味？

Experiment 5   Description，Identification and Test of Typical TCM

1. Purposes

1.1   To study the identification of traditional Chinese medicine（TCM）by thin-layer chromatography（TLC）.

1.2   To know about the procedure and features of microscopical identification.

2. Instruments and chemical reagents

2.1   Instruments

Microscope，heating refulgence equipment，silica gel G thin layer plate（CMC-Na as the adhesive）, ultraviolet lamp，chromatographic chamber water bath，funnel，filter-paper，evaporating dish.

2.2   Chemcal reagents

Sanhuang tablets，fructus evodiae，poria，radix ginseng，sophorae flos，berberine hydrochloride CRS，baicalin CRS，Radix et Rhizoma Rhei reference material，chrysophanol CRS，emodin CRS，methanol，ethyl acetate，butanone，formic acid，water，diluted hydrochloric acid，solution of ferric chloride in ethanol，ether，petroleum ether（30 ~ 60℃）, ethyl formate，ammonia vapour，ethanol，magnesium powder，chlorhydric acid.

3. Procedures and methods

3.1   Physical and chemical identification of Chinese medicinal material

3.1.1   Identification of alkaloid and volatile oil in fructus evodiae

Add 0.5g powder in a 10ml test tube with stopper，add hydrochloric acid（1→100）8ml，shake it for a few minutes，then filter. To 2ml of the filtrate add one drop of potassium mercuric iodide，then a yellow-white precipitate is produced after shaking. In addition，to 1ml of the filtrate add 2ml para-amino benzaldehyde，heat it in a water bath（do not shake）, a brunneus crico-band is produced between the liquid interface.

Take some powder and get the oily substance through microsublimation，add 2 drops of sulphuric acid and some crystal of vanillin，observe the change of color. In addition，dissolve the oily substance in ethyl ether，apply it to the plate using silica gel G as the coating substance and a mixture of petroleum ether and ethyl acetate（8: 1）as the mobile phase. After developing and removing of the plate，dry it in air，spray with vanillin-concentrated sulfuric acid，observe the spot of volatile oil（You can correspond it with the volatile oil obtained through wet distillation）.

3.1.2   Identification of pachymaran in poria

Add 0.5g powder and 10ml distilled water to a test tube，extract with shaking in a hot water bath for a few minutes，filter，to 2ml of the filtrate add a few drops of 5% α-naphthol alcohol solution which is freshly prepared. Add 0. 5ml sulphuric acid along the test tube wall slowly. Allow standing for a moment, a prunosus band is produced between the liquid interface. After heating and shaking, the liquid in the test tube shows purple nephelo-state, and a purple precipitate is produced after standing for a few hours.

3. 1. 3　Identification of panaxsaponin in radix ginseng

To 0. 2g of the powder of radix ginseng, add 2ml acetic anhydride, heat it in a water bath for 2min, filter. To 1ml of the filtrate, add 0. 5ml concentrated sulfuric acid slowly, the color between the liquid interface will change from red to marron, and become dark brown finally.

Take the powder of radix ginseng 0. 5g, add 5ml alcohol, shake for 5min, filter. Put a small amount of the filtrate to a evaporating dish and evaporate it to dryness, add antimony trichloride-trichlormethane saturated solution by dripping, purple is produced after evaporating to dryness.

3. 1. 4　Identification of sophorae flos

To 0. 1g of the powder add 10ml of ethanol, heat for 5min and filter. To 1ml of the filtrate, add a small quantity of magnesium powder and 2 ~ 3 drops of hydrochloric acid, a cherry red colour is produced.

3. 2　Identification of sanhuang tablets

3. 2. 1　Ingredients

1000 tablets: Radix et Phizoma Rhei 300g; berberine hydrochloride 5g; extractum scutellariae 21g.

3. 2. 2　Description

Sugar coated or film coated tablets with brown core; taste, bitter and slightly astringent.

3. 2. 3　Identification

a. Microscopical method for Radix et Phizoma Rhei: Finely powdered 2 ~ 3 tablets, and then spread a small quantity of the powder on a slide. Examine after treated with glycerol-acetic TS, chloral hydrate TS or other suitable teat solution, cover the cover glass: clusters of calcium oxalate large, 60 ~ 140μm in diameter.

b. Berberine hydrochloride and Baicalin: Weigh 5 tablets, removed the coats and finely powdered, then ultrasonicate 0. 25g powder with 5ml of methanol for 5 minutes, filter, and use the filtrate as the test solution. Dissolve berberine hydrochloride CRS in methanol to produce a solution containing 0. 2mg/ml as the reference solution. And dissolve baicalin CRS in methanol to produce a solution containing 1mg/ml as the reference solution. Carry out the method for thin-layer chromatography, using silica gel G as the coating substance and mixture of ethyl acetate, butanone, formic acid and water(10 : 7 : 1 : 1) as the mobile phase. Apply separately 3 ~ 5μl of each of the test solution and the test reference solution to the plate. After developing and removing of the plate, dry in air, examine under ultraviolet lamp at 365nm and ultraviolet lamp at 254nm. For berberine hydrochloride, the fluorescent spot in the chromatogram obtained with the test solution corresponds in position and color to the spot in the chromatogram obtained with the reference solution under ultraviolet lamp at 365nm. For baicalin, the fluorescent spot in the chromatogram obtained with the test solution corresponds in position and color to the spot in the chromatogram obtained with the reference solution under ultraviolet lamp at 254nm.

c. Radix et Rhizoma Rhei: Obtained under 3. 2 b as the test solution. Ultrasonicate 0. 2 g of Radix et Rhizoma Rhei reference material with 3ml of methanol for 5 minutes, filter, and use the filtrate as the reference solution. Carry out the method for thin-layer chromatography, using silica gel G mixed with sodium carboxymethylcellulose as the coating substance and the cyclohexane and ethyl acetate and formic acid(12 : 3 : 0. 1) as the mobile phase. Apply separately 5μl of each of the test solution to the plate. After developing and removing of the plate, dry in air, examine under ultraviolet light at 365nm. The fluorescent spots in the chromatogram obtained with the test solution correspond in position and color to the spots in the chromatogram obtained with the reference solution.

4. Prepare lessons before class

4. 1　How to use microscope correctly?

4. 2　Which methods can be employed in identification of Traditional Chinese Medicine?

4. 3　How to prepare TLC plates? What should be pay attention to during TLC procedure?

5. Guide for experiment

5. 1　Selection of the ingredients in prescription

In principle, the identification of each ingredient in prescription should be studied for TCM preparation. And the ingredients as much as possible should be identified in standard. Sanhuang tablet is composed of Radix et Phizoma Rhei, berberine hydrochloride and Extractum Scutellariae. Therefore these three ingredients are identified in quality criteria. Sanhuang tablet contains the powder of Radix et Phizoma Rhei(Procedure of sanhuang tablet), thus, microscopic can be used to identify Radix et Phizoma Rhei. The berberine hydrochloride, the baicalin in Extractum Scutellariae and Radix et Rhizoma Rhei reference material are identified with TLC method. These TLC methods are recorded in Ch. P.

Procedure of sanhuang tablet: Decoct Radix Scutellariae with water for 3 times, 1. 5 hours for the first time, 1 hour for the second time and 40 minutes for the third time respectively, combine the decoctions and filter. Adjust the filtrate to pH 1 – 2 with hydrochloric acid; allow standing for 1 hour. Wash the precipitate with water to pH 5 – 7, heat to dryness and pulverize to fine powder. Pulverize 150g of Radix et Rhizoma Rhei to fine powder and sift. Heat under reflux the rest of Radix et Rhizoma Rhei, in coarse powder, with 30% ethanol for 3 times filter, combine the filtrate, recover ethanol and concentrate on vacuum to a thick extract. Add the fine powders of Radix et Rhizoma Rhei, berberine hydrochloride, Extractum Scutellariae and a quantity of excipient, mix thoroughtly, make granules, dry, and compress into 1000 tablets and coat with sugar or film.

5. 2　Microscopical identification

Microscopical identification is a method with the application of the microscope to identify the characters of tissues, cells or cell contents in sections, powders, disintegrated tissues or surface slide of crude drugs and dosage forms including powder of crude drugs. Representative samples are chosen to be identified and slides are prepared to meet the requirements of identification for each other. The slides can be treated with glycerol-acetic TS or chloral hydrate, and be covered with the cover glass. Heat until it is transparent as the method above if necessary.

5.3 TLC indentificaiton

5.3.1 Election of reference substance in TLC

Reference substance consists of two kinds: One is reference substance (It primarily refers to the monomer of active ingredients and specific composition), the other is reference material. The setting of reference substance has the following four ways.

a. Reference substance control   To detect a certain kind active ingredients or specific component of the standard substance in Traditional Chinese Medicine, dilute to reference solution, and carry out the method for chromatography with substance examined in the same condition. According to spot in the chromatogram obtained with the test solution corresponding in position and color to the spot in the chromatogram obtained with the reference solution or not, identify whether samples containing crude drug. Set one or more kinds of reference simultaneously.

b. Reference material control   The single reference substance does not represent the overall characteristics of Traditional Chinese Medicine, and the specificity of chemical composition is poor when many herbs coexist. So the reference drug control is a better method, it can be identified by integrity of the reference material.

c. Reference material and reference substance control simultaneously   To detect the authenticity of medicine preparation accurately, sometimes using reference substance only is failed to make perfect identification. At this moment, the original medicinal materials are added as reference drug. The spot in the chromatogram obtained with the test solution corresponds in position and color to the spot in the chromatogram obtained with the reference solution, thus it has improved specificity and integrity significantly.

d. Negative and positive control   Traditional Chinese Medicine consists of enormous chemical composition and active ingredients which may not clear, or which has been clear but there is no reference substance. Consequently, negative and positive control can be applied to identification.

5.3.2 The visualization and detection in thin-layer chromatography (TLC)

For the ordinary thin-layer plates, the color substance can be detected visually. The colorless substance can be detected by spraying chemical reagent on the plate or immersing the plate in the chemical reagent solution. The fluorescence chromatogram obtained under ultraviolet light at 365nm can be used for the detection of fluorescent substance. The fluorescence quenching method can be used for the fluorescence thin-layer plate. In the present experiment, berberine hydrochloride, baicalin and dihydrodiketoanthracene of Radix et Rhizoma Rhei can emit fluorescence, the fluorescent spots in the chromatogram can be detected at 254nm and 365nm.

6. Discussions

6.1   How to ensure the specificity of TLC due to the complex constituents in the Traditional Chinese Medicine?

6.2   Which kind of TCM preparation can be evaluated with microscopical identification?

6.3   How to select the identified ingredients in TCM preparation?

（徐新军）

第三章　药物的含量测定

Chapter 3　Determination of Drugs

实验六　硫酸奎尼丁及其片剂的含量测定

一、目的

（1）掌握非水滴定法的原理与应用。

（2）掌握硫酸奎尼丁及其片剂的非水滴定法原理及操作方法。

二、仪器与试药

1. 仪器

分析天平、水浴锅、研钵、锥形瓶、量筒、5ml 移液管、10ml 滴定管（宜选用分度值较精密者，建议选用分度值为 0.05ml 的）。

2. 试药

硫酸奎尼丁原料、硫酸奎尼丁片、高氯酸滴定液（0.1mol/L）、冰乙酸、乙酐、结晶紫指示液。

（1）高氯酸滴定液的制备与标定（0.1mol/L）

① 制备　取冰乙酸 500ml，加入高氯酸（70% ~72%）8.5ml，摇匀，在室温下缓缓滴加乙酐 21ml，边加边摇，加完后再振摇均匀，放冷，加冰乙酸适量使成 1000ml，摇匀，放置 24h。若所测供试品易乙酰化，则须用水分测定法测定本液的含水量，再用水和乙酐调节至本液的含水量为 0.01% ~0.2%。

本液也可用二氧六环配制。取高氯酸（70% ~ 72%）8.5ml，加二氧六环稀释至 1000ml。标定时，取在 105℃ 干燥至恒重的基准邻苯二甲酸氢钾约 0.16g，精密称定，加冰乙酸 20ml 溶解，加结晶紫指示液 1 滴，用本液滴定至由绿色变为蓝绿色，并将滴定的结果用空白试验校正。即得。

② 标定　取在 105℃ 干燥至恒重的基准邻苯二甲酸氢钾约 0.16g，精密称定，加冰乙酸 20ml 溶解，加结晶紫指示液 1 滴，用本液缓缓滴定至蓝绿色，并将滴定的结果用空白试验校正。每毫升高氯酸滴定液（0.1mol/L）相当于 20.42mg 的邻苯二甲酸氢钾。根据本液的消耗量与邻苯二甲酸氢钾的取用量算出本液的浓度，即得。

③ 贮藏　置棕色玻璃瓶中，密闭保存。

（2）结晶紫指示液的制备

取结晶紫 0.5g，加冰乙酸 100ml 溶解，即得。

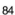

84

三、实验方法

（一）硫酸奎尼丁的含量测定

1. 硫酸奎尼丁的结构、分子式相对分子质量

$$[(C_{20}H_{24}N_2O_2)_2 \cdot H_2SO_4 \cdot 2H_2O, \; Mw = 782.96]$$

本品为（9S）－6′－甲氧基－脱氧辛可宁－9－醇硫酸盐二水合物。按干燥品计算，含 $(C_{20}H_{24}N_2O_2)_2 \cdot H_2SO_4$ 不得少于 99.0%。

2. 含量测定

取本品约 0.2g，精密称定，加冰乙酸 5ml 溶解，加乙酐 20ml 与结晶紫指示液 1 滴，用高氯酸滴定液（0.1mol/L）滴定至溶液显绿色，并将滴定的结果用空白试验校正。每毫升高氯酸滴定液（0.1mol/L）相当于 24.90mg 的 $(C_{20}H_{24}N_2O_2)_2 \cdot H_2SO_4$。

（二）硫酸奎尼丁片的含量测定

1. 性状与规格

本品为糖衣片，除去糖衣后显白色。规格为 0.2g。本品含硫酸奎尼丁 $[(C_{20}H_{24}N_2O_2)_2 \cdot H_2SO_4 \cdot 2H_2O]$ 应为标示量的 93.0% ~ 107.0%。

2. 含量测定

取本品 20 片，除去包衣，精密称定，研细，精密称取适量（约相当于硫酸奎尼丁 0.2g），加乙酐 20ml，加热使硫酸奎尼丁完全溶解后，加结晶紫指示液 1 滴，用高氯酸滴定液（0.1mol/L）滴定至溶液显绿色，并将滴定的结果用空白试验校正。每毫升高氯酸滴定液（0.1mol/L）相当于 26.10mg 的 $(C_{20}H_{24}N_2O_2)_2 \cdot H_2SO_4 \cdot 2H_2O$。

四、预习提要

（1）非水滴定法与水溶液中滴定法的滴定管有什么不同？

（2）硫酸奎尼丁属哪种结构类型的药物？依据该类药物的结构特点与理化性质，为什么可采用非水滴定法测定含量？

（3）非水溶液滴定法测定弱酸性与弱碱性药物的分析条件有何不同？

（4）非水滴定法测定生物碱类药物的盐类时，应注意哪些问题？

（5）硫酸奎尼丁及其片剂的含量测定方法有哪些异同？各自的滴定度如何计算？

五、实验指导

（一）非水溶液滴定法

非水溶液滴定法是在非水溶剂中进行滴定的分析方法（《中国药典》2015 年版二部）。以非水溶液为滴定介质，能改变物质的化学性质（主要是酸碱强度），使在水中不能反应完全的滴定反应能在非水溶剂中顺利进行，有时还能增大有机化合物的溶解度。选择的非水溶剂应能溶解试样并使滴定反应进行完全、不引起副反应，有适宜的极性使终点明显突跃。可使用单一或混合溶剂。非水溶液滴定法主要用来测定有机碱及其氢卤酸盐、磷酸盐、硫酸盐或有机酸盐，以及有机酸碱金属盐类药物的含量，也用于测定某些有机弱酸的含量。

1. 非水溶剂的种类

（1）酸性溶剂　有机弱碱在酸性溶剂中可显著地增强其相对碱度，最常用的酸性溶剂为冰乙酸。

（2）碱性溶剂　有机弱酸在碱性溶剂中可显著地增强其相对酸度，最常用的碱性溶剂为二甲基甲酰胺。

（3）两性溶剂　兼有酸、碱两种性能，最常用的为甲醇。

（4）惰性溶剂　这一类溶剂没有酸性、碱性，如苯、三氯甲烷等。

2. 非水滴定的方法

（1）第一法　除另有规定外，精密称取供试品适量（约消耗 0.1mol/L 高氯酸滴定液 8ml），加冰乙酸 10~30ml 溶解，加各品种项规定的指示液 1~2 滴，用高氯酸滴定液（0.1mol/L）滴定。终点颜色应以电位滴定时的突跃点为准，并将滴定的结果用空白试验校正。

若滴定供试品与标定高氯酸滴定液时的温度差别超过 10℃，则应重新标定；若未超过 10℃，则可根据下式将高氯酸滴定液的浓度加以校正。

$$N_1 = \frac{N_0}{1 + 0.0011(t_1 - t_0)}$$

式中，0.0011 为冰乙酸的膨胀系数；t_0 为标定高氯酸滴定液时的温度；t_1 为滴定样品时的温度；N_0 为 t_0 时高氯酸滴定液的浓度；N_1 为 t_1 时高氯酸滴定液的浓度。

供试品如为氢卤酸盐，应在加入乙酸汞试液 3~5ml 后，再进行滴定；供试品如为磷酸盐，可以直接滴定；硫酸盐也可直接滴定，但滴定至其成为硫酸氢盐为止；供试品如为硝酸盐时，因硝酸可使指示剂褪色，终点极难观察，遇此情况应以电位滴定法指示终点为宜。

电位滴定时用玻璃电极为指示电极，饱和甘汞电极（玻璃套管内装氯化钾的饱和无水甲醇溶液）为参比电极。

（2）第二法　除另有规定外，精密称取供试品适量（约消耗 0.1mol/L 碱滴定液 8ml），加各品种项规定的溶剂溶解，再加规定的指示液 1~2 滴，用规定的碱滴定液（0.1mol/L）滴定。终点颜色应以电位滴定时的突跃点为准，并将滴定的结果用空白试验校正。

在滴定过程中，应注意防止溶剂和碱滴定液吸收大气中的二氧化碳和水蒸汽，防止滴定液中的溶剂挥发。

电位滴定时所用的电极同第一法。

3. 注意事项

（1）酸碱滴定液标定时，同一操作者标定不得少于 3 份，第二操作者复标亦不得少于 3 份；酸滴定液标定和复标的相对偏差均不得过 0.1%。

（2）高氯酸有腐蚀性，配制时要注意防护，并应将高氯酸先用冰乙酸稀释，在搅拌下缓缓加入乙酐。如高氯酸滴定液颜色变黄，即说明高氯酸部分分解，不能使用。

（3）配制高氯酸滴定液和溶剂所用的冰乙酸，或非水滴定用的其他溶剂，含有少量水分时，对滴定突跃和指示剂变色敏锐程度均有影响，因此常加入计算量的乙酐，使与水反应后生成乙酸，以除去水分。为避免过剩的乙酐，应测定含水量后加乙酐。

（4）供试品一般宜用干燥样品，含水分较少的样品也可采用在最后计算中除去水分的方法。对含水量高的碱性样品，应干燥后测定，必要时亦可加适量乙酐脱水，但应注意避免试样的乙酰化。

（5）指示剂不宜多加，以 1~2 滴为宜，指示终点的颜色由电位滴定突跃来确定。

（6）滴定操作应在 18℃ 以上室温进行，因冰乙酸流动较慢，滴定到终点应稍待片刻再读数。

（7）供试品每次测定应在 2 份以上。

（8）原料药用高氯酸液直接滴定者，相对偏差不得过 0.15%；用碱滴定液直接滴定者，相对偏差不超过 0.3%。

（9）制剂须提取后用高氯酸液滴定者，相对偏差不得过 0.3%。

（二）硫酸奎尼丁的含量测定

奎尼丁是一种从金鸡纳树皮中提取出来的生物碱，临床用于治疗心房颤动、阵发性心动过速和心房扑动等。奎尼丁的分子结构包括喹啉环和喹核碱两部分，各含一个氮原子，均有碱性。喹核碱的碱性较强，可与硫酸成盐，而喹啉环上的氮原子碱性较弱，不能与硫酸成盐而始终保持游离状态。硫酸奎尼丁在水溶液中显示的碱性较弱，不能直接进行中和滴定；在非水的酸性介质中，能显出较强的碱性，可以顺利地进行中和滴定。《中国药典》规定采用高氯酸非水溶液滴定法测定硫酸奎尼丁及其片剂的含量。

在冰乙酸中，硫酸奎尼丁的喹啉环碱性变强，用高氯酸滴定时，也能和质子结合，1mol 硫酸奎尼丁含 2mol 喹核碱，可结合 2mol 质子。由于硫酸的酸性强，用非水滴定法测定有机碱的硫酸盐时，只能滴定至 HSO_4^- 的程度，即在滴定过程中，SO_4^{2-} 作为共轭碱，只能结合 1 个 H^+ 成 HSO_4^-。其反应式为

$$(C_{20}H_{24}N_2O_2 \cdot H^+)_2SO_4^{2-} + 3HClO_4 \longrightarrow (C_{20}H_{24}N_2O_2 \cdot 2H^+) \cdot 2ClO_4^- +$$
$$(C_{20}H_{24}N_2O_2 \cdot 2H^+) \cdot HSO_4^- \cdot ClO_4^-$$

从上式可知，1mol 的硫酸奎尼丁可消耗 3mol 的高氯酸。无水硫酸奎尼丁的相对分子量为 746.93，所以 1ml 的高氯酸滴定液（0.1mol/L）相当于 24.90mg 的无水硫酸奎尼丁 $[(C_{20}H_{24}N_2O_2)_2 \cdot H_2SO_4]$。

$$含量（\%） = \frac{(V - V_0) \times 24.90 \times 10^{-3} \times F}{W} \times 100\%$$

式中，V 和 V_0 分别为滴定供试品和空白试验时消耗滴定液的体积，ml；W 为样品的称样量，g；F 为浓度换算因数，$F = \dfrac{C}{0.1}$，其中 C 为高氯酸滴定液的实际浓度，mol/L。

非水溶液滴定法可用指示剂或电位法指示终点。非水减量法常用的指示剂是结晶紫，结晶紫分子中的氮原子能结合多个质子而表现为多元碱。滴定时，随着溶液酸度增加，结晶紫由紫色（碱式色）变至蓝紫、蓝、蓝绿、绿、黄绿，最后转为黄色（酸式色）。在滴定不同强度的碱时，终点颜色不同：滴定较强碱时，终点为蓝色或蓝绿色；滴定极弱碱时，终点为蓝绿色或绿色。

除结晶紫外，有时也使用 α-萘酚苯甲醇、喹哪啶红等指示剂。

（三）硫酸奎尼丁片的含量测定

本品须经提取分离等步骤处理，因为片剂中有许多附加成分，如硬脂酸镁、羧甲基纤维素钠等在滴定中都能消耗高氯酸，须经碱化、有机溶剂提取分离后才能测定奎宁游离碱。反应方程式为

$$(BH^+)_2 \cdot SO_4^{2-} + 2NaOH \longrightarrow 2B + Na_2SO_4 + 2H_2O$$
$$2B + 4HClO_4 \rightleftharpoons 2(BH_2^{2+} \cdot 2ClO_4^-)$$

由反应式可知，1mol 的硫酸奎宁相当于 4mol 的高氯酸。因此片剂分析时的滴定度与原料药的滴定度不同。

六、讨论

（1）写出高氯酸滴定硫酸奎尼丁的滴定反应方程式并计算滴定度，写出硫酸奎尼丁含量测定结果的计算公式。

（2）非水溶液滴定法测定生物碱类药物的盐类时，应注意哪些问题？

（3）非水溶液滴定法测定碱性药物的注意事项有哪些？常用的终点指示方法是什么？

Experiment 6　Assay of Quinidine Sulfate and Quinidine Sulfate Tablets

1. Purposes

1.1　To learn nonaqueous titration and its application for assay of basic drugs.

1.2　To understand principles and procedures for assay of quinidine sulfate and its tablets.

2. Instruments and chemical reagents

2.1　Instruments

Analytic balance,water bath,agate mortar,conical flask,volumetric cylinder,5ml pipette,10ml burette(0.05ml scale is preferred).

2.2　Chemical reagents

Quinidine sulfate,quinidine sulfate tablets,perchloric acid(0.1mol/L)VS,glacial acetic acid,acetic anhydride,crystal violet IS.

2.2.1　Perchloric acid VS(0.1mol/L,in glacial acetic acid)

a. Preparation　Mix 8.5ml perchloric acid with 500ml glacial acetic acid and 21ml acetic anhydride,cool,and add glacial acetic acid to make 1000ml. Alternatively,the solution may be prepared as follows. Mix 11ml 60 percent perchloric acid with 500ml glacial acetic acid and 30ml acetic anhydride,cool,and add glacial acetic acid to make 1000ml.

Allow the prepared solution to stand for 1 day for the excessive acetic anhydride to be combined,and determine the water content to use a test specimen of about 5g of the 0.1mg/L perchloric acid that is expected to contain approximately 1mg water and the reagent diluted such that 1ml is equivalent to about 1 to 2mg water. If the water content exceeds 0.5%, add more acetic anhydride. If the solution contains no titratable water, add sufficient water to obtain a content of between 0.02% and 0.5% water. Allow the solution to stand for 1 day, and again titrate the water content. The solution so obtained contains between 0.02% and 0.5% water, indicating freedom from acetic anhydride.

b. Standardize ation weigh accurately about 0.16 g of potassium biphthalate, dried at 105℃, and dissolve it in 20ml glacial acetic acid. Add 1 drop of crystal violet TS, and titrate with the perchloric acid solution until the violet color changes to blue-green. Deduct the volume of the perchloric acid consumed by 20ml the glacial acetic acid, and calculate the normality. Each 20.42mg of potassium biphthalate is equivalent to 1ml of 0.1mol/L perchloric acid.

c. The solution is sealed in brown glass bottle.

2.2.2 Crystal violet IS

Dissolve 0.5g of crystal violet in 100ml glacial acetic acid.

3. Procedures and methods

3.1 Assay of quinidine sulfate

3.1.1 Structure, molecular formula and molecular weight of quinidine sulfate

$$[(C_{20}H_{24}N_2O_2)_2 \cdot H_2SO_4 \cdot 2H_2O, Mw = 782.96]$$

Quinidine sulfate is (9S)-6′-Methoxy-cinchonane-9-ol sulfate (2 : 1, salt) dihydrate. It contains not less than 99.0% of $(C_{20}H_{24}N_2O_2)_2 \cdot H_2SO_4$, calculated on the dried basis.

3.1.2 Assay

Dissolve 0.2g, accurately weighed, in 5ml glacial acetic acid, add 20ml acetic anhydride and a drop of crystal violet IS. Titrate with perchloric acid (0.1mol/L) VS until the colour changes to green. Perform a blank determination and make any necessary correction. Each 1 milliliter of perchloric acid (0.1mol/L) VS is equivalent to 24.90mg ($C_{20}H_{24}N_2O_2$)$_2 \cdot H_2SO_4$.

3.2 Assay of quinidine sulfate tablets

3.2.1 Description and specification

Quinidine sulfate tablets are sugar-coated with white core. Quinidine sulfate tablets contain not less than 93.0% and not more than 107.0% of the labeled amount of quinidine sulfate $[(C_{20}H_{24}N_2O_2)_2 \cdot H_2SO_4 \cdot 2H_2O]$. Labeled strength: 0.2g.

3.2.2 Assay

Weigh accurately and powder 20 tablets with the sugar coating removed. To an accurately weighed quantity of the powdered tablets equivalent to about 0.2g of quinidine sulfate add 20ml acetic anhydride, warm to dissolve quinidine sulfate. Add 1 drop of crystal violet IS. Titrate with perchloric acid(0.1mol/L) VS until the solution changes to green. Perform a blank determination and make any necessary correction. Each 1 milliliter of perchloric acid(0.1mol/L) VS is equivalent to 26.10mg[$(C_{20}H_{24}N_2O_2)_2 \cdot H_2SO_4 \cdot 2H_2O$].

4. Prepare lessons before class

4.1   Explain the differences on buret used for nonaqueous titration and aqueous titration.

4.2   What type of drug does quinidine sulfate belong to? Based on its physicochemical properties, why can nonaqueous titration be used for assay of quinidine sulfate?

4.3   Figure out conditions of non-aqueous titration for both weak base and acid respectively.

4.4   How to avoid interference for halide ion in determination of alkali salts of halogen acids in nonaqueous titration?

4.5   Why are procedures for determination of quinidine sulfate different from those of its tablet? Try to calculate their equivalent factors respectively.

5. Guide for experiment

5.1   Nonaqueous titration

Nonaqueous titration is the titration of substances dissolved in nonaqueous solvents. In nonaqueous solvent, the apparent strength of a weak acid or base is determined by the extent of its reaction with a solvent. As a result, they can behave as strong acids or bases and make the titration work well. Sometimes, water-insoluble compounds acquire enhanced solubility when dissolved in organic solvents. Solvent used in nonaqueous titration should dissolve the analyte thoroughly and protect from side-reaction, with appropriate polarity and yield apparent sudden change at endpoint. Nonaqueous titration is generally employed for determination of organic bases, organic salts of hydrohalic acid, phosphoric acid and sulfuric acid or organic acids and the alkali metal salts of organic acids, as well as weak organic acids.

5.1.1   Nonaqueous solvents

a. Acidic solvents   The relative alkalinity of weak organic bases can be remarkably enhanced in acidic solvents. The most commonly used acidic solvent is glacial acetic acid.

b. Basic solvents   The relative acidity of weak organic acids can be remarkably enhanced in basic solvents. The most commonly used basic solvent is dimethylformamide.

c. Amphiprotic solvents   They have the properties of acids and bases. The most commonly used amphiprotic solvent is methanol.

d. Aprotic solvents   They are neither acidic nor basic, such as benzene, chloroform etc.

5.1.2   Nonaqueous titration methods

Method 1   Unless otherwise specified, dissolve an accurately weighed quantity, equivalent to about 8ml of perchloric acid(0.1mol/L) VS, of the substance being examined in 10 ~ 30ml of glacial acetic acid, add 1 ~ 2 drops of the indicator solution as specified in the monograph and titrate with perchloric acid(0.1mol/L) VS. The color change of the indicator should be checked by potentiometric method and a blank determination performed to make any necessary correction.

If the temperature at which the titration is performed differs by more than 10°C from the temperature at which the perchloric acid VS was standardized, the titrant must be standardized again. If the difference does not exceed $10°C$, the concentration of the titrant can be corrected as follows.

$$N_1 = \frac{N_0}{1 + 0.0011(t_1 - t_0)}$$

Where 0.0011 is the volume expansion coefficient of glacial acetic acid; t_0 is the temperature at which perchloric acid VS was standardized; t_1 is the temperature at which the titration is performed; N_0 is the concentration of perchloric acid VS at t_0; N_1 is the concentration of perchloric acid VS at t_1.

When the substance being examined is a salt of hydrohalic acids, the titration should be carried out after the addition of 3 ~ 5ml mercuric acetate TS. Phosphates and sulfates can be titrated directly, but in the case of sulfates, the reaction stops when bisulfate is formed. In the titration of nitrates, the end point should be determined by potentiometric method, because the indicator can be discolored by nitric acid.

In nonaqueous potentiometric titration, the indicator electrode is a glass electrode and the reference electrode is a saturated calomel electrode using a saturated solution of potassium chloride in dehydrated methanol as the salt bridge.

Method 2 Unless otherwise specified, dissolve an accurately weighed quantity, equivalent to 8ml the titrant (0.1mol/L), of the substance being examined in a solvent specified in the monograph, add 1 ~ 2 drops of the specified indicator solution and titrate with the specified basic titrant(0.1mol/L). The colour change of the indicator should be checked by potentiometric method and a blank determination performed to make any necessary correction.

In the course of the titration, protect the solvent, titrant from atmospheric carbon dioxide and moisture, and avoid the evaporation of the titrant. The electrodes used in potentiometric titration is the same as that described in method 1.

5.1.3 Notes

a. While standardizing the volume solution, 3 specimens should be conducted concomitantly either for the analyst or for auditor, with their relative deviation not more than 0.1%.

b. Perchlorid acid is corrosive and should dilute with glacial acetic acid first, then add acetic anhydride carefully. It is unable to use if it has turned yellow.

c. Water in the glacial acetic acid may make the endpoint uneasy to observe, so appropriate acetic anhydrous need to be add to react with the water. The water content should be tested first to help to calculate the quantity of acetic anhydrous needed.

d. Samples should be dried previously. Samples with a little amount of water can be titrated first and calculate anhydrously. Samples with more water can add acetic anhydrous to move water out, but acetylate reaction should be prevented.

e. Indicator had better be added no more than 1 ~ 2 drops, which is result of potentiometric titration.

f. Titration should be done in condition over 18℃, and low temperature makes glacial acetic acid more sticky. It is better to stand for a while before recording the volume.

g. More than 2 specimens of testing samples should be determined to minimize errors.

h. Relative deviation for drug raw material contents should not more than 0.15%, which not more than 0.3% for samples titrated with basic solution.

i. Relative deviation for drug dosage form contents should not more than 0.3% titrated directly with perchlorid acid.

5.2　Assay of quinidine sulfate

Quinidine sulfate is an alkaloid extracted from the bark of cinchona tree, and used in the treatment of atrial fibrillation, paroxysmal tachycardia, atrial flutter and so on. Quinidine contains two alkalic centers, i.e. quinuclidine and quinoline. Quinuclidine is an alkaloid stronger than quinoline, and only quinuclidine can obtain a proton to produce quinidine sulfate. The alkalinity of quinidine sulfate in aqueous solution is weak, and is not suitable for neutralization titration directly. When quinidine sulfate dissolves in glacial acetate acid, apparent strength of quinoline is enhanced by the extent of its reaction with the solvent, and can obtain a proton. Hence, in Ch. P, quinidine sulfate and quinidine sulfate tables are assayed by nonaqueous titration with perchloric acid VS.

When quinidine sulfate dissolves in glacial acetate acid, apparent strength of quinoline is enhanced by the extent of its reaction with the solvent, and can obtain a proton. In this case, 1 mol quinidine sulfate contains 2 mol quinoline, which needs 2 mol perchlorid acid to donate protons. In addition, SO_4^{2-} calls for 1 mol of perchlorid acid to be titrated to HSO_4^-. The reaction equation is as follows.

$$(C_{20}H_{24}N_2O_2 \cdot H^+)_2 SO_4^{2-} + 3HClO_4 \longrightarrow (C_{20}H_{24}N_2O_2 \cdot 2H^+) \cdot 2ClO_4^- +$$
$$(C_{20}H_{24}N_2O_2 \cdot 2H^+) \cdot HSO_4^- \cdot ClO_4^-$$

As a result, 1 mol quinidine sulfate can react with 3 mol perchlorid acid. Formula weight for anhydrous quinidine sulfate is 746.93, 1 ml perchloric acid(0.1 mol/L) VS is equivalent to 24.90 mg quinidine sulfate $[(C_{20}H_{24}N_2O_2)_2 \cdot H_2SO_4]$.

$$\text{Content}(\%) = \frac{(V - V_0) \times 24.90 \times 10^{-3} \times F}{W} \times 100\%$$

Where, V and V_0 are titrant volumes(ml) for sample and blank respectively; W is the quantity of sample(g); F is the correction factor for concentration of VS, $F = \dfrac{C}{0.1}$, in which C is the concentration(mol/L) of perchlorid acid in titration.

In nonaqueous titration, endpoint can be determined either by color change, or potentiometry. Indicator of crystal violet is commonly used since it can combines with several protons and become multi-conjugate base. When adding acid in solutions, crystal violet changes its color from purple(basic color) to blue-purple, blue, blue-green, green, yellow-green, and finally to yellow (acid color). Crystal violet shows different colors for different alkalinity, in which the strong bases yield blue or blue-green endpoint and weak ones blue-green or green.

Other indicators, such as α-naphthol in benzyl alcohol or quinaldine red are often used besides crystal violet.

5. 3 Assay of quinidine sulfate tablets

For assay of quinidine sulfate tablets, grind not less than 20 tablets to fine powder, weigh accurately a portion of the powder, equivalent to the quantity of drug specified in the individual monograph. In order to circumvent interference from excipients (such as magnesium stearate, carboxymethylcellulose sodium etc), sodium hydroxide is added to liberate quinidine, which can be extracted with organic solvent. The reacted equation is as follows.

$$(BH^+)_2 \cdot SO_4^{2-} + 2NaOH \longrightarrow 2B + Na_2SO_4 + 2H_2O$$

$$2B + 4HClO_4 \Longleftrightarrow 2(BH_2^{2+} \cdot 2ClO_4^-)$$

As a result, 1mol quinidine sulfate can react with 4mol of perchloric acid. Quinidine Tablet shows different equivalence factor with its raw material.

6. Discussions

6. 1　Figure out the reaction equation of quinidine sulfate with perchloric acid and calculate the equivalent factor for titration of raw material. Give the formula for calculating percentage of quinidine sulfate in the portion of sample taken.

6. 2　What cautions should be taken during the nonaqueous titration of salts of alkaloids?

6. 3　What cautions should be taken during the nonaqueous titration of basic drugs? What are the common methods to indicate the end-point.

（曹丽娟）

实验七　盐酸普鲁卡因或注射用盐酸普鲁卡因的含量测定

一、目的

（1）掌握永停滴定法测定含量的方法与原理。

（2）掌握盐酸普鲁卡因测定的操作条件及要点。

二、仪器与试药

1. 仪器

分析天平、电位计、10ml 滴定管、100ml 量筒、100ml 烧杯、电磁搅拌器。

2. 试药

（1）盐酸普鲁卡因原料、注射用盐酸普鲁卡因、溴化钾、亚硝酸钠滴定液（0.1mol/L）、水。

（2）亚硝酸钠滴定液（0.1mol/L）

配制：取亚硝酸钠 6.9g，加水适量溶解成 1000ml，摇匀，0.05mol/L 的滴定液由此稀释制得。

标定：取在 120℃ 干燥至恒重的基准物质对氨基苯磺酸约 0.5g，精密称定，加水 30ml 与浓氨试液 3ml，溶解后加盐酸（1→2）20ml，搅拌，在 30℃ 以下用本液迅速滴定，滴定时将滴定管尖端插入液面下约 2/3 处，随滴随搅拌，至近终点时，将滴定管尖端提出液面，用少量水洗涤尖端，洗液并入溶液中，继续缓缓滴定，用永停法指示终点。每毫升亚硝酸钠滴定液（0.1mol/L）相当于17.32mg的对氨基苯磺酸。根据本液的消耗量与对氨基苯磺酸的取用量算出本液的浓度，即得。

三、实验方法

（一）盐酸普鲁卡因的含量测定

1. 盐酸普鲁卡因的结构、分子式、相对分子质量

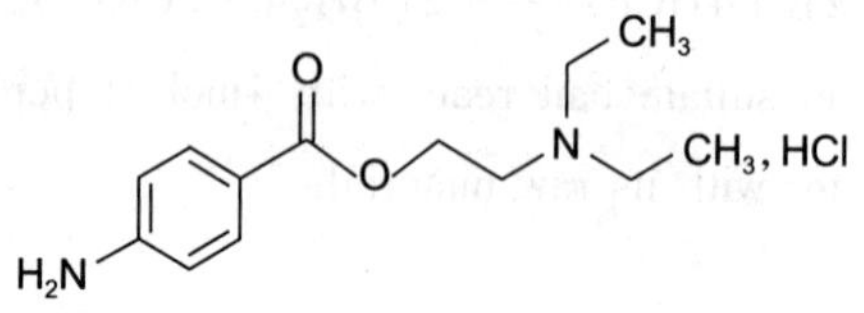

$$（C_{13}H_{20}N_2O_2 \cdot HCl，M_w = 272.77）$$

本品为4-氨基苯甲酸-2-（二乙氨基）乙酯盐酸盐。按干燥品计算，含$C_{13}H_{20}N_2O_2 \cdot HCl$不得少于99.0%。

2. 含量测定

取本品约0.6g，精密称定，照永停滴定法（《中国药典》2015年版二部），在15~25℃，用亚硝酸钠滴定液（0.1mol/L）滴定。每毫升亚硝酸钠滴定液（0.1mol/L）相当于27.28mg的$C_{13}H_{20}N_2O_2 \cdot HCl$。

（二）注射用盐酸普鲁卡的含量测定

1. 性状与规格

本品为盐酸普鲁卡因的灭菌粉末。按平均装量计算，含盐酸普鲁卡因（$C_{13}H_{20}N_2O_2 \cdot HCl$）应为标示量的95.0%~105.0%。

2. 含量测定

取装量差异项的内容物，混合均匀，精密称取适量（约相当于盐酸普鲁卡因0.6g），照永停滴定法，在15~20℃，用亚硝酸钠滴定液（0.1mol/L）滴定。每毫升亚硝酸钠滴定液（0.1mol/L）相当于27.28mg的$C_{13}H_{20}N_2O_2 \cdot HCl$。

四、预习提要

（1）盐酸普鲁卡因是临床广泛使用的局部麻醉药，具有良好的局部麻醉作用，毒性低，无成瘾性。该药物属于对氨基苯甲酸酯类局麻药物，分子结构中具有芳伯氨基，在酸性溶液中可与亚硝酸钠反应。《中国药典》规定采用亚硝酸钠滴定法测定盐酸普鲁卡因及其注射用无菌粉末的含量。

（2）永停滴定法是容量分析中用以确定终点或选择核对指示剂变色的方法，可用于重氮化法的终点指示。永停滴定法采用两支相同的铂电极，在电极间加一低电压（如50mV）时，若电极在溶液中极化，则在未到滴定终点时，仅有很小或无电流通过；当到达终点时，滴定液略有过剩，使电极去极化，溶液中即有电流通过，电流计指针突然偏转，不再回复。若电极由去极化变为极化，则电流计指针从有偏转回到零点，不再变动。

五、实验指导

（一）亚硝酸钠滴定法

1. 基本原理

以亚硝酸钠液为滴定液的容量分析法称为重氮化法，也即亚硝酸钠法。亚硝酸钠是重氮化反应最常用试剂，它在酸性环境中释放亚硝酸。芳伯氨基或水解后生成芳伯氨基的药物在酸性溶液中能定量与亚硝酸钠产生重氮化反应，生成重氮盐。依此，用已知浓度的亚硝酸钠滴定液用永停法或外指示剂法指示终点，根据消耗的亚硝酸钠滴定液的浓度和体积，可计算出芳伯胺类药物的含量。反应式如下。

$$Ar—NHCOR + H_2O \xrightarrow{H^+} Ar—NH_2 + RCOOH$$

$$Ar—NH_2 + NaNO_2 + 2HCl \longrightarrow Ar—N_2^+Cl^- + NaCl + 2H_2O$$

2. 测定的主要条件

（1）加入适量溴化钾，加快反应速度。

（2）加过量盐酸，加速反应。

（3）反应温度：可在室温（10~30℃）下进行，其中15℃以下结果较准确。

（4）滴定速度。

3. 指示终点的方法

有电位滴定法、永停滴定法、外指示剂法和内指示剂法等。《中国药典》主要采用永停法指示终点。

（二）永停滴定法

1. 仪器装置

永停滴定法（《中国药典》四部通则）可用永停滴定仪或如图3-1所示的装置。

亚硝酸钠滴定时，电流计的灵敏度除另有规定

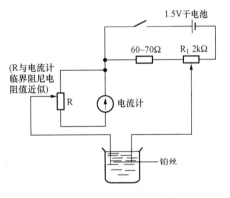

图3-1 永停滴定法的装置

外，为 10^{-9} A per graduation。永停滴定法采用两支相同的铂电极，注意铂电极使用含少量三氯化铁的硝酸或铬酸清洁液浸洗。

2. 操作方法

调节永停滴定装置 R_1，使加于电极上的电压约为50mV。取供试品适量，精密称定，置烧杯中，除另有规定外，可加水40ml与盐酸溶液（1→2）15ml，而后置电磁搅拌器上，搅拌使溶解，再加溴化钾2g，插入铂—铂电极后将滴定管的尖端插入液面下约2/3处，用亚硝酸钠滴定液（0.1mol/L或0.05mol/L）迅速滴定，随滴随搅拌，至近终点时，将滴定管的尖端提出液面，用少量水淋洗尖端，洗液并入溶液中，继续缓缓滴定，至电流计指针突然偏转，并不再回复，即为滴定终点。

（三）外指示剂法

反应到终点时加入稍过量的亚硝酸钠滴定液，即可产生亚硝酸，使得外指示剂淀粉试纸或淀粉糊变色。淀粉–碘化钾试纸或糊通过淀粉溶液加入等量的5%碘化钾溶液制得，指示终点反应如下。

$$KI + HCl \longrightarrow HI + KCl$$

$$2HI + 2HNO_2 \longrightarrow I_2 + 2NO + 2H_2O$$

过量（碘）+ 淀粉 ⟶ 蓝色（指示终点）

游离出的单质碘遇淀粉显蓝色。重氮化反应只有在无机酸存在的条件下才能定量发生。在滴定的终点测试酸度是很重要的，如果没有过量的酸存在，淀粉–碘化钾试纸就不能检出过量的亚硝酸，也即不能指示终点。

六、讨论

（1）写出亚硝酸钠滴定盐酸普鲁卡因的滴定反应式并计算滴定度。

（2）在亚硝酸钠滴定法中，永停滴定法指示终点的适用范围是什么？

（3）实验注意事项有哪些？常用终点指示方法有哪些？

Experiment 7　Assay of Procaine Hydrochloride or Procaine Hydrochloride for Injection

1. Purposes

1.1　To study the principle and procedure of dead-stop titration.

1.2　To experiment on the assay of procaine hydrochloride.

2. Instruments and chemical reagents

2.1　Instruments

Analytic balance, potentiometer, 10ml burette, 100ml volumetric cylinder, 100ml beaker, electromagnetic stirrer.

2.2　Chemical reagents

2.2.1　Procaine hydrochloride material, procaine hydrochloride for injection, potassium bromide, sodium nitrite(0.1mol/L)VS, water.

2.2.2　Sodium nitrite(0.1mol/L)VS

Preparation　Sodium nitrite R, dissolved in water to contain 6.9g of $NaNO_2$ in 1000ml. The solution could be diluted to yield the concentration of 0.05mol/L.

Standardization　Weigh accurately about 0.5g of sulfanilic acid primary standard, previously dried to constant weight at 120℃, and dissolve it in 30ml water and 3ml　concentrated ammonia TS. Add 20ml hydrochloric acid solution(1→2)with stirring, plunge the burette into the solution so that about 2/3 of the tip is under the liquid surface, titrate with sodium nitrite VS quickly with stirring at a temperature below 30℃. Withdraw the burette tip towards the endpoint of titration, rinse it with water and add the washings to the solution, continue the titration slowly, and adopt the dead-stop method for endpoint determination. Each 1ml of sodium nitrite(0.1mol/L)VS is equivalent to 17.32mg of sulfanilic acid.

3. Procedures and methods

3.1 Assay of procaine hydrochloride

3.1.1 Structure, molecular formula and molecular weight of procaine hydrochloride

$$(C_{13}H_{20}N_2O_2 \cdot HCl, M_w = 272.77)$$

Procaine hydrochloride is 2 - (diethylamino) ethyl 4 - aminobenzoate monohydrochloride. It contains not less than 99.0% of $C_{13}H_{20}N_2O_2 \cdot HCl$, calculated on the dried basis.

3.1.2 Assay

Weigh accurately about 0.6g, and carry out the method for dead-stop titration. Titrate at 15 ~ 25℃ with sodium nitrite(0.1mol/L) VS. Each 1ml of sodium nitrite(0.1mol/L) VS is equivalent to 27.28mg of $C_{13}H_{20}N_2O_2 \cdot HCl$.

3.2 Assay of procaine hydrochloride for injection

3.2.1 Description and specification

Procaine hydrochloride for injection is a sterile powder of procaine hydrochloride. It contains not less than 95.0% and not more than 105.0% of the labeled amount of procaine hydrochloride ($C_{13}H_{20}N_2O_2 \cdot HCl$), calculated on the basis of the average weight of contents.

3.2.2 Assay

Weigh accurately a quantity of the mixed contents obtained in the test for weight variation of contents, equivalent to 0.6g of procaine hydrochloride, carry out the method for dead-stop titration, and titrate with sodium nitrite(0.1mol/L) VS at 15 ~ 25°C. Each 1ml of sodium nitrite(0.1mol/L) VS is equivalent to 27.28mg of $C_{13}H_{20}N_2O_2 \cdot HCl$.

4. Prepare lessons before class

4.1 Procaine hydrochloride is a commonly used local anesthetics. It possesses good local anesthetic effect, low toxicity and no addiction. Procaine hydrochloride is classified as the para-aminobenzoic esters anesthesia drugs. There is an aromatic primary amine in the molecular structure, which could react with sodium nitrite in acidic solution. In Ch. P, procaine hydrochloride and procaine hydrochloride for injection are assayed by nitrite titration.

4.2 The dead-stop method may be used for the confirmation of endpoint or the color change of indicators at the endpoint. Using a suitable electrode system, these methods can be applied to nitrite titrations. In the dead-stop titration, a low voltage of about 50mV is applied across two same platinum electrodes. Since the electrodes are polarized, there is no current or only very weak current flows. When the endpoint is reached, a slight excess of the titrant depolarizes the electrodes and current flows, causing a permanent deflection of the galvanometer needle. On the other hand, if non-polarized electrodes are polarized, the deflected galvanometer needle turns back to zero permanently.

5. Guide for experiment

5.1 Nitrite titration

5.1.1 Principle

Nitrite titration (diazotization) is used in the analysis of aromatic compounds containing an amino group in the molecules. Sodium nitrite is generally used in direct method of diazotization, and it gives nitric acid in acidic solution. This analysis is based on the reaction between aromatic primary amine and sodium nitrite, in presence of excessive mineral or inorganic acids. Hence, many aromatic primary amines with free amino group can be analyzed quantitatively by measuring the volume of sodium nitrite solution required to convert them into diazonium salts. The typical reaction of diazotization reaction in presence of HCl is given as follows.

$$Ar-NHCOR + H_2O \xrightarrow{H^+} Ar-NH_2 + RCOOH$$

$$Ar-NH_2 + NaNO_2 + 2HCl \longrightarrow Ar-N_2^+Cl^- + NaCl + 2H_2O$$

5.1.2 Main conditions for assay

a. Adding suitable amount of potassium bromide to speed up the reaction.

b. Adding excessive hydrochloric acid to accelerate the rate of response.

c. Reaction temperature: the reaction may be performed at room temperature ($10 \sim 30°C$), results obtained below $15°C$ are relative accurate.

d. Speed of titration.

5.1.3 Methods for indicating the end point

There are potentiometric titration, dead-stop titration, visual endpoint determination method and so on for indicating the endpoint. The dead-stop titration was adopted by Ch. P.

5.2 Potentiometric titration and dead-stop titration

5.2.1 Apparatus

In dead-stop titration, any model of a dead-stop titration apparatus or an assembly illustrated in the following figure may be used (Figure 3 – 1).

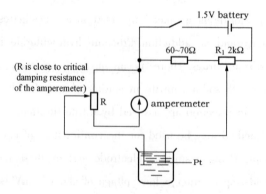

Figure 3 – 1　Model of a dead-stop titration apparatus

Unless otherwise specified, the sensitivity of galvanometer is 10^{-9} A per graduation for nitrite titration. Please note the platinum electrodes should be cleaned with nitric acid containing a small quantity of ferric chloride, or with chromic acid cleaning solution.

5.2.2 Operate method

For the indication of the endpoint of diazotization reaction by a nitrite titration, apply a voltage of about 50mV across the electrodes by adjusion R_1. Place an accurately weighed quantity of the substance being examined in a beaker on a magnetic stirrer, add 40ml water and 15ml of hydrochloric acid solution($1 \rightarrow 2$), unless otherwise specified, stir to effect dissolution. Add 2g of potassium bromide, dip the electrodes into the solution, plunge the burette into the solution so that about 2/3 of the tip is under the liquid surface, and titrate with sodium nitrite(0.1mol/L or 0.05mol/L) VS quickly with stirring. Withdraw the burette tip when the endpoint is nearly reached, rinse it with water and add the washings to the solution, and continue the titration slowly until the galvanometer needle is permanently deflected.

5.3 Visual endpoint determination method

When all the aromatic amine has reacted with $NaNO_2$ then next portion(slightly excessive) of $NaNO_2$ is added to the solution under test, converted to HNO_2 that remain in the solution and can be detected by the starch paper or paste as an external indicator. This appearance of free HNO_2 in solution indicates that diazotization reaction is complete and equivalence point is attained.

Starch iodide paper or paste is the starch solution plus equivalent volume of 5% KI solution in H_2O. Starch iodide paste with reaction mixture is as follows.

$$KI + HCl \longrightarrow HI + KCl$$
$$2HI + 2HNO_2 \longrightarrow I_2 + 2NO + 2H_2O$$
$$(excessive)I_2 + Starch \longrightarrow blue\ color(endpoint)$$

The liberated I_2 reacts with starch to give blue color. The diazotization proceeds quantitatively only in presence of inorganic acid. It is important to check the acidity at the end of the titration. If there is no excess of acid present, starch-iodide paper will not detect excess HNO_2 and so will not indicate the end point.

6. Discussion

6.1　Figure out the chemical reaction equation of procaine hydrochloride with sodium nitrite and the equivalent relationship.

6.2　What type of compounds may be assayed with the dead-stop titration by sodium nitrite?

6.3　What precautions should be taken in the dead-stop titration? What other end-point indicating methods are there?

（曹丽娟）

实验八　维生素 C 片的含量测定

一、目的

（1）掌握剩余碘量法的基本原理。

（2）熟悉剩余碘量法测定维生素 C 片含量的操作方法。

二、仪器与试药

1. 仪器

分析天平，研钵，量筒，50ml 移液管，25ml 移液管，100mL 棕色容量瓶，25mL 聚四氟乙烯活塞滴定管，250mL 碘量瓶，玻璃漏斗，滤纸。

2. 试药

（1）维生素 C 片（规格 0.1 克）。

（2）硫代硫酸钠滴定液（0.1mol/L）

①配制　取硫代硫酸钠 26g 与无水碳酸钠 0.20g，加新沸过的冷水适量使溶解成 1000ml，摇匀，放置 1 个月后滤过。

②标定　取在 120℃ 干燥至恒重的基准重铬酸钾 0.15g，精密称定，置碘瓶中，加水 50ml 使溶解，加碘化钾 2.0g，轻轻振摇使溶解，加稀硫酸 40ml，摇匀，密塞；在暗处放置 10 分钟后，加水 250ml 稀释，用本液滴定至近终点时，加淀粉指示液 3ml，继续滴定至蓝色消失而显亮绿色，并将滴定的结果用空白试验校正。每 1ml 硫代硫酸钠滴定液（0.1mol/L）相当于 4.903mg 的重铬酸钾。根据本液的消耗量与重铬酸钾的取用量，算出本液的浓度，即得。

（3）碘滴定液（0.05mol/L）　取碘 13.0 g，加碘化钾 36g 与水 50ml 溶解后，加盐酸 3 滴与水适量使成 1000ml，摇匀，用垂熔玻璃滤器滤过。

（4）淀粉指示液　取可溶性淀粉 0.5g，加水 5ml 搅匀后，缓缓倾入 100ml 沸水中，随加随搅拌，继续煮沸 2 分钟，放冷，倾取上层清液，即得。本液应临用新制。

（5）稀醋酸溶液　取冰醋酸 60ml，加水稀释至 1000ml 即得。

三、实验方法

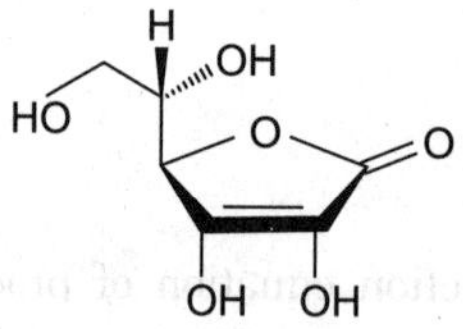

（$C_6H_8O_6$, $Mw = 176.13$）

本品为 L - 维生素 C。含 $C_6H_8O_6$ 不得少于 99.0%。

本品为白色结晶或结晶性粉末；无臭，味酸；久置色渐变微黄；水溶液显酸性反应。本品在水中易溶，在乙醇中略溶，在三氯甲烷或乙醚中不溶。

含量测定　本品 20 片（规格 0.1 克），精密称定，研细，精密称取适量（约相当于维生素 C 0.2g），置 100mL 容量瓶中，加新沸过的冷水 100ml 与稀醋酸 10ml 的混合液适量，振摇使维生素 C 溶解并稀释至刻度，摇匀，经干燥滤纸迅速滤过；精密量取续滤液 50ml，置碘量瓶中，再精密加碘滴定液（0.05 mol/L）25ml，密塞，瓶口加少许水，置暗处放置 5 分钟后，用硫代硫酸钠滴定液（0.1 mol/L）滴定至溶液呈浅黄色后，加淀粉指示液 1ml，继续滴定至蓝色刚好消失。并将滴定的结果用空白试验校正。每 1ml 的碘滴定液

（0.05mol/L）相当于 8.806mg 的 $C_6H_8O_6$。

四、预习提要

1. 剩余滴定法中先加入定量过量的滴定液 A，使其与被测物定量反应，待反应完全后，再用另一滴定液 B 会滴定反应剩余的滴定液 A，实际操作时 A 滴定液是否需要标定？为什么？

2. 依据维生素 C 的结构特点，说明剩余碘量法含量测定的原理。

3. 除了剩余碘量法，维生素 C 的含量测定方法还有哪些方法？

五、实验指导

（一）维生素 C 的测定

1. 原理

维生素 C 在醋酸酸性条件下，可与碘发生氧化还原反应，过量的碘用硫代硫酸钠标准液滴定，碘与淀粉结合所显的蓝色消失即为终点，反应式如下：

$$I_2 + 2Na_2S_2O_3 \rightarrow Na_2S_4O_6 + 2NaI$$

2. 注意事项

（1）因在酸性介质中维生素 C 受空气中氧的氧化速度减慢，所以滴定时，须加入稀醋酸 10ml 使滴定在酸性溶液中进行。但样品溶于稀酸后仍需立即进行滴定。

（2）加新沸过的冷水，目的是为减少水中溶解的氧对测定的影响。

（3）为消除片剂中辅料对测定的干扰，在片粉中的维生素 C 溶解后应采用干燥滤纸滤过，取续滤液测定。

（4）碘量瓶是为碘量法测定中专用的一种锥形瓶，其构造不同于一般的锥形瓶。加入反应物后，应立即盖紧塞子，并在塞子外加上适量水作密封，防止碘挥发，静置反应一定时间后，慢慢打开塞子，让密封水沿瓶塞流入锥形瓶，再用水将瓶口及塞子上的碘液洗入瓶中。

（二）碘量法

碘量法是以碘作为氧化剂，或以碘化物（如碘化钾）作为还原剂进行滴定的方法。碘量法根据滴定的方式不同分为直接碘量法和间接碘量法，间接碘量法又分为置换碘量法和剩余碘量法两种。

1. 直接碘量法　直接碘量法是用碘滴定液直接滴定还原性物质的方法。在滴定过程中，I_2 被还原为 I^-：

$$I_2 + 2e \rightleftharpoons 2I^-$$

直接碘量法只能在酸性、中性或弱碱性溶液中进行，如果溶液 $pH > 9$，可发生副反应使测定结果不准确。

直接碘量法可用淀粉指示剂指示终点。淀粉遇碘显蓝色，反应极为灵敏。化学计量点稍后，溶液中有过量的碘，碘与淀粉结合显蓝色而指示终点到达。直接碘量法还可利用碘自身的颜色指示终点，化学计量点后，溶液中稍过量的碘显黄色而指示终点。

2. 剩余碘量法　剩余碘量法是在供试品（还原性物质）溶液中先加入定量、过量的碘滴定液，待 I_2 与测定组分反应完全后，然后用硫代硫酸钠滴定液滴定剩余的碘，以求出待测组分含量的方法。滴定反应为：

$$I_2（定量过量）+ 还原性物质 \longrightarrow 2I^- + I_2（剩余）$$

$$I_2（剩余）+ 2S_2O_3^{2-} \longrightarrow S_4O_6^{2-} + 2I^-$$

使用剩余碘量法时，用淀粉作指示剂。淀粉指示剂应在近终点时加入，因为当溶液中有大量碘存在时，碘易吸附在淀粉表面，影响终点的正确判断。

3. 置换碘量法　置换碘量法是先在供试品（氧化性物质）溶液中加入碘化钾，供试品将碘化钾氧化析出定量的碘，碘再用硫代硫酸钠滴定液滴定，从而可求出待测组分含量。滴定反应为：

$$氧化性物质 + 2I^- \longrightarrow I_2$$

$$I_2 + 2S_2O_3^{2-} \longrightarrow S_4O_6^{2-} + 2I^-$$

4. 注意事项

（1）配制本滴定液所用的水必须经过煮沸后放冷，以除去水中溶解的二氧化碳和氧，并杀灭微生物；在配制中还应加入 0.02% 的无水碳酸钠作为稳定剂，使溶液的 pH 值保持在 9~10，以防止硫代硫酸钠的分解。

（2）配制后应在避光处贮放一个月以上，待浓度稳定，再经滤过，而后标定。

（3）标定时，如照药典的规定量称取基准重铬酸钾，则消耗本滴定液约为 30ml，须用 50ml 的滴定管；如拟以常用的 25ml 滴定管进行标定，则基准重铬酸钾的称取量为 0.11~0.12g。

（4）碘化钾的强酸性溶液，在静置过程中遇光也会释出微量的碘，因此在标定中的放置过程应置于暗处，并用空白试验予以校正。本滴定液在贮存中如出现浑浊，即不得再供使用。

六、讨论

1. 碘量法的基本原理与主要操作方式有哪些？
2. 写出剩余碘量法测定维生素 C 片含量测定结果的计算公式。

扫码"看一看"

Experiment 8　Assay of Vitamin C Tablets

1. Purposes

1.1　To understand principles of residual iodimetric titration.

1.2　To learn proceduresof residual iodimetric titration for assay of vitamin C.

2. Instruments and chemical reagents

2.1 Instrumets

Analytical balance, agate mortar, volumetric cylinder, 50ml pipette, 25ml pipette, 100ml brown volumetric flask, 25ml polytetrafluoroethylene burette, 250ml iodine flask, glass funnel, filter paper.

2.2 Chemical reagents

2.2.1 Vitamin C Tablets (labeled strength: 0.1g).

2.2.2 Sodium Thiosulfate VS (0.1mol/L)

Dissolve about 26 g of sodium thiosulfate and 200 mg of sodium carbonate in 1000 ml of recently boiled and cooled water. Mix well and filter after one month.

Standardize the solution as follows. Accurately weigh about 150 mg of primary standard potassium dichromate dried to constant weight at 120℃ into a iodine flask, and dissolve in 50ml of water. Add 2 g of potassium iodide and gently shake to dissolve. Mix well after adding sulphuric acid 40ml and make a seal; put it in the dark for 10 minutes and add 250ml of water to dilute. Add starch indicator solution 3ml when titrating to near the end point and continue the titration until the blue color is discharged and the solution is yellowish green in color. Perform a blank determination and make any necessary correction. Each 1ml of sodium thiosulfate (0.1 mol/L) VS is equivalent to 4.903 mg potassium dichromate.

2.2.3 Iodine VS (0.05mol/L) Dissolve 13.0 g of iodine, and 36 g of potassium iodine into 50ml of water, add 3 drops of hydrochloric acid and dilute to 1000ml with water. Mix well and filter with sintered glass filter.

2.2.4 Starch IS Dissolve 0.5g of soluble starch into 5ml of water, mix well and pour suspension slowly into 100ml of boiling water with stirring, boil for 2 min, cool and decant the supernatant liquid. The test solution should be freshly prepared.

2.2.5 Dilute acetic acid solution Dilute 60 ml of glacial acetic acid in water to make a volume of 1000 ml.

3. Procedure and methods

$(C_6H_8O_6, Mw = 176.13)$

Vitamin C is L – ascorbic acid. It contains not less than 99.0% of $C_6H_8O_6$.

Vitamin C iswhite crystalline or crystalline powder, odorless, acid flavor; it turns yellow gradually; acidic reaction is carried out in aqueous solution. It is very soluble in water, slightly soluble in ethanol, insoluble in chloroform or ether.

Assay Weigh accurately and powder 20 tablets (labeled strength 0.1g). Weigh accurately a quantity of the powder equivalent to about 200 mg of vitamin C into a 100 ml volumetric flask and add a quantity of recently boiled and cooled water 100ml and 10ml of dilute acetic acid solution. Shake to dissolve vitamin C and dilute to volume and shake well. Filter quickly with drying filter paper. Accurately transfer 50 ml of the successive filtrate into a iodine flask and precisely add 25ml of iodine VS (0. 05mol/L), add a little water to the bottle mouth to make a seal. Put it in the dark for 5 minutes and titrate with sodium thiosulfate titration solution (0. 1 mol/L) until the solution is light yellow in color. Add 1ml of starch indicator solution and continue the titration until the blue color is just discharged. Perform a blank determination and make any necessary correction. Each 1ml of iodine (0. 05mol/L) VS is equivalent to 8. 806 mg $C_6H_8O_6$.

4. Prepare lessons before class

4. 1   Residual iodimetric titration requires the addition of a measured volume of titration solution A, in excess of the amount actually needed to react with the substance being assayed, the excess of this solution then is titrated with another titration solution B. Does the titration solution A need to be standardized in practice? Why?

4. 2   Figure out the physicochemical properties of vitamin C and the principle for its determination.

4. 3   In addition to the residual iodimetric titration method, what other methods are available for the assay of vitamin C?

5. Guide experimental

5. 1   Assay of vitamin C

5. 1. 1   Principle

Vitamin C can react with iodine in acidic acetic acid. Titrate excess iodine with sodium thiosulfate VS until the blue color is discharged. The reaction equation is as follows:

$$I_2 + 2Na_2S_2O_3 \rightarrow Na_2S_4O_6 + 2NaI$$

5. 1. 2   Cautions

a. Affected by oxygen, oxidation of vitamin C in acidic medium slows down. 10 ml of acetic acidis necessary to make sure that the titration is carried out under acidic conditions. However, the sample should be titrated immediately after dissolving in dilute acetic acid solution.

b. The cooled boiled water is required to reduce the influence on the determination caused by dissolving O2 in water.

c. In order to eliminate the interference of excipients in tablets, filter vitamin C in tablet powder with dry filter paper after dissolution and use the the successive filtrate for determination.

d. Structurally different from common erlenmeyer flask, iodimetry flask is a special erlenmeyer flask for iodimetry. After adding the reactant, immediately plunge the stopper, add a little water around the rim of stopper to make a seal in case of iodine volatilization. Open the stopper slowly after reaction, so that the sealed water flows into the erlenmeyer flask along the stopper, and then wash the iodine solution around the bottle mouth and stopper into the flask.

5.2 Iodimetric Titration

Iodimetric titration is established upon oxidative ability of iodine and reductive ability of

iodide ion. Accordingly, there are direct and indirect titrations, and indirect titrations include

replacement and residual methods.

5.2.1 Direct iodimetric titration

Dissolve reductive analyte in solution in a suitable vessel and titrate with iodine VS (the titrant), the endpoint being determined with the aid of a starch indicator. In the process, iodine is reduced to iodide ion:

$$I_2 + 2e \Longleftrightarrow 2I^-$$

The method is performedin acid neutral or weak basic solutions. Iodine may take place side reaction with pH > 9, which makes it less accurate.

Starch is used as the indicator in direct method and becomes blue with iodine. The endpoint is easily detected by the appearance of blue color. Iodine can serve as its own indicator, since a slight excess of iodine can easily be detected by its yellow color.

5.2.2 Residual iodimetric titration

Residual iodimetric titration requires the addition of a measured volume of a iodine VS, in excess of the amount actually needed to react with the substance being assayed, the excess of this solution then is titrated with a thiosulfate volumetric solution. The equation is:

$$I_2 (\text{measured and excess}) + \text{reducing agent} \longrightarrow 2I^- + I_2 (\text{excess})$$

$$I_2 (\text{excess}) + 2S_2O_3^{2-} \longrightarrow S_4O_6^{2-} + 2I^-$$

When starch serves as indicator, it should be added till the titration is near the endpoint, for large quantity of iodine is absorbed to surface of starch and lead to an endpoint error.

5.2.3 Replacement iodimetric titration

Replacementiodimetric titration is processed by addition of potassium iodide, which can liberate same quantity of free iodine, which is titrated with sodium thiosulfate. The equation is as follows:

$$\text{Oxidizing agent} + 2I^- \longrightarrow I_2$$

$$I_2 + 2S_2O_3^{2-} \longrightarrow S_4O_6^{2-} + 2I^-$$

5.2.4 Cautions

a. The volumetric solution requires the cooled boiled water, in order to remove the dissolving CO_2 and kill the microbes; anhydrous $NaHCO_3$ (soda ash) as stabilizer was added to be 0.02% of the weigh, to keep the pH 9 - 10 and prevent $Na_2S_2O_4$ from decomposition during the preparation.

b. The volumetric solution should be stored in the dark for over one month, and then filtered, standardized after stabilization.

c. In the standardization, the K_2CrO_4 would consume about 30ml volumetric solution, thus the volume buret of 50ml was needed according to the Pharmacopeia; if the one of 25ml was used, the weight of reference K_2CrO_4 should be 0.11 – 0.12g.

d. The slight I_2 would be released during storage if the highly acidic KI solution meets with light, thus it should be stored in the dark, and then corrected by the blank solution. What's more, the solution would not be used if some cloudiness appeares.

6. Discussion

6.1　What are the principles and titration methods foriodimetric titration?

6.2　Give the formula for calculating percentage of iophendylate in the portion of sample taken.

（苏梦翔）

实验九　头孢拉定及其片剂的含量测定

一、目的

（1）掌握高效液相色谱法（HPLC）的原理及其在药物分析中的应用。

（2）掌握头孢拉定及其片剂的高效液相色谱测定方法。

二、仪器与试药

高效液相色谱仪按国家计量检定规程中液相色谱仪的规定定期检定，应符合规定，按仪器操作说明使用。若无特别说明，所有试剂应该分析纯，用于色谱的试剂应该是 HPLC 级，超纯水。

三、实验方法

（一）HPLC 测定头孢拉定的含量

1. 头孢拉定的结构、分子式、相对分子质量

$$(C_{16}H_{19}N_3O_4S,\ Mw = 349.40)$$

本品为（6R, 7R）－7［（R）－2－氨基－2－（1, 4－环己烯基）乙酰氨基］－3－甲基－8－氧代－5－硫杂－1－氮杂双环 ［4.2.0］ 辛－2－烯－2－羧酸。

2. 性状

白色或类白色结晶性粉末，微臭。在水中略溶，在乙醇、三氯甲烷或乙醚中几乎不溶。按无水物计算，含头孢拉定（$C_{16}H_{19}N_3O_4S$）不得少于 90.0%。

3. 含量测定

（1）色谱条件与系统适用性试验　用十八烷基硅烷键合硅胶为填充剂；水－甲醇－3.86%醋酸钠溶液－4%醋酸溶液（1564∶400∶30∶6）为流动相；流速为每分钟0.7～0.9ml；检测波长为254nm。取头孢拉定对照品溶液10份和头孢氨苄对照品贮备液（0.4mg/ml）1份，混匀，取10μl注入液相色谱仪测定，头孢拉定峰和头孢氨苄峰的分离度应符合规定。理论板数按头孢拉定峰计算应不小于2500。

（2）对照品溶液的制备　取头孢拉定对照品适量（相当于头孢拉定约35mg），精密称定，置50ml量瓶中，加水约6ml，置超声波浴中溶解，再加流动相稀释至刻度，摇匀。

（3）供试品溶液的制备与测定　取供试品约70mg，精密称定，置100ml量瓶中，加流动相约70ml，置超声波浴中溶解，再加流动相稀释至刻度，摇匀，同时取10μl注入液相色谱仪，记录色谱图。另取头孢拉定对照品溶液同法测定作对照，计算出供试品中$C_{16}H_{19}N_3O_4S$的含量。

（二）头孢拉定片的测定

头孢拉定片为薄膜衣片，除去包衣后显类白色或微黄色。本品含头孢拉定（$C_{16}H_{19}N_3O_4S$）应为标示量的90.0%～110.0%。本品规格为0.25g和0.5g。

测定法　取本品10片，精密称定，研细，精密称取适量（约相当于头孢拉定70mg），置100ml量瓶中，加流动相［水－甲醇－3.86%醋酸钠溶液－4%醋酸溶液（1564∶400∶30∶6）］70ml，置超声波浴中15min，再振摇10min，使头孢拉定溶解，加流动相稀释至刻度，摇匀，过滤，取续滤液10μl，照头孢拉定项下的方法测定。

四、预习提要

（1）简述头孢拉定的结构特点与理化性质。
（2）高效液相色谱法的定量方法有哪些？
（3）高效液相色谱法系统适用性实验的内容有哪些？
（4）高效液相色谱法测定头孢拉定的流动相与固定相分别是什么？
（5）高效液相色谱法常用的检测器有哪些？

五、实验指导

高效液相色谱法系采用高压输液泵将规定的流动相泵入装有填充剂的色谱柱，对供试品进行分离测定的色谱方法。注入的供试品由流动相带入柱内，各组分在柱内被分离，并依次进入检测器，由积分仪或数据处理系统记录和处理色谱信号（图3-2）。

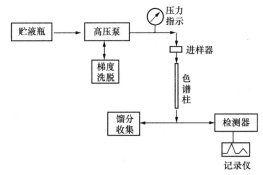

图3-2　高效液相色谱仪示意图

（一）对仪器的一般要求

高效液相色谱法所用的仪器为高效液相色谱仪。仪器应定期检定并符合有关规定。

1. 色谱柱

最常用的色谱柱填充剂为化学键合硅胶。反相色谱系统使用非极性填充剂，以十八烷基硅烷键合硅胶最为常用，辛基硅烷键合硅胶和其他类型的硅烷键合硅胶（如氰基键合硅烷和氨基键合硅烷等）也有使用。正相色谱系统使用极性填充剂，常用的填充剂有硅胶等。离子交换色谱系统使用离子交换填充剂；分子排阻色谱系统使用凝胶或高分子多孔微球等填充剂；对映异构体的分离通常使用手性填充剂。

填充剂的性能（如载体的形状、粒径、孔径、表面积、键合基团的表面覆盖度、含碳量和键合类型等）及色谱柱填充直接影响供试品的保留行为和分离效果。孔径在 15nm（1nm = 10Å）以下的填料适合于分析相对分子质量小于 2000 的化合物，相对分子质量大于 2000 的化合物则应选择孔径在 30nm 以上的填料。除另有规定外，分析柱的填充剂粒径一般在 3~10μm 之间。粒径更小（约 2μm）的填充剂常用于填装微径柱（内径约 2mm），使用微径柱时，输液泵的性能、进样体积、检测池体积和系统的死体积等必须与之匹配。如有必要，色谱条件也须作适当调整。对其测定结果产生争议，应以品种正文规定的色谱条件的测定结果为准。

以硅胶为载体的普通键合固定相的使用温度通常不超过 40℃，为改善分离效果可适当提高色谱柱的使用温度，但不能超过 60℃。流动相的 pH 值应控制在 2~8 之间。当 pH 值大于 8 时，可使载体硅胶溶解；当 pH 值小于 2 时，与硅胶相连的化学键合相易水解脱落。当色谱系统中须使用 pH 值大于 8 的流动相时，应选用耐碱的填充剂，如采用高纯硅胶为载体并具有高表面覆盖度的键合硅胶填充剂、包覆聚合物填充剂、有机 – 无机杂化填充剂或非硅胶填充剂等；当须使用 pH 值小于 2 的流动相时，应选用耐酸的填充剂，如具有大体积侧链能产生空间位阻保护作用的二异丙基或二异丁基取代十八烷基硅烷键合硅胶填充剂，或有机 – 无机杂化填充剂等。

2. 检测器

最常用的检测器为紫外检测器，包括二极管阵列检测器，其他常见的检测器有荧光检测器、蒸发光散射检测器、示差折光检测器、电化学检测器和质谱检测器等（图 3 – 3）。

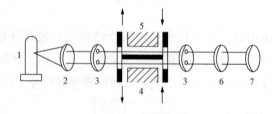

图 3 – 3　紫外检测器光路图

1. 低压汞灯；2. 透镜；3. 遮光板；4. 测量池；5. 参比池；6. 紫外滤光片；7. 双紫外光敏电阻

紫外检测器、荧光检测器、电化学检测器为选择型检测器，其响应值不仅与待测溶液的浓度有关，还与化合物的结构有关；蒸发光散射检测器和示差折光检测器为通用型检测器，对所有的化合物均有响应；蒸发光散射检测器对结构类似化合物的响应值几乎仅与待测物的质量有关；二极管阵列检测器可以同时记录待测物的吸收光谱，故可用于待测物的光谱鉴定和色谱峰的纯度检查。

紫外检测器、荧光检测器、电化学检测器和示差折光检测器的响应值与待测溶液的浓度在一定范围内呈线性关系，但蒸发光散射检测器响应值与待测溶液的浓度通常呈指数关系，故进行计算时，一般须经对数转换。

不同的检测器对流动相的要求不同。如采用紫外检测器，所用流动相应符合紫外 – 可见分光光度法对溶剂的要求；采用低波长检测时，还应考虑有机相中有机溶剂的截止使用波长，并选用色谱级有机溶剂。蒸发光散射检测器和质谱检测器通常不允许使用含不挥发性盐组分的流动相。

3. 流动相

反相色谱系统的流动相首选甲醇 – 水系统（采用紫外末端波长检测时，首选乙腈 – 水系统），如经试用不适合时，再选用其他溶剂系统。应尽可能少用含有缓冲液的流动相，必须使用时，应尽可能选用含较低浓度缓冲液的流动相。由于 C18 链在水相环境中不易保持伸展状态，故对于十八烷基硅烷键合硅胶为固定相的反相色谱系统，流动相中有机溶剂的比例通常应不低于 5%，否则 C18 链的随机卷曲导致组分保留值变化，造成色谱系统不稳定。

各品种项规定的条件除固定相种类、流动相组分、检测器类型不得改变外，其余如色谱柱内径、长度、载体粒度、流动相流速、混合流动相各组分的比例、柱温、进样量、检测器的灵敏度等均可适当改变，以适应供试品并达到系统适用性试验的要求。其中，调整流动相组分比例时，以组分比例较低者（小于或等于 50%）相对改变量不超过 ±30% 且绝对改变量不超过 ±10% 为限，如 30% 相对改变量的数值超过 10% 时，则改变量以 ±10% 为限。对于必须使用特定牌号的填充剂方能满足分离要求的品种，可在该品种项下注明。

（二）系统适用性试验

高效液相色谱法用高压输液泵将具有不同极性的单一溶剂或不同比例的混合溶剂、缓冲液等流动相泵入装有固定相的色谱柱，经进样阀注入供试品，由流动相带入柱内，在柱内各成分被分离后，依次进入检测器，色谱信号由记录仪或积分仪记录。高效液相色谱法是在经典的液相色谱法基础上发展起来的一种在线分离分析方法，具有分离效能高、分析速度快、应用范围广等特点，是在药品检验中应用非常广泛的一种仪器分析方法。

色谱系统适用性试验系指按各品种项要求对仪器进行适用性试验，即用规定的对照品对仪器进行试验和调整，应达到规定的要求。色谱系统适用性试验通常包括：理论板数、分离度、重复率和拖尾因子等四个指标。其中分离度和重复率是系统适用性试验中更具实用意义的参数。

在各品种项下规定的条件除固定相种类、流动相组成、检测器类型不得改变外，其余如色谱柱内径、色谱柱长度、固定相牌号、载体粒度、流动相流速、混合流动相各组成的比例、柱温、进样量、检测器的灵敏度等均可适当改变，以适应具体的色谱系统并达到色谱系统适用性试验的要求。

1. 色谱柱的理论板数

在选定的条件下，注入供试品溶液或各品种项规定的内标物质溶液，记录色谱图，量出供试品主成分或内标物质峰的保留时间 t_R（以分钟或长度计，下同，但应取相同单位）和半峰高宽（$W_{h/2}$），按

$$n = 5.54 \left(t_R / W_{h/2} \right)^2$$

计算色谱柱的理论板数（n）。如果测得理论板数低于各品种项规定的最小理论板数，应改变色谱柱的某些条件（如柱长、载体性能、色谱柱充填的优劣等），使理论板数达到要求。

2. 分离度

定量分析时，为便于准确测量，要求定量峰与其他峰或内标峰之间有较好的分离度（图 3 – 4）。分离度（R）的计算公式为

$$R = \frac{2(t_{R_2} - t_{R_1})}{W_1 + W_2}$$

式中，t_{R_2} 为相邻两峰中后一峰的保留时间；t_{R_1} 为相邻两峰中前一峰的保留时间；W_1 及 W_2 为此相邻两峰的峰宽。除另有规定外，分离度应大于 1.5。

3. 重复率

取各品种项的对照溶液，连续进样 5 次，除另有规定外，其峰面积测量值的相对标准偏差应不大于 2.0%。可按各品种校正因子测定项配制相当于 80%、100% 和 120% 的对照品溶液，加入规定量的内标溶液，配成 3 种不同浓度的溶液，分别进样 3 次，计算平均校正因子，其相对标准偏差也应不大于 2.0%。

4. 拖尾因子

为保证测量精度，特别当采用峰高法测量时，应检查待测峰的拖尾因子（T）是否符合各品种项的规定，或不同浓度进样的校正因子误差是否符合要求（图 3 –5）。

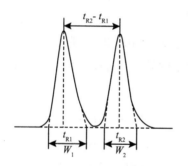

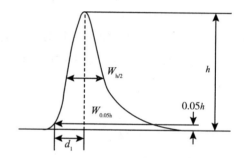

图 3 – 4　分离度计算示意图　　图 3 – 5　拖尾因子计算示意图

拖尾因子计算公式为

$$T = \frac{W_{0.05h}}{2d_1}$$

式中，$W_{0.05h}$ 为 0.05 峰高处的峰宽；d_1 为峰极大至峰前沿之间的距离。除另有规定外，T 应在 0.95 ~ 1.05 之间。峰面积法测定时，T 值偏离过大，也会影响小峰的检测和定量的准确度。

（三）测定法

1. 内标法加校正因子测定供试品中某个杂质或主成分含量

按各品种项下的规定，精密称（量）取对照品和内标物质，分别配成溶液，精密量取各溶液，配成校正因子测定用的对照溶液。取一定量注入仪器，记录色谱图。测量对照品和内标的峰面积或峰高，按

$$f = \frac{A_S / C_S}{A_R / C_R}$$

计算校正因子（f）。式中，A_S 为内标物质的峰面积或峰高；A_R 为对照品的峰面积或峰高；

C_S 为内标物质的浓度；C_R 为对照品的浓度。

再取各品种项含有内标物质的供试品溶液，注入仪器，记录色谱图，测量供试品中待测成分（或其杂质）和内标物质的峰面积或峰高，按

$$C_X = f \cdot \frac{A_X}{A_S / C_S}$$

计算含量（C_X）。式中，A_X 为供试品（或其杂质）峰面积或峰高；C_X 为供试品（或其杂质）的浓度。f、A_S 和 C_S 的意义同上。

当配制校正因子测定用的对照溶液和含有内标物质的供试品溶液使用同一份内标物质溶液时，则配制内标物质溶液不必精密称（量）取。

2. 外标法测定供试品中某个杂质或主成分含量

按各品种项的规定，精密称（量）取对照品和供试品，配制成溶液，分别精密取一定量，注入仪器，记录色谱图，测量对照品和供试品待测成分的峰面积（或峰高），按

$$C_X = C_R \cdot \frac{A_X}{A_R}$$

计算含量（C_X），式中各符号意义同上。

在测定杂质或主成分含量时，若手动操作的微量注射器不能准确定量控制进样量，可采用定量环或自动进样器。

3. 加校正因子的主成分自身对照法

测定杂质含量时，可采用加校正因子的主成分自身对照法。在建立方法时，按各品种项的规定精密称（量）取杂质对照品和待测成分对照品各适量，配制测定杂质校正因子的溶液，并记录色谱图，按上述 1 法计算杂质的校正因子。此校正因子可直接载入各品种正文中，用于校正杂质的实测峰面积。

测定杂质含量时，按各品种项规定的杂质限度将供试品溶液稀释成与杂质限度相当的溶液作为对照溶液，进样，调节仪器灵敏度（以噪音水平可接受为限）或进样量（以柱子不过载为限），使对照溶液的主成分色谱峰高达满量程的 10%～25% 或其峰面积能准确积分（面积约为通常条件下满量程峰积分值的 10%）。然后，取供试品溶液和对照品溶液适量，分别进样，供试品溶液的记录时间除另有规定外，应为主成分保留时间的若干倍，测量供试品溶液色谱图上各杂质的峰面积，分别乘以相应的校正因子后与对照溶液主成分的峰面积比较，依法计算各杂质含量。

4. 不加校正因子的主成分自身对照法

当没有杂质对照品时，可采用不加校正因子的主成分自身对照法。同上述 3 法配制对照溶液并调节仪器灵敏度后，取供试品溶液和对照溶液适量，分别进样，前者的记录时间除另有规定外，应为主成分保留时间的若干倍，测量供试品溶液色谱图上各杂质的峰面积并与对照溶液主成分的峰面积比较，计算杂质含量。

若供试品所含的部分杂质未与溶剂峰完全分离，则按规定先记录供试品溶液的色谱图 Ⅰ，再记录等体积纯溶剂的色谱图 Ⅱ。色谱图 Ⅰ 上杂质峰的总面积（包括溶剂峰）减去色谱图 Ⅱ 上的溶剂峰面积即为总杂质峰的校正面积，然后依法计算。

5. 面积归一化法

由于峰面积归一化法测定误差大，因此，本法通常只能用于粗略考察供试品中的杂质含量。除另有规定外，一般不宜用于微量杂质的检查。方法是测量各杂质峰的面积和色谱

图上除溶剂峰以外的总色谱峰面积，并计算各峰面积占总峰面积的百分率，即得。

（四）注意事项

（1）缓冲盐任何时候不能快速加入纯有机洗脱剂以防盐析出；流动相用前必须过滤。建议采用色谱纯试剂制备流动相。每次更换流动相后首先要排管路气泡。

（2）不要使系统超过最高限压。建议在低压下工作，高压时会增加色谱仪部件的负担。

（3）供试品溶液与流动相的 pH 必须在色谱柱允许的范围内。

（4）保证储液瓶有足够的溶液以防色谱柱流干。

（5）分析柱须用柱体积（约 11ml）5 倍量，制备柱须用柱体积（约 182ml）10 倍量平衡。

（6）过高的系统压力说明系统局部（如预柱）有堵塞现象；过低的压力则说明系统局部（如柱连接处）有漏液现象。

（7）注意系统压力的波动，不正常的压力波动预示色谱泵须检修。

（8）注意观察系统漏液情况，任何情况下的漏液都应及时处理。

（9）应放缓流速后停泵，瞬间停泵可能损害色谱柱。

（10）UV 检测器应平衡半小时，未分析样品时，紫外灯应关闭。

六、讨论

（1）简述头孢拉定及其片剂的含量测定方法及结果计算原理。

（2）简述高效液相色谱法系统适用性试验的内容。

（3）简述头孢拉定片剂测定的样品前处理的方法。

Experiment 9   Assay of Cefradine and Cefradine Tablets

1. Purposes

1.1   To learn the principles of high performance liquid chromatography (HPLC) and its application in pharmaceutical analysis.

1.2   To learn the assay method for cefradine and cefradine tablets by HPLC.

2. Instruments and chemical reagents

High performance liquid chromatography should be checked and calibrated periodically and meet all requirements. The instruction manual should be followed closely on such matters as care, cleaning and calibration of the instrument as well as instructions for operation. All reagents should be of analytical reagent grade unless otherwise stated. For accurate quantitative work, high-purity reagents and HPLC grade organic solvents must be used. Water of suitable quality should have low conductivity and low UV absorption and be appropriate to the intended use.

3. Procedures and methods

3.1   Assay of cefradine by HPLC

3.1.1   Structure, molecular formula and molecular weight of cefradine

$$(C_{16}H_{19}N_3O_4S, Mw = 349.40)$$

Cefradine is $(6R,7R) - 7 - [[(2R) - 2 - amino - 2 - (1 - cyclohexa - 1,4 - dienyl) acetyl]$ amino $] - 3 - methyl - 8 - oxo - 5 - thia - 1 - azabicyclo [4.2.0] oct - 2 - ene - 2 - carboxylic acid.

3.1.2　Description

It is a white or almost white crystalline powder, slightly odourous. It is sparingly soluble in water, practically insoluble in ethanol, chloroform or ether. Cefradine contains not less than 90.0% of $C_{16}H_{19}N_3O_4S$, calculated on the anhydrous basis.

3.1.3　Assay

Chromatographic system　Carry out the method for high performance liquid chromatography, using a column packed with an octadecylsilane bonded silica gel and a mixture of water : methanol : 3.86% solution of sodium acetate − 4% solution of acetic acid (1564 : 400 : 30 : 6) as the mobile phase. The flow rate is 0.7 ~ 0.9ml per minute and the detection wavelength is 254nm. Inject 10μl of the resulting solution of 10 parts of cefradine and 1 part of cefalexin CRS stocking solution (0.4mg/ml) into the column and record the chromatograms. The resolution factor between peaks of cefradine and cefalexin complies with the related requirements. The number of theoretical plates of column is not less than 2500, calculated with reference to the peak of cefradine.

Procedure　Dissolve about 70mg of substance to be examined, accurately weighed in mobile phase by ultrasonic treatment and dilute to 100ml, mix well. Inject 10μl into column and record the chromatogram. Repeat the operation, using cefradine CRS preparation instead of the substance being examined. Calculate the content of cefradine ($C_{16}H_{19}N_3O_4S$) by external stand method.

3.2　Assay of Cefradine tablets

Cefradine tablets are film coated tablets with almost white or slight yellow cores. They contain not less than 90.0% and not more than 110.0% of the labeled amount of cefradine ($C_{16}H_{19}N_3O_4S$). Their labeled strength are 0.25g and 0.5g.

Assay　accurately weigh and powder 10 tablets, weigh accurately a quantity of powder equivalent to about 70mg of cefradine and dissolve it in a 100ml volumetric flask with 70ml of mobile phase by ultrasonic treatment for 15min and shaking for 10min, then dilute to volume with mobile phase, and mix well and filter. Inject 10μl of the successive filtrate into the column. Carry out the assay described under cefradine.

4. Prepare lessons before class

4.1　What are the physicochemical properties of cefradine?

4.2　List the quantitative methods for drug assay by HPLC.

4.3　Explain the contents of system suitability test for HPLC.

4.4 Figure out the stationary phase and mobile phase for the assay of cefradine by HPLC.

4.5 List the types of detectors commonly used in HPLC.

5. Guide for experiment

High performance liquid chromatography(HPLC)is a method of chromatographic separation in which the mobile phase is pumped into a column containing stationary phase by a high-pressure pump system. The test solution injected is carried into the column by the mobile phase. All the components are separated in the column and pass through the detector sequentially. The recorder, integrator or data acquisition system thus records the chromatographic signals(Figure 3 – 2).

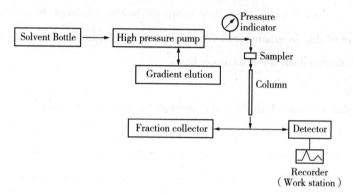

Figure 3 – 2   HPLC equipment

5.1   General requirement for apparatus

The HPLC instrument is used here, which should be checked periodically and meet the requirements of relative specification.

5.1.1   Chromatographic column

The most widely used packing material is the chemically bonded silica gel. Reverse-phase chromatographic system uses nonpolar packing material, in which the most frequently used is octadecyl-chemically bonded silica gel. Octylsilane silica gel and other types of chemically bonded silical gels (such as cyano and amino group bonded silica gel) are also used. Positive-phase chromatographic system uses polar packing material, of which the most widely used is silica gel. The ion-exchange resin is used in ion-exchange chromatography. The gel and macromolecular porous microsphere are used in size exclusion chromatography. Chiral bonded packing materials are used in the separation of enantiomers(chiral chromatography).

The characteristics of packing materials(the shape of the support, the particle size, the pore diameter, the surface area, the surface coverage of the bonded functional group, the carbon content and the bonding mode, ect.) and the packing of the chromatographic column directly affect the retention behavior and separation performance. The packing material with pore diameter less than 15nm(1nm = 10Å)is suitable for the analysis of compound whose molecular weight is less than 2000, and that with a pore diameter of more than 30nm is suitable for analysis of compound whose molecular weight is more than 2000.

The mobile phase in which the pH value is 2 ~ 8 is suitable for the stationary phase with silica gel as the support. If the pH value is more than 8, the silica gel may be dissolved and if the pH value is less than 2, the phase chemically bonded with the silica gel may be broken off. In the case when the mobile phase in which the pH value is more than 8 should be used, the packing material, which is alkali-proof, should be chosen, such as bonded silica gel with high purity silicon as support and a high surface coverage, polymer coated packing material, the organic and inorganic hybridized packing materials and the non-silica gel packing material. In the case when the mobile phase in which the pH value is less than 2, should be used, the packing material, which is acid-proof, may be chosen; the octadecylsilane modified silica gel with diisopropyl or diisobutyl substitution, which has a bulk mass and thus results in a protection through a steric hindrance, or organic and inorganic hybridized packing material, ect.

5. 1. 2　Detector

The most commonly used detector is the ultraviolet (UV) spectrophotometers. Besides, diode array differential refractometers, evaporative light scattering detectors are all available detector (Figure 3 − 3). The response value is related not only to the concentration of the test solution, but also to the structure of the compound. On the contrary, the differential refractometers and evaporative light scattering detector are general-purpose detectors, they will respond to all compounds. The response value of the evaporative light scattering detectors for compounds with similar structure is almost related to the mass of the test compound. Diode array detector may record the absorption spectrum within the prescribed wavelength range simultaneously, thus it can be used to measure the spectrum and inspect the purity of the chromatographic peaks.

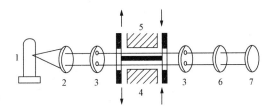

Figure 3 − 3　UV detector optical path diagram

1. Low pressure mercury lamp; 2. Lens; 3. Hood; 4. Sample cell; 5. Reference cell;

6. Ultra − violet filter; 7. Double ultra − violet photoresistance

The response value of the UV spectrophotometers, fluorescence spectrophotometers, electrochemical detectors and differential refractometers is linear with the concentration of the test solution within a certain range, while the response value of the evaporative light scattering detectors is not always linear with the concentration of the test solution; if necessary, it should be transferred mathematically before calculating.

Different detectors have different requirements for the mobile phase. For example, if the UV spectrophotometer is used in the experiment, the mobile phase should at least meet the requirements for the solvent described in UV spectrophotometry. When the light of lower wavelength is applied for detection, the cut-off wavelength of the organic solvent should be considered and it is better to use chromatographic grade organic solvent. The evaporative light scattering detectors and the mass spectrometers generally do not allow using the mobile phase that contains non-volatile salts.

5. 1. 3　Mobile phase

As the C18 chain is not able to keep a spreading state in the water solution, the ratio of the organic solvent of the mobile phase should not be less than 5%, in the reverse phase chromatographic system of which the stationary phase is octadecylsilane bonded silica gel. Otherwise the random curl of the C18 chain will lead to the change of the retention value of the component, which may result in the instability of the chromatographic system.

The type of the stationary phase, the composition of the mobile phase and the mode of the detectors specified under the monograph should not be changed. Others, such as the inner diameter, the length, the brand of the stationary phase and the particle size of the support, the flow rate of the mobile phase and the ratio of each component in the mixed mobile phase, the time span in the gradient elution program, the temperature of the column, the injection volume and the sensitivity of the detectors could be changed appropriately to meet the requirement of the system suitability test. But for some monographs, in which only the specific brand of packing material is able to satisfy the requirement of the separation, clear indications should be given under them.

5.2　System suitability test

The suitability test of the chromatographic system generally includes four indexes, number of theoretical plates, resolution, repeatability and tailing factors, in which the resolution and the repeatability are more practical indexes. To carry out the suitability test of the chromatographic system according to the requirement under the individual monograph is to test the chromatographic system by using specific reference substance. The separation conditions of the chromatography should be adjusted in case the requirement cannot be met.

5.2.1　Theoretical plates of the column

Inject the test solution or the internal standard specified under the monograph into the system according to the prescribed chromatographic conditions. Record the chromatogram and measure the retention time t_R (in minutes or length units, the same as below, which should be in the same unit) and the peak width at half peak height ($W_{h/2}$) of the principal component peak of the test solution or that of the internal standard. Calculate the theoretical plates of the chromatographic column (n) by the equation.

$$n = 5.54(t_R/W_{h/2})^2$$

5.2.2　Resolution

In either in qualitative analysis or quantitative analysis, the peak of substance being examined and other peaks, such as internal standard peak or specific impurity peak, must have good resolution Figure 3−4. The equation for calculating the resolution (R) is as follow.

$$R = \frac{2(t_{R_2} - t_{R_1})}{W_1 + W_2}$$

Where t_{R_2} is the retention time of the latter of the two adjacent peaks, t_{R_1} is the retention time of the former of the two adjacent peaks. W_1 and W_2 are the peak width of the two adjacent peaks.

Unless otherwise specified, the resolution value should not be less than 1.5 in quantitative analysis.

5.2.3　Repeatability

Inject the reference solution described under the monograph for 5 times successively. Unless otherwise specified, the relative standard deviation of the measured value of the peak areas should be no more than 2.0%.

According to the measurement of the correction factor specified under each monograph, prepare a series of reference solutions equivalent to 80%, 100% and 120% of the content of the substance being examined, each containing a definite amount of internal standard substance. Inject each solution at least 2 times, calculating the average correction factors, the relative standard deviation of which should be no more than 2.0%.

5.2.4 Tailing factor

In order to guarantee the performance of the separation and the precision of the measurement, the tailing factor (T) should be inspected to see whether it meets the prescription under each monograph. The equation for calculating the tailing factor is as follows.

$$T = \frac{W_{0.05h}}{2d_1}$$

Where $W_{0.05h}$ is the peak width at 5% of the peak height, d_1 is the distance between the perpendicular line passing through the peak maximum and that of the leading edge of the peak (Figure 3 – 5).

Unless otherwise specified, the T value should be within 0.95 ~ 1.05 in quantitative analysis using peak height. In the quantitative analysis using peak area, over deviation of T value will also affect the detection and the quantification precision of the small peak.

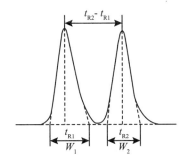

Figure 3 – 4　The calculation of Resolution　　**Figure 3 – 5　The calculation of Tailing factor**

5.3　Quantitative method

5.3.1　Correcting internal standard method for the determination of individual impurities or the main components

Prepare solutions containing an accurately weighed quantity of the reference substance and the internal standard respectively as specified in the monograph. Accurately measure each solution and prepare the reference solution for determining the correction factors. Inject a certain amount of solution into the equipment and record the chromatogram. Measure the peak area of height of the reference substance and the internal standard and calculated the correction factors according to the following equation.

$$f = \frac{A_S/C_S}{A_R/C_R}$$

Where A_S is the peak area or the peak height of the internal standard; A_R is the peak area or the peak height of the reference substance; C_S is the concentration of the internal standard; C_R is the concentration of the reference standard.

Prepare solutions containing the substance being examined and the internal standard as described in the monograph. Inject the solution into the equipment and record the chromatogram.

Measure the peak area or the peak height of the substance being examined and that of the internal standard. Calculate the content is as follows.

$$C_X = f\frac{A_X}{A_S/C_S}$$

Where A_X is the peak area or the peak height of the substance being examined (or its impurity) ; C_x is the concentration of the solution of the substance being examined (or its impurity) ; f, A_S, C_S have the same meaning as that mentioned above.

If an equal amount of the internal standard of the same concentration is used both in preparing the reference solution for measuring the correction factors and in preparing the test solution, that is $C_S = C'_S$. In this case accurate weighing is not necessary for preparing the internal standard solution.

5. 3. 2   External standard method for the determination of the individual impurity of the main component

Prepare solutions containing an accurately weighed quantity of the reference substance and the substance being examined respectively and inject a certain amount of each solution into the equipment. Record the chromatogram and measure the peak area (or peak height). Calculate the content is as follows.

$$C_X = C_R\frac{A_X}{A_R}$$

Where each symbol has the same meaning as that mentioned above.

As the micro syringe is not able to control the amount of solution being injected precisely, the sampling loop or automatic sampler may be used in measuring the content of the impurity and main components in the substance being examined.

5. 3. 3   Correcting peak areas of impurities compared with that produced by the main peak of a diluted solution of substance being examined

This method could be used to measure the content of the impurity. Prepare solutions containing an accurately weighed quantity of the reference substances of impurities and the main component as specified in the monograph. Inject a volume and record the chromatogram. Calculate the correction factor of the impurity according to the method described in 5. 3. 1. The correction factor could be directly recorded in the individual monograph and used for the correction of the measured peak areas of impurities.

When measuring the content of the impurities, dilute the solution of the substance being examined to a concentration as specified in the individual monograph so that its peak area is around that produced by the impurities in the original concentration. Inject and adjust the attenuation of the detector (limited by the noise level that can be accepted) or vary the injection volume (limited by the loading ability of the column) until the peak height of the main component is 10% ~25% of the full scale or the peak area which could be accurately measured (generally, for the impurity, the content is lower than 0.5%, the RSD of the peak area should be less than 10%, while for the impurity, the content of which is between 0.5% ~ 2%, the RSD of peak area should be less than 5%, for the impurity whose content is higher than 2%, the RSD of the peak area should be less than 2%). Inject separately an appropriate amount of the test solution and reference solution. The recorded time span of the test solution, unless otherwise specified, should be 2 times that of the main component. Measure the peak areas of each impurity on the chromatogram of the test solution. Multiply them by the respective correction factors and then compare them with the peak area of the main component of the reference solution and calculate the content of the impurities accordingly.

5.3.4　Peak areas of impurities compared with that produced by the main peak of a diluted solution of substance being examined

This method could be used when the impurity reference substance is not available. Prepare the reference solution according to method 5.2.3 and adjust the attenuation of the detector. Inject separately an appropriate volume of the test solution and reference solution. The record time span of the former should be 2 times the retention time of the main areas of the impurities on the chromatogram of the test solution and compare them with those of the main component of the reference solution and calculate the content of the impurities.

If there are some impurities in the substance being examined which are not completely separated from the solvent peak, record chromatogram Ⅰ of the substance being examined according to the specification and then record chromatogram Ⅱ of the pure solvent solution. Then, the corresponding peak area of solvent in chromatogram Ⅱ is subtracted from chromatogram Ⅰ (including the solvent peak). The result is equal to the correction peak area of the total impurities. Calculate the content of the impurities accordingly.

5.3.5　Peak area normalization method

The deviation of this method is so large that it can only be used to roughly inspect the contents of impurities in the substance being examined. It is not suitable for the determination of minute impurities, unless otherwise specified in this method; the peak area of the impurities and the total peak area on the chromatogram except the solvent peak are measured. Calculate the peak area of each impurity and the percentage of their sum in the total peak area.

5.4　Notes

5.4.1　At any time buffer solution should not switch to a pure organic solvent quickly. All samples must be filtered. HPLC grade solvents are highly recommended. Exhaust bubbles in pipes after changing mobile phase.

5.4.2　Do not exceed the maximum pressure for each column. It is recommended to use the lowest pressure for the separations. High pressures may increase wear on the components.

5.4.3　The pH value of samples and eluent must be within the working range of a column.

5.4.4　Never run the column dry. Make sure there is enough solvent in the reservoir.

5.4.5　Equilibrate the columns by running 5-fold and 20-fold the column volume full of solvent for RP and NP columns, respectively. The column volumes are approximately 11ml and 182ml for the small and large columns.

5.4.6　Too high pressure of the HPLC indicates a blocked guard column. A too low pressure of the HPLC hints that solvent delivery system has an opening.

5.4.7　Watch the fluctuation of the pressure. Irregular ups and downs indicate that pumps need to be serviced.

5.4.8　Watch out any possible leaking. Any leaking needs to be taken care immediately.

5.4.9　Ramp the pumps up or down over a period of time(<5ml/min). Do not suddenly shut them off, which may damage the column.

5.4.10　Equilibrate the UV detector for 0.5 hour. When not running a sample, turn the UV lamp OFF.

6. Discussions

6.1　Explain the quantitative methods for the assay of cefradine and its tablet.

6.2　Explain the principles of system suitability test.

6.3　Explain the sample treatment for the assay of cefradine tablet.

（曹丽娟）

第四章　药物质量的全检验

Chapter 4　Drug Analysis

实验十　维生素 E 或维生素 E 软胶囊的质量检查

一、目的

（1）掌握维生素 E 及其软胶囊分析的原理、操作条件及注意事项。
（2）掌握气相色谱法测定的原理与方法。

二、仪器与试药

1. 仪器

旋光仪、折光仪、紫外 – 分光光度计、红外光谱仪、气相色谱仪、分析天平、分液漏斗、滴定管、毛细管柱（100% 二甲基聚硅氧烷为固定液）、固定液硅酮（OV – 17）、移液管、量瓶、棕色具塞锥形瓶。

2. 试药

维生素 E 原料、维生素 E 对照品、维生素 E 软胶囊、α – 生育酚、正三十二烷、正己烷、乙醇、乙醚、二苯胺试液、硫酸铈滴定液、氢氧化钠滴定液。

三、实验方法

（一）维生素 E 的质量分析

1. 维生素 E 的结构、分子式、相对分子质量

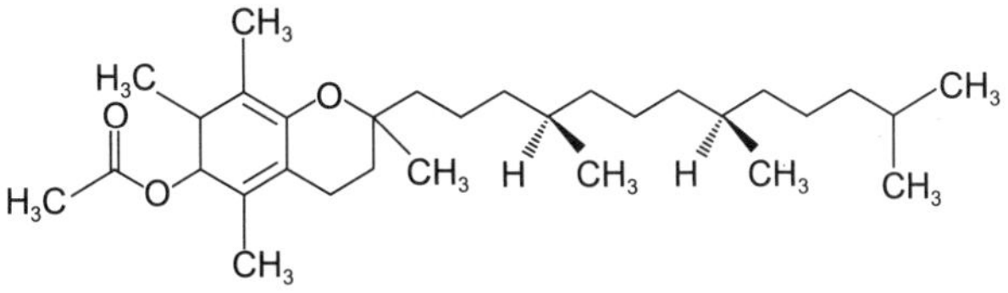

合成型

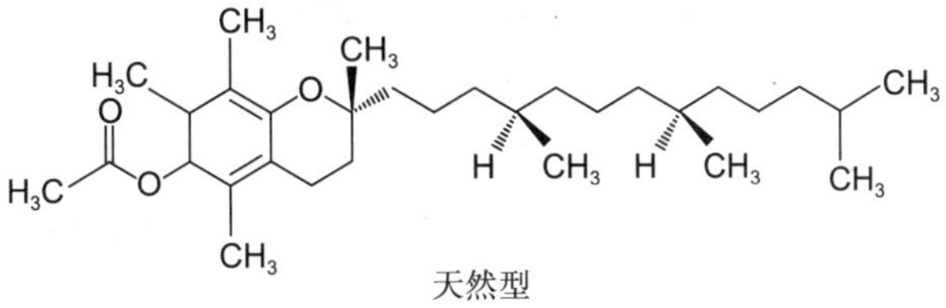

天然型

（$C_{31}H_{52}O_3$，$Mw = 472.75$）

本品为合成型或天然型维生素 E；合成型为（±）-2，5，7，8-四甲基-2-（4，8，12-三甲基十三烷基）-6-苯并二氢吡喃醇乙酸酯或 dl-α-生育酚乙酸酯，天然型为（+）-2，5，7，8-四甲基-2-（4，8，12-三甲基十三烷基）-6-苯并二氢吡喃醇乙酸酯或 d-α-生育酚乙酸酯。含 $C_{31}H_{52}O_3$ 应为 96.0% ~102.0%。

2. 性状

本品为微黄色至黄色或黄绿色澄清的黏稠液体；几乎无臭；遇光色渐变深；天然型放置会固化，25℃左右熔化。

本品在无水乙醇、丙酮、乙醚或植物油中易溶，在水中不溶。

（1）比旋度　避光操作。取本品 0.4g，精密称定，置 150ml 具塞圆底烧瓶中，加无水乙醇 25ml 溶解，加硫酸乙醇溶液（1→7）20ml，置水浴上回流 3h，放冷，用硫酸乙醇溶液（1→72）定量转移至 200ml 量瓶中并稀释至刻度，摇匀。精密量取 100ml，置分液漏斗中，加水 200ml，用乙醚提取两次（75ml，25ml），合并乙醚液，加铁氰化钾氢氧化钠溶液 [取铁氰化钾 50g，加氢氧化钠溶液（1→125）溶解并稀释至 500ml]50ml，振摇 3min；取乙醚层，用水洗涤 4 次，每次 50ml，弃去洗涤液，乙醚液经无水硫酸钠脱水后置水浴上减压或在氮气流下蒸干至 7~8ml 时，停止加热，继续挥干乙醚，残渣立即加异辛烷溶解并定量转移至 25ml 量瓶中，用异辛烷稀释至刻度，摇匀，依法测定，比旋度（按 d-α-生育酚计，即测得结果除以换算系数 0.911）不得低于 +24°（天然型）。

（2）折光率　本品的折光率为 1.494~1.499。

（3）吸收系数　取本品，精密称定，加无水乙醇溶解并定量稀释制成每毫升中约含 0.1mg 的溶液，照紫外-可见分光光度法，在 284nm 的波长处测定吸光度，吸收系数（$E_{1cm}^{1\%}$）为 41.0~45.0。

3. 鉴别

（1）取本品约 30mg，加无水乙醇 10ml 溶解，加硝酸 2ml，摇匀，在 75℃ 加热约 15min，溶液显橙红色。

（2）本品的红外吸收图谱应与对照的图谱（光谱集 1206 图）一致。

（3）在含量测定项下记录的色谱图中，供试品溶液主峰的保留时间应与对照品溶液主峰的保留时间一致。

4. 检查

（1）酸度　取乙醇与乙醚各 15ml，置锥形瓶中，加酚酞指示液 0.5ml，滴加氢氧化钠滴定液（0.1mol/L）至微显粉红色，加本品 1.0g，溶解后用氢氧化钠滴定液（0.1mol/L）滴定，消耗的氢氧化钠滴定液（0.1mol/L）不得过 0.5ml。

（2）生育酚（天然型）　取本品 0.10g，加无水乙醇 5ml 溶解后加二苯胺试液 1 滴，用硫酸铈滴定液（0.01mol/L）滴定，消耗的硫酸铈滴定液（0.01mol/L）不得过 1.0ml。

（3）有关物质（合成型）　取本品，用正己烷稀释制成每毫升中约含 2.5mg 的溶液，作为供试品溶液；精密量取适量，用正己烷定量稀释制成每毫升中含 25μg 的溶液，作为对照溶液。照含量测定项的色谱条件，取对照溶液 1μl 注入气相色谱仪，调节检测灵敏度，使主成分色谱峰的峰高约为满量程的 30%，再精密量取供试品溶液与对照溶液各 1μl，分别注入气相色谱仪，记录色谱图至主成分峰保留时间的两倍，供试品溶液的色谱图中如有杂质峰，α-生育酚（相对保留时间约为 0.87）的峰面积不得大于对照溶液主峰面积（1.0%），其他单个杂质峰面积不得大于对照溶液主峰面积的 1.5 倍（1.5%），各杂质峰面积的和不得大于对照溶液主峰面积的 2.5 倍（2.5%）。

（4）残留溶剂　正己烷（天然型）取本品，精密称定，加 N,N – 二甲基甲酰胺溶解并定量稀释制成每毫升中约含 50mg 的溶液，作为供试品溶液；另取正己烷，加 N,N – 二甲基甲酰胺定量稀释制成每毫升中约含 10μg 的溶液，作为对照品溶液。照残留溶剂测定法试验，以 5% 苯基甲基聚硅氧烷为固定液（或极性相近的固定液），起始柱温为 50℃，维持 8min，然后以每分钟 45℃ 的速率上升至 260℃，维持 15min。含正己烷应符合规定。

5. 含量测定

照气相色谱法测定。

色谱条件与系统适用性试验　用硅酮（OV – 17）为固定液，涂布浓度为 2% 的填充柱，或用 100% 二甲基聚硅氧烷为固定液的毛细管柱；柱温为 265℃。理论塔板数按维生素 E 峰计算不低于 500（填充柱）或 5000（毛细管柱），维生素 E 峰与内标物质峰的分离度应符合要求。

校正因子的测定　取正三十二烷适量，加正己烷溶解并稀释成每毫升中含 1.0mg 的溶液，作为内标溶液。另取维生素 E 对照品约 20mg，精密称定，置棕色具塞瓶中，精密加内标溶液 10ml，密塞，振摇使溶解，取 1～3μl 注入气相色谱仪，计算校正因子。

测定法　取本品约 20mg，精密称定，置棕色具塞瓶中，精密加内标溶液 10ml，密塞，振摇使溶解，取 1～3μl 注入气相色谱仪，测定，计算，即得。

（二）维生素 E 软胶囊的质量分析

1. 规格与描述

5mg，10mg，50mg，100mg。

本品含合成型或天然型维生素 E（$C_{31}H_{52}O_3$）应为标示量的 90.0%～110.0%。

2. 性状

本品内容物为淡黄色至黄色的油状液体。

3. 鉴别

（1）取本品的内容物，照维生素 E 鉴别（1）项试验，显相同的反应。

（2）在含量测定项记录的色谱图中，供试品溶液主峰的保留时间应与对照品溶液主峰的保留时间一致。

4. 检查

（1）比旋度　避光操作。取本品的内容物适量（约相当于维生素 E 400mg），精密称定，照维生素 E 比旋度项的方法测定，比旋度（按 d – α – 生育酚计）不得低于 +24°（天然型）。

（2）有关物质　取本品内容物适量（相当于维生素 E 25mg），加正己烷 10ml，振摇使维生素 E 溶解，滤过，取滤液作为供试品溶液，精密量取 1ml，至 100ml 棕色量瓶中，用正己烷稀释至刻度，摇匀，作为对照溶液。照维生素 E 有关物质项的方法试验，供试品溶液的色谱图中如有杂质峰，α – 生育酚（相对于保留时间约为 0.87）峰面积不得大于对照溶液主峰面积（1.0%），其他单个杂质峰面积不得大于对照溶液主峰面积的 1.5 倍（1.5%），各杂质峰面积的和不得大于对照溶液主峰面积的 2.5 倍（2.5%）。

（3）其他　应符合胶囊剂项下有关的各项规定。

5. 含量测定

取装量差异项的内容物，混合均匀，取适量（约相当于维生素 E 20mg），精密称定，照维生素 E 含量测定项的方法测定，计算，即得。

四、预习提要

（1）生育酚的来源和检查目的是什么？

（2）了解折光率的测定方法及注意事项。

（3）残留溶剂的检查目的和原理是什么？

（4）通过分析维生素 E 的理化性质，试说明维生素 E 和维生素 E 软胶囊含量测定的依据。

五、实验指导

（一）折光率测定

光线自一种透明介质进入另一透明介质时，由于光线在两种介质中的传播速度不同，使光线在两种介质的平滑界面上发生折射。常用的折光率系指光线在空气中进行的速度与在供试品中进行速度的比值。根据折射定律，折光率是光线入射角的正弦与折射角的正弦的比值，即

$$n = \frac{\sin i}{\sin r}$$

式中，n 为折光率；$\sin i$ 为光线入射角的正弦；$\sin r$ 为光线折射角的正弦。

物质的折光率因温度或入射光波长不同而改变，透光物质的温度升高，折光率变小；入射光的波长越短，折光率越大。折光率以 n_D^t 表示，D 为钠光谱的 D 线，t 为测定时的温度。折光率可以区别不同的油类或检查某些药品的纯杂程度。

本法系采用钠光谱的 D 线（589.3nm），测定供试品相对于空气的折光率（如阿贝折光计，可用白光光源），除另有规定外，供试品温度为 20℃。测定用的折光计须能读数至 0.0001，测量范围为 1.3~1.7，如用阿贝折光计或与其相当的仪器，测定时应调节温度至 20℃±0.5℃（或各品种项规定的温度），测量后再重复读数 2 次，3 次读数的平均值即为供试品的折光率。

测定前，折光计读数应使用校正用棱镜或水进行校正，水的折光率 20℃时为 1.3330，25℃时为 1.3325，40℃时为 1.3305。

（二）残留溶剂检查

药物中的残留溶剂是在原料或赋形剂的生产中，以及在制剂制备过程中产生或使用的有机挥发性化合物，它们在工艺中不能完全除尽。

在溶剂残留量的限度要求中，按有机溶剂的毒性程度分为以下四类。

（1）第一类溶剂　应避免的溶剂，为人体致癌物、疑为人体致癌物或环境危害物。

（2）第二类溶剂　应限制的溶剂，非遗传毒性动物致癌或可能至其他不可逆毒性如神经毒性或致畸性的试剂。

（3）第三类溶剂　低毒性溶剂，对人体低毒的溶剂，无须制定接触限度；第三类溶剂的允许日接触量为每天 50mg 或 50mg 以上。

除另有规定外，第一类、二类、三类溶剂的残留量应符合《中国药典》中的规定。对于其他溶剂（第四类等），应根据生产工艺的特点，制定相应的限度，使其符合产品规范、

GMP 或其他基本的质量要求。

残留溶剂通常采用色谱技术，如 GC 法测定，如可能对药典上规定要检测的残留溶剂应采用统一的测定方法。生产厂家也可选用更合适、经论证的方法来测定。若仅存在第三类溶剂，可用非专属性的方法如干燥失重来检查。

（三）气相色谱法

气相色谱法系采用气体为流动相（载气）流经装有填充剂的色谱柱进行分离测定的色谱方法。物质或其衍生物气化后，被载气带入色谱柱进行分离，各组分先后进入检测器，用记录仪、积分仪或数据处理系统记录色谱处理信号。

1. 仪器组成及功能

气相色谱仪由载气源、进样部分、色谱柱、柱温箱、检测器和数据处理系统组成。进样部分、色谱柱和检测器的温度均在控制状态。

（1）载气源气相色谱法的流动相为气体，称为载气，氦气、氮气和氢气可用作载气，可由高压钢瓶或高纯度气体发生器提供，经过适当的减压装置，以一定的流速经过进样器和色谱柱。根据供试品的性质和检测器种类选择载气，除另有规定外，常用载气为氮气。

（2）进样部分进样方式一般采用溶液直接进样方式或顶空进样方式。

溶液直接进样方式采用微量注射器、微量进样阀或有分流装置的气化室进样；采用溶液直接进样时，进样口温度应高于柱温 30～50℃；进样量一般不超过数微升；柱径越细，进样量应越少；采用毛细管柱时，一般应分流以免过载。

顶空进样方式适用于固体和液体供试品中挥发性组分分离和测定。将固态或液态的供试品制成供试液后置于密闭小瓶中，在恒温控制的加热室中加热至供试品中挥发性组分在非气态和气态达至平衡后由进样器自动吸取一定体积的顶空气注入色谱柱中。

（3）色谱柱为填充柱或毛细管柱。填充柱的材质为不锈钢或玻璃，内径为2～4mm，柱长为2～4m，内装吸附剂、高分子多孔小球或涂渍固定液的载体，粒径为 0.25～0.18mm，0.18～0.15mm 或 0.15～0.125mm。常用载体为经酸洗并硅烷化处理的硅藻土或高分子多孔小球，常用固定液有甲基聚硅氧烷、聚乙二醇等。毛细管柱的材质为玻璃或石英，内壁或载体经涂渍或交联固定液，内径一般为 0.25mm、0.32mm 或 0.53mm，柱长 5～60m，固定液膜厚 0.1～5.0μm，常用的固定液有甲基聚硅氧烷、不同比例组成的苯基甲基聚硅氧烷、聚乙二醇等。

新填充柱和毛细管柱在使用前须老化以除去残留溶剂及低相对分子质量的聚合物。色谱柱如长期未用，使用前应老化处理，使基线稳定。

（4）由于柱温箱温度的波动会影响色谱分析结果的重现性，因此柱温箱控温精确度应在 ±1℃，且温度波动小于每小时 0.1℃，温度控制系统分为恒温和程序升温两种。

（5）适合气相色谱法的检测器有火焰离子化检测器（FID）、热导检测器（TCD）、氮磷检测器（NPD）、火焰光度检测器（FPD）、电子捕获检测器（ECD）、质谱检测器（MSD）等。火焰离子化检测器对碳氢化合物响应良好，适合检测大多数药物；氮磷检测器对含氮、磷元素的化合物灵敏度高；火焰光度检测器对含磷、硫元素的化合物灵敏度高；电子捕获检测器适用于含卤素的化合物；质谱检测器还能给出供试品某个相应成分的结构信息，可用于结构确证。除另有规定外，一般用火焰离子化检测器，用氢气作为燃气，空气作为助燃气。在使用火焰离子化检测器时，检测器温度一般应高于柱温，并不得低于

150℃，以免水汽凝结，通常为250~350℃。

（6）数据处理系统可分为记录仪、积分仪以及计算机工作站等。

各品种项规定的色谱条件，除检测器种类、固定液品种及特殊指定的色谱柱材料不得改变外，其余如色谱柱内径、长度、载体牌号、粒度、固定液涂布浓度、载气流速、柱温、进样量、检测器的灵敏度等，均可适当改变，以适应具体品种并符合系统适用性试验的要求。色谱图一般约于30min内记录完毕。

除另有规定外，应参照高效液相色谱法的规定。

2. 常用的洗脱模式

气相色谱法中常用的洗脱模式为程序升温，系指色谱柱的温度按设置的程序连续地随时间线性或非线性逐渐升高，以使低沸点组分和高沸点组分在色谱柱中都适宜地保留，色谱峰分布均匀且峰形对称。程序升温具有改进分离、使峰变窄、检测限下降及节约时间等优点。相比恒温而言，可使后出峰的高沸点物质保留时间缩短，减小扩散量，而对于前面组分也更大地保留，利于分离。故针对沸点范围宽的混合物，可采用程序升温法进行分析。缺点是稳定状态差，等待降温使分析时间加长，所以有一些外标或内标用恒温检测也有一定的优势。

3. 内标法中校正因子的计算

按各品种项的规定，精密称（量）取对照品和内标物质，分别配成溶液，精密量取各试液，混合配成测定校正因子用的对照溶液。取一定量注入仪器，记录色谱图。测量对照品和内标物质的峰面积或峰高，按

$$校正因子\ (f) = \frac{A_S/c_S}{A_R/c_R}$$

计算校正因子。式中，A_S 为内标物质的峰面积或峰高；A_R 为对照品的峰面积或峰高；c_S 为内标物质的浓度；c_R 为对照品的浓度。

再取各品种项含有内标物质的供试品溶液，注入仪器，记录色谱图，测量供试品中待测成分和内标物质的峰面积或峰高，按

$$含量\ (c_X) = f\frac{A_X}{A'_s/c'_s}$$

计算含量。式中，A_X 为供试品的峰面积或峰高；c_X 为供试品的浓度；A'_s 为内标物质的峰面积或峰高；c'_s 为内标物质的浓度；f 为校正因子。

4. 气相色谱法的定量计算方法

（1）内标加校正因子测定供试品中某个杂质或主成分含量。

（2）外标法测定供试品中某个杂质或主成分含量。

（3）面积归一化法。上述各法的具体内容均同高效液相色谱法项的规定。

（4）标准溶液加入法测定供试品中某个杂质或主成分含量。精密称（量）取某个杂质或待测成分对照品适量，配制成适当浓度的对照品溶液，取一定量，精密加入到供试品溶液中，根据外标法或内标法测定杂质或主成分含量，再扣除加入的对照品溶液含量，即得供试溶液中杂质和主成分含量。

可按公式进行计算，加入对照品溶液前后校正因子应相同，即

$$\frac{A_{is}}{A_x} = \frac{c_x + \Delta c_x}{c_x}$$

则待测组分的浓度 c_x 可通过

$$c_x = \frac{\Delta c_x}{(A_{is}/A_x) - 1}$$

进行计算。

式中，c_x 为供试品中组分 X 的浓度；A_x 为供试品中组分 X 的色谱峰面积；Δc_x 为所加入已知浓度的待测组分对照品的浓度；A_{is} 为加入对照品后组分 X 的色谱峰面积。

对于气相色谱法定量分析，采用手工进样时，由于留针时间和室温等对进样量的影响，使进样量不宜精确控制，故最好采用内标法定量；采用自动进样器时由于进样重复率提高，在保证进样误差的前提下，也可采用外标法定量。采用顶空进样技术时，由于供试品和对照品处于不完全相同的基质中，故可采用标准溶液加入法以消除基质效应的影响；当标准溶液加入法与其他定量方法不一致时，应以标准溶液加入法结果为准。

六、讨论

（1）气相色谱法测定维生素 E 含量时为什么使用内标法？

（2）试述气相色谱法的特点及分析适用范围。

（3）维生素 E 含量测定中除气相色谱法，还可采用哪些方法？各有什么特点？

Experiment 10　Analysis of Vitamin E or Vitamin E Soft Capsules

1. Purposes

1.1　To experiment on the analysis of Vitamin E and Vitamin E Soft Capsules.

1.2　To study the principles and procedures of gas chromatography for the assay of volatile drugs.

2. Instruments and chemical reagents

2.1　Instruments

Polarimeter, refractometer, UV spectrophotometer, infrared spectrometer, gas chromatography, analytical balances, separating funnel, buret, capillary column (100% dimethyl polysiloxane), silicone(OV – 17), pipette, brown stoppered erlenmeyer flask.

2.2　Chemical reagents

Vitamin E material, Vitamin E reference, vitamin E soft capsules, α-tocopherol, dotriacontane, n-hexane, dehydrated ethanol, ethylether, diphenylamine TS, sodium hydroxide VS, ceric sulfate VS.

3. Procedures and methods

3.1　Analysis of Vitamin E(Alpha tocopheryl acetate)

3.1.1　Structure, molecular formula and molecular weight of vitamin E

Vitamin E is $dl - 2,5,7,8$ – tetramethyl – 2 – (4,8,12 – trimethyl tridecyl) chromakey – 6 – acetate. It contains not less than 96.0% and not more than 102% of $C_{31}H_{52}O_3$.

Synthetic Type

Natural Type

$(C_{31}H_{52}O_3, Mw = 472.75)$

3.1.2 Description

A clear pale yellow to pale or greenish-yellow, viscous, oily liquid, almost odourless, the color deepens on exposure to light.

Freely soluble in dehydrated ethanol, acetone, ether or plant oil, insoluble in water.

Specific Optical Rotation　Protect from light throughout the procedure. Dissolve about 0.4g, accurately weighed, into a conical flask, in 25ml of dehydrated ethanol, and 20ml of ethanolic solution of sulfuric acid. Reflux in water both for 3 hours and cool, transfer to 200ml volumetric flask and dilute to volume with ethanolic solution of sulfuric acid, and mix well. Measure accurately 100ml into a separator, add 200ml of water, extract twice with ether(75ml, 25ml), combine the extracts, add 50ml of sodium hydroxide solution of potassium ferricyanide (dissolve 50 g potassium ferricyanide with solution hydroxide solution(1→125) and dilute to 500ml), shake for 3 minutes, transfer the other layer and wash with four portions of 50ml each of water, discard the washings, and dry with anhydrous sodium sulfate. When evaporate to 7 ~ 8ml on water both in vacuum or in a current of nitrogen, stop heating evaporate either to dry. Dissolve the residue with isooctane and transfer to 25ml volumetric flask carefully, dilute to volume. Not less than +24°(calculate on d-α-tocopherol, the result divide by coefficient 0.911, natural).

Refractive index　1.494 ~ 1.499.

Specific absorbance　Measure the absorbance of a solution of 0.1mg per milliliter in dehydrated ethanol at 284nm, the value of A(1%, 1 cm) is 41.0 ~ 45.0.

3.1.3 Identification

a. Dissolve about 30mg in 10ml of dehydrated ethanol, add 2ml of nitric acid, mix well, heat at 75℃ for 15 minutes, then an orange-red color is produced.

b. The infrared absorption spectrum(1206) is concordant with the reference spectrum of vitamin E CRS.

c. The retention time of the principal peak obtained with the test solution is identical with that of the peak obtained with vitamin E CRS.

3.1.4 Test

Acidity　Dissolve 1.0g in 15ml of a mixture of ethanol and ether which has been neutralized to pale pink with sodium hydroxide(0.1mol/L) VS and 0.5ml of phenolphthalein titrate with sodium hydroxide(0.1mol/L) VS, not more than 0.5ml is consumed.

Tocopherol　Dissolve 0.1g in 5ml of dehydrated ethanol, add 1 drop of diphenylamine TS, titrate with ceric sulfate(0.1mol/L) VS, not more than 1.0ml is consumed.

Related substance(synthetil compound)　Dissolve a quantity of the substance being examined, accurately weighed, in n-hexane to procedure the test solution about 2.5mg per milliliter as sample solution, then diluting to 25μg per milliliter with n-hexane as the reference solution. According to the chromatographic conditions of content determination, inject 1μl of reference solution into the column, and adjust the detectability so that the principal peak height in the chromatogram is about 30% of full scale of the chart. Inject separately accurately 1μl each of the sample solution and reference solution into the column, and record the chromatogram for double the retention time of the principal peak. If there are any other impurity peaks in the chromatogram of test solution, α-tocopherol peak area (relative retention time is about 0.87) is not greater than principal peak area(1%) of reference solution, any single impurity peak area is not greater than 1.5 times of principal peak area(1.5%) and the sum of the areas of all peaks other than the principal peak is not greater than 2.5 times of area(2.5%) of the major peak of reference solution.

Residual solvents　n-Hexane Carry out the method for determination of residual solvents, using an HP-5 capillary column(5% polydimethylsiloxane) and flaring sensation detector. Maintaining the temperature of the column at 50℃ for 8min, then raising the temperature at a rate of 45℃ every minute to 260℃ and maintaining it at 260℃ for 15min. Dissolve an accurately weighed quantity and dilute to produce a solution of 50mg perml with dimethylformamide, as the test solution. To a quantity of n-hexane, dilute to produce a solution of 10μg per milliliter with dimethylformamide as the reference solution. Calculate the content of n-hexane completes with the related requirements (natural vitamin E).

3.1.5　Assay

a. Carry out the method for gas chromatography, using a column packed with 2% silicone (OV-17) as the stationary phase and maintain the column temperature at 265℃. The number of theoretical plates of the column is not less than 500(packed column) or 5000(capillary column), calculated with reference to the peak of vitamin E, and the resolution factor between the peaks of vitamin E and internal standard compiles with the requirement.

b. Dissolve a quantity of dotriacontane in n-hexane to produce a solution of 1.0mg per 1 millilite as the internal standard solution. To 20mg of vitamin E CRS, accurately weighed, in an amber colored flask with stopper, add 10ml of internal standard solution, accurately measured, stopper the flask, shake well. Inject 1~3μl into the column and calculate the correction factor.

c. Procedure　To about 20mg, accurately weighed, in an amber colored volumetric flask with stopper, add 10ml of internal standard solution, accurately measured, stopper the flask and shake well. Inject 1~3μl into the column and calculate the content of $C_{31}H_{52}O_3$.

3.2　Analysis of vitamin E soft capsules

3.2.1　Strength and description

a. 5mg, 10mg, 50mg, 100mg.

b. Vitamin E soft capsules contain not less than 90.0% and not more than 110.0% of the labelled amount of vitamin E(natural or synthetic vitamin E)($C_{31}H_{52}O_3$).

3.2.2　Description

Soft capsules containing yellow to pale yellow only liquid.

3.2.3　Identification

a. Its contents comply with the test(3.1.3a) for identification described under Vitamin E.

b. The retention time of the principal peak obtained with the test solution is identical with that of the peak obtained with vitamin E CRS.

3.2.4　Test

a. Specific optical rotation　Protect from light throughout the procedure. Accurately weighed about 400mg, not less than $+24°$(natural type), in a solution for preparation described under vitamin E.

b. Related substance　Weigh a propriate amount content of this product(it equals to 25mg vitamin E), add 10ml n-hexane, shake for a period of time to make the vitamin E dissolve, filtrate, and take the filtration as test solution. Measure accurately 1ml the test solution into a 100ml brown volumetric flask and dilute to the volume with n-hexane, and mix well as the reference solution. Carry out the method for relevant substance of vitamin E, if there are any other impurity peaks in the chromatogram of test solution, α-tocopherol peak area(relative retention time is about 0.87) is not greater than principal peak area(1%) of reference solution, any single impurity peak area is not greater than 1.5 times of principal peak area(1.5%) and the sum of the areas of all peaks other than the principal peak is not greater than 2.5 times of area(2.5%) of the principal peak of reference solution.

Other requirements comply with the general requirements for capsules.

3.2.5　Assay

Mix well the contents obtained in the test for weight variation. Weigh accurately a propriate amount of the mixed contents equaling to 20mg of vitamin E. Carry out the method stated under vitamin E. Calculate the content of $C_{31}H_{52}O_3$.

4. Prepare lessons before class

4.1　Where is α-tocopherol from? What is the principle of its test?

4.2　How to determine refractive index?

4.3　Why is the test of residual solvents carried out in the analysis of aspirin?

4.4　Please describe the principles of assay for vitamin E and its soft capsules.

5. Guide for experiment

5.1　Determination of refractive

Refraction takes place when a beam of light is transmitted from a transparent medium into another transparent medium, since the velocity of light changes in a medium of different density. The refractive index of a substance is the ratio of velocity of light in air to its velocity in the substance. The refractive index may also be defined as the ratio of the sine of the angle of the incidence to the sine of the angle of refraction, namely

$$n = \frac{\sin i}{\sin r}$$

Where n is the refractive index, i is the angle of incidence, r is the angle of refraction.

The refractive index varies with the temperature of the substance being examined and the wavelength of incident light. It decreases with the increase of temperature. The shorter the wavelength of incident light, the larger refractive index. Refractive indices are usually stated in terms of sodium line D at a temperature of t and symbolised by n_D^t. The measurement of refractive index is employed to establish the identity of oils and test for purity of the substance being examined.

Unless otherwise specified, the values of refractive index cited in this method are measured at 20℃ with sodium D line(589. 3nm) against air(while light may be use if an Abbe refractometer is available).

The refractometer should be able to give readings accurate to 0. 0001 in the range of 1. 3 ~ 1. 7. An Abbe refractometer or other equivalent instrument is used, the measurement should be conducted at 20℃ ± 0. 5℃ (or in an accordance with the temperature stated under individual monograph). Three readings should be taken and the mean value is used as the refractive index of the substance being examined. The readings of the refractometer should be calibrated before use with a prism or against water. The refractive index of water is 1. 3330 at 20℃, 1. 3325 at 25℃ and 1. 3305 at 40℃.

5. 2 Residual solvents

Residual solvents in pharmaceuticals are defined here as organic volatile chemicals that are used or produced in the manufacture of drug substances or excipients, or in the preparation of drug products. The solvents are not completely removed by practical manufacturing techniques.

They were evaluated for their toxicity and placed into one of four classes as follows:

Class 1 solvents: solvents to be avoided. Known human carcinogens, strongly suspected human carcinogens, and environmental hazards.

Class 2 solvents: solvents to be limited. Non-genotoxic animal carcinogens or possible causative agents of other irreversible toxicity such as neurotoxicity or teratogenicity. Solvents suspected of other significant but reversible toxicities.

Class 3 solvents: solvents with low toxic potential. Solvents with low toxic potential to man; no health-based exposure limit is needed. Class 3 solvents have PDEs of 50mg or more per day.

Unless otherwise specified, the residual quantity of Class 1, 2, 3 solvents must meet the requirements stated in Ch. P. For other solvents (such as Class 4 solvents), according to the characteristics of manufacturing technique, establish corresponding limitation, in order to make it comply with product practice, GMP or other basic quality requirements.

Residual solvents are typically determined using chromatographic techniques such as gas chromatography. Any harmonised procedures for determining levels of residual solvents as described in the pharmacopoeias should be used, if feasible. Otherwise, manufacturers would be free to select the most appropriate validated analytical procedure for a particular application. If only Class 3 solvents are present, a non-specific method such as loss on drying may be used.

5.3　Gas chromatography

Gas chromatography(GC) is a separation technique in which the mobile phase, an inert gas known as carrier gas, is passing through the chromatographic column packed with packing materials for separation and determination. The substance or its derivatives are injected into the vaporizer with a micro-syringe and vaporized, separated on the stationary phase. Each component passes through the detector in succession and a chromatogram is thus recorded by integrator, recorder or data acquisition system.

5.3.1　Configuration of the instrument

The apparatus consists of a carrier gas source, an injector port, a chromatographic column conditioned in an oven, a detector and a data acquisition system. The injection part, column, and detector are temperature-controlled.

a. Carrier gas source　　The mobile phase of gas chromatography is gas, known as carrier gas. Carrier gases used are usually nitrogen, helium and hydrogen. The gas is supplied by a high-pressure steel cylinder or high-purity gas generator and passes through suitable pressure-reducing valve and a flow meter to the injector port and column. The gas selection depends on the properties of the substances being examined and the species of the detector. The commonly used carrier gas is nitrogen, unless otherwise specified.

b. Injection part　　Direct injection of solutions and headspace injection are the usual modes of injection.

Direct injection may be carried out using a syringe or an injection valve, or into a vaporization chamber which may be equipped with a stream splitter. The temperature of the equipment is usually 30 ~ 50℃ higher than that of the column when using direct injection. The volume of solution injected is not more than several microliter. The smaller the diameter, the less the volume of injected solutions. Capillary column used with injections is able to split samples into two fractions to avoid overloading.

Headspace injectors are suitable for the separation and determination of volatile components in solid or liquid substance being examined. The test solutions produced with solid or liquid substance being examined and stored in a tightly closed container are heated in the chamber for a period of time, allowing the volatile components in the test solution to reach a equilibrium between the nongaseous phase and the gaseous phase. A predetermined amount of the head-space of the vial is flushed into the column by automatic syringe.

c. The charmatographic column　　The charmatographic columns are classified into the packed columns and capillary columns. The packed columns, which are made of stainless steel or glass, are 2 ~ 4mm in internal diameter and 2 ~ 4m in length. The columns are packed with the sorbent, porous polymer beads or the supports coated with liquid phase, the particle size of which is 0.25 ~ 0.18mm, 0.18 ~ 0.15mm or 0.15 ~ 0.125mm. The support usually used is acid washed and silanized diatomaceous earth or porous polymer beads; the liquid phase commonly used is methylpolysiloxane, polysilphenylene of different consist, polyethyleneglycol etc. The capillary columns are made of glass or quartz. The inner wall of the column is coated or cross-linked with stationary liquid; the internal diameter is usually 0.25mm, 0.32mm or 0.53mm, the length is 5 ~

60m, and the film thickness of the stationary liquid is 0. 1 ~ 5. 0 μm. The stationary liquid commonly used are methyl polysiloxane, phenylmethylpolysiloxane with different ratio of composition and carbowax, etc. New packed and capillary column must be conditioned before use to remove oxygen and residual solvents. The charmatographic column must be conditioned before use until the baseline is stable if the column has not been in use for a long time.

d. The column oven   The temperature-controlled precision of the oven should be ± 1℃ and fluctuation of temperature should be less than 0. 1℃ per hour, as the temperature fluctuation of the oven will influence the reproducibility of charmatographic analysis result. Temperature-controlled system may be classified into constant temperature and temperature programming.

e. Detector   The detector suitable for the gas charmatography include flame-ionization detector(FID), thermal conductivity detector(TCD), nitrogen-phosphorus detector(NPD), flame-photometer detector (FPD), electron-capture detector (ECD), and mass spectrometric detector (MSD) etc. FID responds well to hydrocarbon and is suitable for the determination of most drug compounds; NPD is sensitive to organic nitrogen and phosphorus compounds; FPD is sensitive to organic sulfur and phosphorus compounds; ECD is suitable for the determination of halogen compounds; MSD can offer chemical construction information of the compounds which is useful for structure vertification. Unless otherwise specified, the detector should be FID, which employs hydrogen as combustion gas and air as combustion-supporting gas. When FID is used, its temperature is higher than that of the column and not less than 150℃ to prevent the condensation of vapour, which usually is 250 ~ 350℃.

f. Data process system   It is classified into recorder, integrator and computer station etc.

If necessary, parameters except for the kind of the detector, the type of the stationary phase and the material of the column are specified under the individual monograph other parameters such as the internal diameter and length of the column, brand and size of the support, concentration of the stationary phase, the flow rate of carrier gas, the temperature of the column, the injection volume, the sensitivity of the detector etc, may be varied to meet the requirement of the system suitability test. Usually the chromatogram is completed within 30min.

For the system suitability test, the requirements are the same as those described under high performance liquid chromatography, unless otherwise specified.

5. 3. 2   The common elution mode

Temperature programming is the common elution mode, it refers to the temperature of chromatography increasing continuously linear or non-linear over time, in order to make low and high boiling point ingredients have appropriate retention, chromatographic peaks distribute uniformly, the shape of chromatographic peaks is symmetric, and each ingredient posseses propriate retention time. Temperature programming has a number of advantages, such as improving separation, narrowing the chromatographic peaks, decreasing limitation of detection   time saving, and so on. While compared with constant temperature, temperature programming makes the peak of high boiling point substance appear in advance and decrease diffusion, Ingredients in front have greater retention and contribute to separation. The method of temperature programming is generally employed to the mixture with wide boiling points range. However, this method is less stable than constant temperature, and after the analysis of an injection sample, also requires waiting for temperature decreasing.

5.3.3   Calculate calibration factor in internal standard method

In order to meet requirements for each other, dissolve an accurately weighed quantity of reference substance and internal standard substance to produce solution respectively, measure accurately, mix well and produce reference solution for determination of calibration factor.

Inject certain quantity of reference solution into the column and record the chromatogram. Measure peak area or height of the reference substance and internal standard substance, the calibration factor may be calculated by the following equation.

$$f = \frac{A_S/c_S}{A_R/c_R}$$

Where A_S is peak area or height of internal standard substance, A_R is peak area or height of reference substance, c_S is the concentration of internal standard substance, c_R is the concentration of reference substance.

Then measure test solution containing internal standard substance, inject into the column, and record the chromatogram. Measure peak area or height of components and internal standard substance, the quantity may be calculated by the following equation.

$$c_X = f \frac{A_X}{A'_S/c'_S}$$

Where A_X is peak area or height of test substance, c_X is the concentration of test solution, A'_S is peak area or height of internal standard substance, c'_S is the concentration of internal standard solution, f is calibration factor.

5.3.4   Data procedure for GC

a. Correcting the internal standard method for the determination of individual impurity or the main component.

b. External standard method for the determination of individual impurity or the main component.

c. Peak area normalization method. The specific content of methods 1 ~ 3 is the same as that described under high performance liquid chromatography.

d. Standard addition method for the determination of individual impurity or the main component. Dissolve an accurately weighed quantity of impurity or reference substance of the substance to be examined to produce reference solution with a suitable concentration. Measure accurately the solution, and add to the test solution, then calculate the content of individual impurities or the main component by internal standard method or extra standard method. Deduct the content of added standard solution and gain the content of individual impurities or the main component in the test solution.

The content may also be calculated by the following equation. The correction factor is the same as that of adding the reference solution.

$$\frac{A_{is}}{A_x} = \frac{c_x + \Delta c_x}{c_x}$$

The concentration c_x of component being examined may be calculated by the following equation.

$$c_x = \frac{\Delta c_x}{(A_{is}/A_x) - 1}$$

Where c_x is the concentration of component X being examined, A_x is the peak area of component X being examined, Δc_x is the concentration of added reference substance of component being examined, A_{is} is the peak area of component X after adding reference substance of component being examined.

In quantitative essay of gas chromatography, a major source of error is the irreproducibility in the amount of sample injected, which is affected by the retaining time of syringe and room temperature, notably when manual injections are made with a syringe. The influence of variability can be minimized by an internal standard. Automatic injectors greatly improve the reproducibility of sample injections and reduce the need for internal standard. When headspace injectors are equipped, the influence on matrix may be eliminated by standard addition method because the test solution and reference solution are in different matrixes, the quantitative result of standard addition method should be adopted even when it is different from that of other methods.

6. Discussions

6.1　Why is the internal reference standard method employed for the assay of Vitamin E for GC?

6.2　Give an explanation of the features and applications of GC method.

6.3　What other methods are there for the assay of Vitamin E? Give an explanation on the features of each method.

（许慧君）

实验十一　阿司匹林与阿司匹林肠溶片的质量分析

一、目的

（1）掌握原料药物和制剂的质量检验项目与方法。

（2）掌握阿司匹林与阿司匹林肠溶片分析的原理、操作方法及要点。

二、仪器与试药

1. 仪器

比色管、坩埚、干燥器、滴定管。

2. 试药

阿司匹林原料及阿司匹林肠溶片、三氯化铁试液、稀硫酸、碳酸钠试液、稀硫酸铁铵溶液、新制的硫酸铁铵指示液、水杨酸、冰乙酸、比色用氯化钴液、比色用重铬酸钾液、比色用硫酸铜液、硫酸、标准铅溶液（10μg Pb/ml）、乙酸盐缓冲液（pH 3.5）、硫代乙酰胺、中性乙醇、酚酞指示液、氢氧化钠滴定液（0.1mol/L）。

3. 试液的配制

三氯化铁试液：取三氯化铁 9g，加水溶解成 100ml，即得。

稀硫酸试液：取硫酸 57ml，加水稀释至 1000ml，即得。本液含 H_2SO_4 应为 9.5% ~ 10.5%。

碳酸钠试液：取一水合碳酸钠 12.5g 或无水碳酸钠 10.5g，加水溶解成 100ml，即得。

硫酸铁铵指示液：取硫酸铁铵 8g，加水 100ml 溶解，即得。

酚酞指示液：取酚酞 1g，加乙醇 100ml 溶解，即得。

三、实验方法

（一）阿司匹林的质量分析

1. 阿司匹林的结构、分子式和相对分子质量

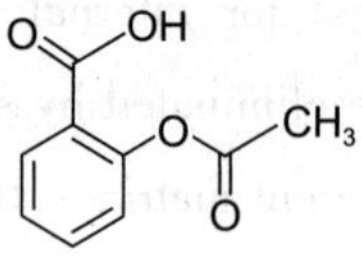

$(C_9H_8O_4, Mw = 180.16)$

本品为 2 - （乙酰氧基）苯甲酸，按干燥品计算，含 $C_9H_8O_4$ 不得少于 99.5%。

2. 性状

本品为白色结晶或结晶性粉末；无臭或微带乙酸臭，味微酸；遇湿气即缓缓水解。

本品在乙醇中易溶，在三氯甲烷或乙醚中溶解，在水或无水乙醚中微溶；在氢氧化钠溶液或碳酸钠溶液中溶解，同时分解。

3. 鉴别

（1）取本品约 0.1g，加水 10ml，煮沸，放冷，加三氯化铁试液 1 滴，即显紫堇色。

（2）取本品约 0.5g，加碳酸钠试液 10ml，煮沸 2min 后放冷，加过量的稀硫酸，即析出白色沉淀，并发生乙酸的臭气。

（3）本品的红外光吸收图谱应与对照的图谱一致。

4. 检查

（1）溶液的澄清度　取本品 0.50g，加温热至约 45℃的碳酸钠试液 10ml 溶解后溶液应澄清。

（2）游离水杨酸　取本品 0.10g，加乙醇 1ml 溶解后加冷水适量成 50ml，立即加新制的稀硫酸铁铵溶液［取盐酸溶液（9→100）1ml，加硫酸铁铵指示液 2ml，加水适量成 100ml］1ml，摇匀；30s 内如显色，与对照液（精密称取水杨酸 0.1g，加水溶解后加冰乙酸 1ml，摇匀，再加水成 1000ml，摇匀，精密量取 1ml，加乙醇 1ml、水 48ml 与上述新制的稀硫酸铁铵溶液 1ml，摇匀）比较，不得更深（0.1%）。

（3）易炭化物　取两支内径一致的比色管，甲管中加入对照液（取比色用氯化钴液 0.25ml、比色用重铬酸钾液 0.25ml、比色用硫酸铜液 0.40ml，加水成 5ml）5ml；乙管中加硫酸（含 H_2SO_4 94.5% ~95.5%，g/g）5ml 后，分次缓缓加入 0.5g 阿司匹林，振摇，溶解。静置 15min 后将甲乙两管同置白色背景前，平视观察，乙管中所显颜色不得较甲管更深。

（4）有关物质　溶液配制：取本品约 0.1g，置 10ml 量瓶中，加 1% 冰乙酸甲醇溶液适量，振摇，溶解并稀释至刻度，摇匀，作为供试品溶液；精密量取 1ml，置 200ml 量瓶中，用1%冰乙酸甲醇溶液稀释至刻度，摇匀，作为对照溶液；精密量取对照溶液1ml，置10ml量瓶中，用1%冰乙酸甲醇溶液稀释至刻度，摇匀，作为灵敏度试验溶液；取水杨酸对照品约10mg，精密称定，置100ml量瓶中，加1%冰乙酸甲醇溶液适量溶解并稀释至刻度，摇匀，精密量取1ml，置10ml量瓶中，用1%冰乙酸甲醇溶液稀释至刻度，摇匀，作为水杨酸对照溶液。

检查：用十八烷基硅烷键合硅胶为填充剂，以乙腈：四氢呋喃：冰乙酸：水（20∶5∶5∶70）为流动相A，乙腈为流动相B进行梯度洗脱：0～60min，20%A～80%A，检测波长为276nm。阿司匹林峰的保留时间约为8min，理论板数按阿司匹林峰计算不低于5000，阿司匹林峰与水杨酸峰的分离度应符合要求。分别精密量取供试品溶液、对照溶液、灵敏度试验溶液及水杨酸对照溶液各10μl，注入液相色谱仪，记录色谱图。供试品溶液色谱图中如有杂质峰，除水杨酸峰外，其他各杂质峰面积的和不得大于对照溶液主峰面积（0.5%），供试品溶液色谱图中任何小于灵敏度试验溶液主峰面积的峰可忽略不计。

（5）干燥失重　取本品约1g，置五氧化二磷为干燥剂的干燥器中，在60℃减压干燥至恒重，减失质量不得过0.5%。

（6）炽灼残渣　取本品1.0g，置已炽灼至恒重的坩埚中，精密称定，缓缓炽灼至完全炭化，放冷至室温；加硫酸0.5～1ml湿润，低温加热至硫酸蒸气除尽后在700～800℃炽灼，使之完全灰化，移置干燥器内，放冷至室温，精密称定后，再在700～800℃炽灼至恒重，炽灼残渣不得过0.1%。

（7）重金属　取25ml纳氏比色管两支，甲管中加标准铅溶液（10μg Pb/ml）1.0ml与乙酸盐缓冲液（pH 3.5）2ml后加乙醇稀释成25ml；乙管中加入本品1.0g，加乙醇23ml溶解后加乙酸盐缓冲液（pH 3.5）2ml。再在甲乙两管中分别加硫代乙酰胺试液各2ml，摇匀，放置2min，同置白纸上，自上向下透视，乙管中显出的颜色与甲管比较，不得更深（含重金属不得过百万分之十）。

5. 含量测定

取本品约0.4g，精密称定，加中性乙醇（对酚酞指示液显中性）20ml溶解后加酚酞指示液3滴，用氢氧化钠滴定液（0.1mol/L）滴定。每毫升氢氧化钠滴定液（0.1mol/L）相当于18.02mg的$C_9H_8O_4$。

（二）阿司匹林肠溶片的质量分析

1. 规格

25mg；40mg；50mg；100mg；300mg。

本品标示量为25mg，含阿司匹林（$C_9H_8O_4$）应为标示量的93.0%～107.0%。

2. 性状

本品为肠溶包衣片，除去包衣后显白色。

3. 鉴别

取本品的细粉适量（约相当于阿司匹林0.1g），加水10ml，煮沸，放冷，加三氯化铁试液1滴，即显紫堇色。

4. 检查

（1）游离水杨酸　取本品60片，研细，用乙醇70ml分次研磨，并移入100ml量瓶中，充分振摇，用水稀释至刻度，摇匀，立即滤过；精密量取续滤液2ml，置50ml纳氏比色管中，用水稀释至 50ml，立即加新制的稀硫酸铁铵溶液［取盐酸溶液（9→100）1ml，加硫酸铁铵指示液 2ml 后再加水适量使成 100ml］3ml，摇匀，30s 内如显色，与对照液（精密量取 0.01% 水杨酸溶液 4.5ml，加乙醇 3ml、0.05% 酒石酸溶液 1ml，用水稀释至 50ml，再加上述新制的稀硫酸铁铵溶液 3ml，摇匀）比较，不得更深（1.5%）。

（2）释放度　照高效液相色谱法测定。

色谱条件与系统适用性试验　用十八烷基硅烷键合硅胶为填充剂，以乙腈：四氢呋喃：冰乙酸：水（20：5：5：70）为流动相，检测波长为 276nm。理论板数按阿司匹林峰计算不低于 3000，阿司匹林峰与水杨酸峰的分离度应符合要求。

酸中释放量　取本品，照溶出度与释放度测定法，采用溶出度测定法第一法装置，以 0.1mol/L 的盐酸溶液 600ml 为溶出介质，转速为每分钟 100 转，依法操作，经 120min 时，取溶液 10ml，滤过，取续滤液作为供试品溶液。另精密称取阿司匹林对照品适量，加 1% 冰乙酸甲醇溶液溶解并稀释制成每毫升中含 4.25μg（25mg 规格）的溶液，作为对照品溶液。精密量取上述溶液各 10μl，注入液相色谱仪，记录色谱图，计算每片中阿司匹林的释放量，限度应小于阿司匹林标示量的 10%。

缓冲液中释放量　在酸中释放量检查项的溶液中继续加入 37℃ 的 0.2mol/L 磷酸钠溶液 200ml，混匀，用 2mol/L 盐酸溶液或 2mol/L 氢氧化钠溶液调节 pH 值至 6.8 ± 0.05，继续溶出 45min，取溶液 10ml，滤过，取续滤液作为供试品溶液。精密称取阿司匹林对照品适量，用 1% 冰乙酸甲醇溶液溶解并稀释制成每毫升中含 22μg（25mg 规格）的溶液，作为阿司匹林对照品溶液。精密称取水杨酸对照品适量，加 1% 冰乙酸甲醇溶液溶解并稀释制成每毫升中含 1.7μg（25mg 规格）的溶液，作为水杨酸对照品溶液。精密量取上述溶液各 10μl，分别注入液相色谱仪，记录色谱图，按外标法计算出每片中阿司匹林和水杨酸的含量，将水杨酸含量乘以 1.304 后与阿司匹林含量相加即得每片缓冲液中释放量。限度为标示量的 70%，应符合规定。

5. 含量测定

取本品 60 片，研细，用中性乙醇 70ml，分数次研磨，并移入 100ml 量瓶中，充分振摇，再用水适量洗涤研钵数次，洗液合并于 100ml 量瓶中，再用水稀释至刻度，摇匀，滤过，精密量取续滤液 10ml（相当于阿司匹林 0.15g），置锥形瓶中，加中性乙醇（对酚酞指示液显中性）20ml，振摇，加酚酞指示液 3 滴，滴加氢氧化钠滴定液（0.1mol/L）至溶液显粉红色，再精密加氢氧化钠滴定液（0.1mol/L）20ml，置水浴上加热 15min 并时时振摇，迅速放冷至室温，用硫酸滴定液（0.05mol/L）滴定，并将滴定的结果用空白试验校正。每毫升氢氧化钠滴定液（0.1mol/L）相当于 18.02mg 的 $C_9H_8O_4$。

四、预习提要

（1）游离水杨酸的来源和检查依据是什么？简述检查时应注意的事项。

（2）通过分析化学性质，简述阿司匹林与阿司匹林肠溶片含量测定的依据。

（3）阿司匹林溶液的澄清度检查的目的是什么？

五、实验指导

1. 游离水杨酸的检查依据与原理

阿司匹林为乙酰水杨酸，在生产过程中乙酰化不完全，或在精制过程及贮藏过程中水解而产生水杨酸。游离水杨酸对人体有毒性，并且其分子中的酚羟基在空气中易被逐渐氧化成一系列醌型有色杂质，因此须对游离水杨酸加以控制。

水杨酸结构的酚羟基可在弱酸性溶液中与高铁盐反应呈紫堇色，而阿司匹林结构中无游离酚羟基，不发生该反应。通过与限度量水杨酸对照液生成的色泽比较，控制游离水杨酸的限量。

2. 阿司匹林的直接酸碱滴定法

（1）原理　阿司匹林结构中有游离羧基，显酸性，K_a 值为 3.27×10^{-4}，可用碱滴定液直接滴定。反应原理如下。

$$\text{COOH-OCOCH}_3 + \text{NaOH} \longrightarrow \text{COONa-OCOCH}_3 + \text{H}_2\text{O}$$

（2）注意事项

① 阿司匹林在水中微溶，易溶于乙醇，故使用乙醇为溶剂。

② 阿司匹林是弱酸，用强碱滴定时，化学计量点偏碱性，故指示剂选用在碱性区变色的酚酞。

③ 乙醇对酚酞指示液显酸性，可消耗氢氧化钠滴定液而使测定结果偏高。所以，乙醇在使用前须用氢氧化钠中和至对酚酞指示液显中性。

④ 在不断振摇下稍快地进行滴定，以防止局部碱浓度过大，致使阿司匹林酯水解。

（3）含量计算

$$含量（\%）= \frac{V \times F \times T}{W \times 1000} \times 100\%$$

式中，V 为消耗氢氧化钠滴定液的体积（ml）；F 为氢氧化钠滴定液的浓度校正系数；T 为氢氧化钠滴定液的滴定度（mg/ml）；W 为阿司匹林供试品的称取量（g）。

3. 阿司匹林肠溶片的两步滴定法

（1）原理　阿司匹林片剂中加入抑制阿司匹林水解的稳定剂酒石酸或枸橼酸，同时在生产或贮存过程中阿司匹林的酯键还有可能水解产生水杨酸和乙酸。这些酸性物质干扰直接酸碱滴定。因此，采用两步滴定法测定：首先中和制剂中的酸性物质（同时中和阿司匹林的游离羧基），以消除其干扰；依据阿司匹林的酯键在碱性条件下定量水解的特性，采用水解后剩余量滴定法测定。反应原理如下。

$$\text{COOH-OCOCH}_3 + \text{NaOH} \longrightarrow \text{COONa-OCOCH}_3 + \text{H}_2\text{O}$$

$$\text{COONa-OCOCH}_3 + \text{NaOH} \xrightarrow{\triangle} \text{COONa-OH} + \text{CH}_3\text{COONa}$$

$$2\text{NaOH} + \text{H}_2\text{SO}_4 \longrightarrow \text{Na}_2\text{SO}_4 + 2\text{H}_2\text{O}$$

（2）注意事项

① 为了消除氢氧化钠滴定液在受热时吸收二氧化碳对实验的影响，须在相同条件下进行空白试验校正。

② 过滤用的漏斗及滤纸应干燥。

（3）含量计算

$$标示量（\%）= \frac{(V_0 - V) \times F \times T \times \overline{W}}{W \times 标示量} \times 100\%$$

式中，V_0 为空白试验时消耗硫酸滴定液的体积（ml）；V 为供试品测定时消耗硫酸滴定液的体积（ml）；F 为硫酸滴定液的浓度校正系数；T 为氢氧化钠滴定液的滴定度（mg/ml）；W 为供试品片粉的称取量（g）；$\overline{W}$ 为供试品的平均片重（g）；标示量为片剂的规格（毫克/片）。

六、讨论

（1）阿司匹林原料及阿司匹林肠溶片在质量检验方面有哪些不同之处？解释原因。

（2）在阿司匹林肠溶片的释放度检查中为何要更换溶剂？

Experiment 11　Analysis of Aspirin and Aspirin Enteric-coated Tablets

1. Purposes

1.1　To master the items and procedures of the analysis of bulk drugs and pharmaceutical formulations.

1.2　To experiment on the analysis of Aspirin and its enteric-coated tablets.

2. Instruments and chemical reagents

2.1　Instruments

Nessler cylinders, crucible, desiccator, buret.

2.2　Chemical reagents

Aspirin bulk drug and aspirin enteric-coated tablets, ferric chloride TS, dilute sulfuric acid, sodium carbonate TS, dilute ferric ammonium sulfate solution, freshly prepared ferric ammonium sulfate IS, salicylic acid, glacial acetic acid, standard cobalt chloride CS, standard potassium dichromate CS, standard copper sulfate CS, sulfuric acid, standard lead solution (10μg Pb/ml), acetate BS(pH 3.5), thioacetamide, neutral ethanol, phenolphthalein IS, sodium hydroxide(0.1mol/L)VS.

2.3　Preparation of TS

Ferric chloride TS　Dissolve 9g ferric chloride in 100ml of water.

Dilute sulfuric acid TS　Measure accurately 57ml of sulfuric acid, and then add water to produce 1000ml. The content of sulfuric acid should be 9.5% ~ 10.5%.

Sodium carbonate TS　Dissolve 12.5g natrium carbonicm monohydratum or 10.5g natronite in 100ml of water.

Ferric ammonium sulfate IS　Dissolve 8g ferric ammonium sulfate in 100ml of water.

Phenolphthalein IS　Dissolve 1g phenolphthalein in 100ml of ethanol.

扫码"学一学"

3. Procedures and methods

3.1 Analysis of aspirin

3.1.1 Structure, molecular formula and molecular weight of aspirin.

$$(C_9H_8O_4, Mw = 180.16)$$

Aspirin, namely 2 - (acetoxy) - benzoic acid, contains not less than 99.5% of $C_9H_8O_4$ (calculated on the anhydrous substance).

3.1.2 Description

White crystals or crystalline powder; odorless or with faint acetic acid odor; slight acid taste; gradually hydrolyzes in moist air.

Freely soluble in ethanol, soluble in chloroform and in ether, slightly soluble in water and in anhydrous ether; soluble in solutions of sodium hydroxide and in sodium carbonate with decomposition.

3.1.3 Identification

a. Boil 0.1g of Aspirin in 10ml of water, cool, and add 1 drop of ferric chloride TS: a violet color is produced.

b. Boil 0.5g of Aspirin in 10ml of sodium carbonate TS for 2 minutes, cool, and add excessive dilute sulfuric acid, a white precipitate is produced and the odor of acetic acid is perceptible.

c. The infrared absorption spectrum is concordant with the reference spectrum of aspirin.

3.1.4 Test

a. Clarity of solution   Dissolve 0.50g of Aspirin in 10ml of sodium carbonate TS previously heated to about 45℃, the solution is clear.

b. Free salicylic acid   Dissolve 0.10g of Aspirin in 1ml of ethanol, add cold water to make 50ml. Add immediately 1ml of a freshly prepared, dilute ferric ammonium sulfate solution [prepared by adding 1ml of hydrochloric acid solution (9→100) to 2ml of ferric ammonium sulfate IS and diluting with water to 100ml] and mix well. Any color produced in 30 seconds is not more intense than that of a reference preparation (dissolve 0.1g of salicylic acid, accurately weighed, in water, and add 1ml of glacial acetic acid and water to make 1000ml. Add 1ml of this solution, 1ml of ethanol and 1ml of freshly prepared dilute ferric ammonium sulfate solution to 48ml of water. Allow to stand for 30 seconds) (0.1%).

c. Readily carbonizable substances   Use two matched color-comparison tubes with the same inner diameter, A and B. To tube A add 5ml of color reference solution (prepared by mixing 0.25ml of standard cobalt chloride CS, 0.25ml of standard potassium dichromate CS, and 0.40ml of standard copper sulfate CS, with water to make 5ml). Dissolve 0.5g of Aspirin in Tube B containing 5ml of sulfuric acid (94.5% ~95.5%, g/g). Mix the contents of each tube: after 15 minutes, any color produced in tube B is not more intense than that in tube A.

141

d. Related substances　Take about 0.1g aspirin in a 10ml volumetric flask, add a quantity of 1% glacial acetic acid in methanol solution, shake to dissolve, dilute to volume and mix well, as the test solution; weigh accurately 1ml of test solution, transfer to a 200ml volumetric flask, dilute with 1% glacial acetic acid in methanol solution to volume and mix well, as the reference solution; accurately take 1ml of the reference solution, transfer to a 10ml volumetric flask, dilute with 1% glacial acetic acid in methanol solution to volume and mix well, as the sensitivity test solution; take about 10mg of salicylic acid reference substance, accurately weighed, transfer to a 100ml volumetric flask, dissolve in a quantity of 1% glacial acetic acid in methanol solution, dilute to volume and mix well, accurately weigh 1ml of the acquired solution, transfer to a 10ml volumetric flask, dilute with 1% glacial acetic acid in methanol solution to volume and mix well, as the salicylic acid reference solution.

Use octadecyl silane bonded silica gel as the filler and perform gradient elution using acetonitrile-tetrahydrofuran-glacial acetic acid-water(20∶5∶5∶70) as the mobile A, acetonitrile as the mobile B:0 ~ 60min, 20% A ~ 80% A. The detect wavelength is set at 276nm. The retention time of aspirin is about 8min, and the number of its theoretical plate is not less than 5000. The resolution of aspirin and salicylic acid should conform to the requirement. Accurately inject 10μl of each test solution, reference solution, sensitivity test solution and salicylic acid reference solution, respectively, into the liquid chromatograph, and record the chromatograms. If there are impurity peaks except the salicylic acid peak in the test solution chromatograph. the peak area sum of other impurity peaks is not more than the peak area of the reference solution(0.5%). Any peak of the test solution whose peak area is less than the main peak area of the sensitivity test solution can be ignored.

e. Loss on drying　Take about 1g aspirin, transfer to a desiccator using phosphorus pentoxide as the desiccant, and dry under reduced pressure at 60℃ to constant weight. The loss on drying is not more than 0.5%.

f. Residue on ignition　Weigh accurately 1.0g of aspirin, in a suitable crucible that previously has been ignited until constant weight is attained. Heat gently until the sample is thoroughly charred, cool, then moisten the residue with 0.5 ~ 1ml of sulfuric acid. Heat gently until white fumes are no longer evolved, and ignite at 700 ~ 800℃ until the incineration is completed. Cool in a desiccator, weigh accurately, repeat igniting at 700 ~ 800℃, until constant weight is attained. The residue on ignition is not more than 0.1%.

g. Heavy metals　Use two 25ml color-comparison tubes, A and B. Into tube A pipet 1.0ml of standard lead solution(10μg of Pb) and add 2ml of acetate BS(pH 3.5), to ethanol to make 25ml. To tube B dissolve 1.0g of aspirin in 23ml of ethanol, and add 2ml of acetate BS(pH 3.5). To each tube add 2ml of thioacetamide TS, mix, allow to stand for 2 minutes, and view downward over a white surface: the color in tube B is not darker than that in tube A(0.001%).

3.1.5 Assay

Dissolve about 0.4g of Aspirin, accurately weighed, in 20ml of neutral ethanol(neutral to phenolphthalein IS) and add 3 drops of phenolphthalein IS. Titrate with sodium hydroxide(0.1mol/ L) VS. Each 1ml of sodium hydroxide(0.1mol/L) VS is equivalent to 18.02mg of $C_9H_8O_4$.

3.2 Analysis of aspirin enteric-coated tablets

3.2.1 Description

25mg;40mg;50mg;100mg;300mg。

Aspirin enteric-coated tablets contain not less than 93.0% and not more than 107.0% of the labeled amount of aspirin(25mg).

3.2.2 Description

Enteric-coated tablets, with white core.

3.2.3 Identification

To a quantity of the powdered tablets equivalent to about 0.1g of Aspirin add 10ml of water, boil, cool and add 1 drop of ferric chloride TS, a violet color is produced.

3.2.4 Test

a. Free salicylic acid   Triturate 60 tablets with 70ml of ethanol in portions and transfer the mixture to a 100ml volumetric flask, shake thoroughly, dilute with water to volume, mix well, and filter immediately. Measure accurately 2ml of the filtrate in a Nessler tube, and add water to produce 50ml. Add immediately 3ml of freshly prepared dilute ferric ammonium sulfate solution(prepared by adding 1ml of 1mol/L hydrochloric acid solution to 2ml of ferric ammonium sulfate IS and diluting with water to 100ml), and mix well. Any color produced in 30 seconds is not more intense than that of a reference preparation(4.5ml of 0.01% salicylic acid solution, accurately measured, add 3ml of ethanol and 1ml of 0.05% tartaric acid solution, dilute with water to produce 50ml, add 3ml of freshly prepared dilute ferric ammonium sulfate solution and mix well, 1.5%).

b. Drug release   Comply with the requirements for high performance liquid chromatography.

Chromatographic system   The separation is carried out using a column packed with octadecylsilane bonded silica gel and a mixture of acetonitrile : tetrahydrofuran : glacial acetic acid : water(20:5:5:70) as the mobile phase. Detection wavelength is 276nm. The number of theoretical plates is not less than 3000, calculated with reference to the peak of aspirin. The resolution factor between the peaks of aspirin and salicylic acid complies with the related requirement.

The amount released in acid solution   Comply with the requirements for drug release test, using the apparatus of the dissolution test method 1 and 600ml of 0.1mol/L hydrochloric acid solution as the dissolution medium. Adjust the rotational speed of basket to 100 rpm. Withdraw 10ml of the solution at 120 minutes, filter, and the successive filtrate was used as the test solution. Dissolve a quantity of aspirin CRS, accurately weighed, in 1% glacial acetic acid solution in methanol to produce a solution of 4.25μg per milliliter. as the reference solution. Separately inject 10μl of the above solutions into the chromatograph, record the chromatograms, and calculate the content of $C_9H_8O_4$ with respect to the peak area. Less than 10% of the labeled amount of $C_9H_8O_4$ is released.

The amount released in buffer solution   Add 200ml of 0.2mol/L sodium phosphate solution previously heated to 37℃ into the solutions obtained for the test of the amount released in acid solution, mix, and adjust to pH 6.8 ± 0.05 with 2mol/L hydrochloric acid solution or 2mol/L sodium hydroxide solution. Withdraw 10ml of the solution after 45 minutes, filter, and the successive filtrate was used as the test solution. Dissolve a quantity of aspirin CRS, accurately weighed, in 1% glacial acetic acid solution in methanol to produce solutions of $22\mu g$ per milliliter as the Aspirin reference solution. Dissolve a quantity of salicylic acid CRS, accurately weighed, in 1% glacial acetic acid solution in methanol to produce solutions of $1.7\mu g$ per milliliter as the salicylic acid reference solution. Separately inject $10\mu l$ of the above solutions into the chromatograph, record the chromatograms, and calculate the contents of aspirin and salicylic acid with respect to the peak area. The release amount equals the sum of the amount of aspirin and 1.304 times of the amount of salicylic acid. Not less than 70% of the labeled amount of $C_9H_8O_4$ is released.

3.2.5 Assay

Weigh accurately and finely powder 60 tablets with divided portions of 70ml neutral ethanol and transfer to a 100ml volumetric flask, shake thoroughly, wash the mortar several times with sufficient water, add the combine washings to the flask, dilute with water to volume, mix well and filter. Measure accurately 10ml of the filtrate equivalent to about 0.15g of aspirin into a conical flask, add 20ml of neutral ethanol (neutral to phenolphthalein IS), shake well. Add 3 drops of phenolphthalein IS and sodium hydroxide (0.1mol/L) VS dropwise until the solution becomes pink. Add 20ml of sodium hydroxide (0.1mol/L) VS, accurately measured, heat on a water bath for 15 minutes with shaking, cool immediately to room temperature and titrate with sulfuric acid (0.05mol/L) VS. Perform a blank determination and make any necessary correction. Each 1ml of sodium hydroxide (0.1mol/L) VS is equivalent to 18.02mg of $C_9H_8O_4$.

4. Prepare lessons before class

4.1 Where does the free salicylic acid come from and how to test it? What should we pay attention to during the analysis?

4.2 Briefly describe the principles for the assay of aspirin bulk drugs and aspirin enteric-coated tablets based on the chemical properties of Aspirin.

4.3 What is the purpose of the test of clarity of solution when analyzing Aspirin bulk drugs?

5. Guide for experiment

5.1 The principle of free salicylic acid test

The salicylic acid is prone to be formed during the production and storage of aspirin due to the incomplete acetylation or the hydrolysis of aspirin. Not only salicylic acid is harmful to the health, but also it is easily oxidized to colored quinone impurities due to the phenolic hydroxyl group in its structure. Therefore, it is necessary to control the amount of the free salicylic acid.

The phenolic hydroxyl group in salicylic acid is able to react with the ferric salt in weak acid solution to generate a violet color, while aspirin has no such reaction because of the absence of the phenolic hydroxyl group. Salicylic acid can be controlled by comparing the color produced from the limit amount of salicylic acid reference with that from Aspirin samples.

5.2 The assay of direct acid-base titration for aspirin

5.2.1 Principle

Aspirin has free carboxyl group, which makes it show acidity and the Ka value is 3.27×10^{-4}.

Thus aspirin can be titrated directly with the alkaline titrant. The reaction is shown as follows.

$$\text{(COOH, OCOCH}_3\text{ benzene)} + \text{NaOH} \longrightarrow \text{(COONa, OCOCH}_3\text{ benzene)} + \text{H}_2\text{O}$$

5.2.2 Attention

a. Since aspirin is slightly soluble in water but freely soluble in ethanol, ethanol is selected as the solvent.

b. As a weak acid, when aspirin is titrated with a strong base, the solution at the stoichiometric point is slightly basic. Thus phenolphthalein which turns colorless in acidic solutions and pink in basic solutions is used as the indicator.

c. When phenolphthalein is used as the indicator, ethanol reacts with sodium hydroxide which will overestimate the result. Therefore, ethanol should be neutralized with sodium hydroxide before using.

d. The titration should be performed with rapid and consecutive shaking in order to avoid the hydrolysis of aspirin due to the locally excessive sodium hydroxide.

5.2.3 The formula for the determination of aspirin is as follows.

$$\text{Content}(\%) = \frac{V \times F \times T}{W \times 1000} \times 100\%$$

Where V is the consumed volume of sodium hydroxide VS (ml), F is the correction factor of sodium hydroxide VS, T is the titer of sodium hydroxide VS (mg/ml), W is the sampling quantity of aspirin.

5.3 Assay of two-step titration for aspirin enteric-coated tablets

5.3.1 Principle

Some stabilizers such as tartaric acid and citric acid are used for the formulation of aspirin tablets. Salicylic acid and acetic acid may be produced due to the hydrolysis of aspirin during its preparation or storage. These acid substances interfere the assay by direct acid-base titration. Thus, two-step titration is used for the assay of aspirin enteric-coated tablets. Firstly, the acid interferences are neutralized, and the carboxyl group of aspirin also reacts with sodium hydroxide. Secondly, the residual titration is used after aspirin is hydrolyzed in the basic solution. The reaction is shown as the following.

$$\text{(COOH, OCOCH}_3\text{ benzene)} + \text{NaOH} \longrightarrow \text{(COONa, OCOCH}_3\text{ benzene)} + \text{H}_2\text{O}$$

$$\text{(COONa, OCOCH}_3\text{ benzene)} + \text{NaOH} \xrightarrow{\triangle} \text{(COONa, OH benzene)} + \text{CH}_3\text{COONa}$$

$$2\text{NaOH} + \text{H}_2\text{SO}_4 \longrightarrow \text{Na}_2\text{SO}_4 + 2\text{H}_2\text{O}$$

5.3.2 Attention

a. Sodium hydroxide can absorb carbon dioxide in the air during heating, which influences the results. Thus, a blank test is necessary.

b. Funnel as well as the filter paper used for filtration should be kept dry.

5.3.3 The formula for determination of aspirin enteric-coated tablets is as follows.

$$Content(\%) = \frac{(V_0 - V) \times F \times T \times \overline{W}}{W \times \text{labelled amount}} \times 100\%$$

Where V_0 is the volume of sulfuric acid VS consumed in the blank test(ml), V is the volume of sulfuric acid VS consumed in the sample determination(ml), F is the correction factor of sulfuric acid VS, T is the titer of sodium hydroxide VS(mg/ml), W is the sampling quantity of Aspirin enteric-coated tablets powder(g), is the average weight of aspirin enteric-coated tablets, and M is the labeled amount of aspirin(mg per tablet).

6. Discussion

6.1 What is the difference between the analysis of aspirin bulk drugs and aspirin enteric-coated tablets?

6.2 Explain the reason of the solvent changing during the drug release test of aspirin enteric-coated tablets.

（许慧君）

实验十二　复方磺胺甲噁唑片的质量分析

一、目的

（1）熟悉复方制剂双波长计算分光光度方法含量测定原理。

（2）掌握复方磺胺甲噁唑片实验的操作条件及要点。

（3）掌握溶剂极性变化对紫外特征吸收带的影响。

二、仪器与试药

1. 仪器

硅胶 GF_{254} 薄层板。

紫外分光光度计：按有关检定规程中紫外分光光度计的规定定期检定，应符合规定。按仪器操作说明使用。

2. 试药

除另有规定外，所有试剂为分析纯级。

三、实验方法

复方磺胺甲噁唑片

本品每片中含磺胺甲噁唑（$C_{10}H_{11}N_3O_3S$）应为 0.360 ~ 0.440g，含甲氧苄啶（$C_{14}H_{18}N_4O_3$）应为 72.0 ~ 88.0mg。磺胺甲噁唑和甲氧苄啶的结构、分子或和相对分子量如下。

$(C_{10}H_{11}N_3O_3S, Mw=253.28)$　　　$(C_{14}H_{18}N_4O_3, Mw=290.32)$

1. 处方

磺胺甲噁唑 400g，甲氧苄啶 80g，制成 1000 片。

2. 性状

本品为白色片。

3. 鉴别

（1）取本品的细粉适量（约相当于磺胺甲噁唑 50mg），显芳香第一胺的鉴别反应。

（2）取本品的细粉适量（约相当于甲氧苄啶 50mg），加稀硫酸 10ml，微热溶解，放冷，滤过，滤液加碘试液 0.5ml，即生成棕褐色沉淀。

（3）取本品的细粉适量（约相当于磺胺甲噁唑 0.2g），加甲醇 10ml，振摇，滤过，取滤液作为供试品溶液；取磺胺甲噁唑 0.2g 与甲氧苄啶 40mg，加甲醇 10ml 溶解，作为对照溶液。照薄层色谱法试验，吸取上述两种溶液各 5μl，分别点于同一硅胶 GF$_{254}$ 薄层板上，以三氯甲烷∶甲醇∶二甲基甲酰胺（20∶2∶1）为展开剂，展开后晾干，置紫外光灯（254nm）下检视。供试品溶液所显两种成分主斑点的位置应与对照溶液的主斑点相同。

（4）称取磺胺甲噁唑对照品约 50mg，置 100ml 量瓶中，加乙醇溶解并稀释至刻度，摇匀。精密量取上述对照品溶液 2ml 置 100ml 量瓶中，加 0.1mol/L 氢氧化钠溶液稀释至刻度，摇匀，得碱性供试品溶液。再精密量取上述对照品溶液 2ml 置 100ml 量瓶中，加 0.01% 盐酸溶液稀释至刻度，摇匀，得酸性供试品溶液。同法分别制备上述碱性和酸性空白溶液，扫描磺胺甲噁唑在碱性和酸性溶液中的紫外吸收曲线，观察最大吸收波长发生的变化。

4. 检查

应符合片剂项有关的各项规定。

5. 含量测定

磺胺甲噁唑　取本品 10 片，精密称定，研细，精密称取适量（约相当于磺胺甲噁唑 50mg 与甲氧苄啶 10mg），置 100ml 量瓶中，加乙醇适量，振摇 15min 使磺胺甲噁唑与甲氧苄啶溶解，加乙醇稀释至刻度，摇匀，滤过，取续滤液作为供试品溶液；精密称取在 105℃ 干燥至恒重的磺胺甲噁唑对照品 50mg 与甲氧苄啶对照品 10mg，分别置 100ml 量瓶中，各加乙醇溶解并稀释至刻度，摇匀，分别作为对照品溶液（1）与对照品溶液（2）。精密量取供试品溶液与对照品溶液（1）和对照品溶液（2）各 2ml，分别置 100ml 量瓶中，各加 0.4% 氢氧化钠溶液稀释至刻度，摇匀，照分光光度法，取对照品溶液（2）的稀释液，以 257nm 为测定波长（λ_2），在 304nm 波长附近（每间隔 0.5nm）选择等吸收点波长为参比波长（λ_1），要求 $\Delta A = A\lambda_2 - A\lambda_1 = 0$。再在 λ_2 与 λ_1 波长处分别测定供试品溶液的稀释液与对照品溶液（1）的稀释液的吸收度，求出各自的吸收度差值（ΔA），计算，即得。

甲氧苄啶　仪器狭缝不得大于 1nm。如使用自动扫描仪，波长重现长度不得大于 0.2nm；如使用手动仪器，波长调节器应同一方向旋转并时时用对照液核对等吸收点波长。精密量取上述供试品溶液与对照品溶液（1）和对照品溶液（2）各 5ml，分别置 100ml 量瓶中，各加盐酸：氯化钾溶液（取 0.1mol/L 盐酸溶液 75ml 与氯化钾 6.9g，加水至 1000ml，摇匀）稀释至刻度，摇匀，照分光光度法，取对照品溶液（1）的稀释液，以 239.0nm 为测定波长（λ_2），在 295nm 波长附近（每间隔 0.2nm）选择等吸收点波长为参比波长（λ_1），要求 $\Delta A = A\lambda_2 - A\lambda_1 = 0$，再在 λ_2 与 λ_1 波长处分别测定供试品溶液的稀释液与对照品溶液（2）的稀释液的吸收度，求出各自的吸收度差值（ΔA），计算，即得。

四、预习提要

（1）简述磺胺甲噁唑和甲氧苄啶的结构特点与理化性质。

（2）本品的三个鉴别试验有何针对性？

（3）本品的检查项包括哪些项目？

（4）说明紫外分光光度计的结构及其操作方法。

（5）说明双波长分光光度法的基本原理及适用的分析对象。

五、实验指导

（一）双波长分光光度法

双波长分光光度法是在传统分光光度法的基础上发展起来的，它的理论基础是差吸光度和等吸收波长。它与传统分光光度法的不同之处在于它采用两个不同的波长，即同时测定一个样品溶液。如果混合物 C 是由 A 和 B 组分组成的，可得下列两个方程式。

$$A_{C_{\lambda_1}} = A_{A_{\lambda_1}} + A_{B_{\lambda_1}} \tag{4-1}$$

$$A_{C_{\lambda_2}} = A_{A_{\lambda_2}} + A_{B_{\lambda_2}} \tag{4-2}$$

式中，$A_{C_{\lambda_1}}$ 和 $A_{C_{\lambda_2}}$ 分别为混合物 C 在 λ_1 和 λ_2 处的吸光度，$A_{A_{\lambda_1}}$ 和 $A_{A_{\lambda_2}}$ 分别为组分 A 在 λ_1 和 λ_2 处的吸光度，$A_{B_{\lambda_1}}$ 和 $A_{B_{\lambda_2}}$ 分别为组分 B 在 λ_1 和 λ_2 处的吸光度。

当 λ_1 和 λ_2 选在组分 A 的等吸收波长处时，不管组分 A 的浓度如何，$A_{A_{\lambda_1}}$ 始终与 $A_{A_{\lambda_2}}$ 相等，式（4-1）和式（4-2）联立，得

$$A_{C_{\lambda_1}} - A_{C_{\lambda_2}} = A_{B_{\lambda_1}} - A_{B_{\lambda_2}} = (\varepsilon_{B_{\lambda_1}} - \varepsilon_{B_{\lambda_2}}) LC_B \tag{4-3}$$

式中，$\varepsilon_{B_{\lambda_1}}$ 和 $\varepsilon_{B_{\lambda_2}}$ 分别为组分 B 在 λ_1 和 λ_2 处的摩尔吸光系数，L 为光径，C_B 为混合物 C 中组分 B 的浓度。由于 $\varepsilon_{B_{\lambda_1}}$，$\varepsilon_{B_{\lambda_2}}$ 和 L 都是常数，式（4-3）说明，混合物 C 待测溶液在 λ_1 和 λ_2 两个波长处测定的差吸光度 $A_{C_{\lambda_1}} - A_{C_{\lambda_2}}$ 与组分 B 的浓度 C_B 成正比。这就是双波长法赖以建立的定量公式。

（二）溶剂极性变化对紫外特征吸收带的影响

在紫外光谱测定时，经常会改变溶剂的极性来考察某些特征基团的吸收带的变化。溶剂极性增加可使吸收光谱的精细结构消失，对吸收峰波长位置和吸收峰强度均有影响，但对波长的影响比对强度的影响更大。

在大多数 $\pi \rightarrow \pi^*$ 跃迁中，由于极性溶剂中的溶剂化作用，分子的 $\pi \rightarrow \pi^*$ 跃迁能（ΔE_2）比在非极性溶剂中分子的 $\pi \rightarrow \pi^*$ 跃迁能（ΔE_1）减小了，所以极性溶剂使 $\pi \rightarrow \pi^*$ 跃迁的吸收峰红移。

在 $n \rightarrow \pi^*$ 跃迁中，在极性溶剂中由于氢键的作用，$n \rightarrow \pi^*$ 跃迁能（ΔE_2）比在非极性

溶剂中 n→π* 跃迁能（ΔE_1）增大了，所以在极性溶剂中 n→π* 跃迁的吸收峰蓝移。

六、讨论

（1）分别说明本品中磺胺甲噁唑和甲氧苄啶双波长法含量测定时波长选择的依据。

（2）为何甲氧苄啶含量测定时供试液的稀释倍数与磺胺甲噁唑测定时不同？

（3）观察磺胺甲噁唑的紫外吸收曲线在碱性条件下和酸性条件下如何变化？试说明为什么会发生这种变化？

Experiment 12 The Analysis of Compound Sulfamethoxazole Tablets

1. Purposes

1.1 To study the spectro-photometric method for the simultaneous determination of drug components in compound formulation.

1.2 To experiment on the assay of compound sulfamethoxazole tablets by the spectro-photometric method.

1.3 To study the effect of the solvent polarity on ultraviolet characteristic absorption bands.

扫码"学一学"

2. Instruments and chemical reagents

2.1 Instruments

Silica gel GF_{254} thin layer plate.

UV spectrophotometer should be checked and calibrated periodically and meet appropriate requirements for intended use. The instruction manual should be followed closely.

2.2 Chemical reagents

All reagents should be of analytical reagent geade unless otherwise stated.

扫码"看一看"

3. Procedures and methods

Compound Sulfamethoxazole Tablets

Compound sulfamethoxazole tablets contains not less than 0.360g and not more than 0.440g of sulfamethoxazole ($C_{10}H_{11}N_3O_3S$), and not less than 72.0mg and not more than 88.0mg of trimethoprim($C_{14}H_{18}N_4O_3$) in each tablet. Structure, molecular formula and molecular weight of sulfame thoxazole and trime thoprim.

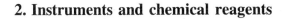

($C_{10}H_{11}N_3O_3S$, Mw=253.28)   ($C_{14}H_{18}N_4O_3$, Mw=290.32)

3.1 Formula

Take sulfamethoxazole 400g, Trimethoprim 80g, to make 1000 tablets.

3.2 Description

White tablets.

3.3 Identification

3.3.1 Yields the reactions characteristic of primary aromatic amines, using a quantity of the powdered tablets equivalent to about 50mg of sulfamethoxazole.

3.3.2 To a quantity of the powdered tablets equivalent to about 50mg of trimethoprim add 10ml of dilute sulfuric acid, heat gently to dissolve, cool and filter. To the filtrate add 0.5ml of iodine TS, a dark brown precipitate is produced.

3.3.3 To a quantity of the powdered tablets equivalent to about 0.2g of sulfamethoxazole add 10ml of methanol, shake and filter, use the filtrate as the test solution. Dissolve 0.2g of sulfamethoxazole and 40mg of trimethoprim in 10ml of methanol and use as the reference solution. Carry out the method for thin layer chromatography, using silica gel GF$_{254}$ as the coating substance and a mixture of chloroform-methanol : dimethylformamide (20 : 2 : 1) as the mobile phase. Apply separately to the plate 5μl each of the two solutions. After developing and removal of the plate, dry it in air and examine under an ultra-violet lamp(254nm). The colour and position of two principal spots in the chromatogram obtained with the test solution correspond to the principal spots obtained with the reference solution.

3.3.4 Weigh about 50mg ofsulfamethoxazole reference substance into a 100mL volumetric flask. Dissolve it in ethanol to volume and mix well. Accurately transfer 2 ml aliquot of this solution into a 100 ml volumetric flask, and fill up to volume with dissolving solution (0.1mol/L sodium hydroxide solution) to make the alkaline test solution. Accurately transfer 2 ml aliquot of this solution into a 100 ml volumetric flask, and fill up to volume with dissolving solution (0.01% hydrochloric acid) to make the acidic test solution. Prepare alkaline and acidic blank solution following the same procedure described above. Test the ultraviolet absorption curve of sulfamethoxazole in alkaline and acidic solutions and observe the change of maximum absorption wavelength.

3.4 Test

Comply with the general requirements for tablets.

3.5 Assay

Sulfamethoxazole Weigh accurately and powder 10 tablets. Weigh accurately a quantity of the powder equivalent to about 50mg of sulfamethoxazol and 10mg of trimethoprim into a 100ml volumetric flask, add a quantity of ethanol and shake for 15 minutes to dissolve sulfamethoxazole and trimethoprim, dilute with ethanol to volume and shake well. Filter and use the successive filtrate as the test solution.

Transfer 50mg of sulfamethoxazole CRS and 10mg of trimethoprim CRS, previously dried to constant weight at 105℃ and accurately weighed, separately to two 100ml volumetric flasks, dissolve in ethanol and dilute to volume, and mix well. The resulting solutions are used as reference solution (1)and solution(2)respectively. Transfer 2ml each of the test solution and reference solutions, accurately measured, to three 100ml volumetric flasks separately, dilute with 0.4% sodium hydroxide solution to volume and mix well. Measure the absorbance of diluted reference solution(2)

at 257nm(λ_2) and find out an isobestic point(λ_1) near 304nm with a stepwise difference of 0.5nm, so that $A_{\lambda_2} - A_{\lambda_1} = 0$. Measure the absorbance of diluted test solution and that of diluted reference solution(1) at wavelengths λ_2 and λ_1, and calculate the difference in absorbance (ΔA) for each solution and the content of $C_{10}H_{11}N_3O_3S$.

Trimethoprim Transfer 5ml each of the test solution and reference solutions, accurately measured, to three 100ml volumetric flasks separately, dilute with hydrochloric acid-potassium chloride solution [To 75ml of hydrochloric acid(0.1mol/L) VS and 6.9 g of potassium chloride add water to produce 1000ml, mix well] to volume and mix well. Measure the absorbance of diluted reference solution(1) at 239nm(λ_2) and find out an isobestic point(λ_1) near 295nm with a stepwise difference of 0.2nm, so that $A_{\lambda_2} - A_{\lambda_1} = 0$. Measure the absorbance of diluted test solution and that of diluted reference solution(2) at wavelengths λ_2 and λ_1, and calculate the difference in absorbance (ΔA) for each solution and the content of $C_{14}H_{18}N_4O_3$.

4. Prepare lessons before class

4.1 Figure out the structure and characteristics of sulfamethoxazole and trimethoprim.

4.2 What are the purposes of the three tests under identification?

4.3 Which items are included in other requirements?

4.4 Explain the structure of UV spectrometer and its operation procedures.

4.5 What is the principle of dual wavelength spectroscopy? Give some examples, analyzed by dual wavelength spectroscopy.

5. Guide for experiment

5.1 Dual wavelength Spectroscopy

Dual wavelength spectroscopy means that we measure two wavelengths at the same time and record the difference of the A values at these wavelengths. On the assumption that sample C is mixture of compound A and B, we can obtain the following two equations.

$$A_{C_{\lambda_1}} = A_{A_{\lambda_1}} + A_{B_{\lambda_1}} \qquad (4-1)$$

$$A_{C_{\lambda_2}} = A_{A_{\lambda_2}} + A_{B_{\lambda_2}} \qquad (4-2)$$

Where $A_{C_{\lambda_1}}$ and $A_{C_{\lambda_2}}$ are the absorbances of mixture C measured at wavelength λ_1 and λ_2, respectively; $A_{A_{\lambda_1}}$ and $A_{A_{\lambda_2}}$ are those of compound A measured at wavelength λ_1 and λ_2, and $A_{B_{\lambda_1}}$ and $A_{B_{\lambda_2}}$ are those of compound B.

If λ_1 and λ_2 are selected where compound A absorbs the same light energy, $A_{A_{\lambda_1}}$ equals to $A_{A_{\lambda_2}}$ regardless of its concentration. The following equation is consequence of subtraction of above equations.

$$A_{C_{\lambda_1}} - A_{C_{\lambda_2}} = A_{B_{\lambda_1}} - A_{B_{\lambda_2}} = (\varepsilon_{B_{\lambda_1}} - \varepsilon_{B_{\lambda_2}})LC_B \qquad (4-3)$$

Where $\varepsilon_{B_{\lambda_1}}$ and $\varepsilon_{B_{\lambda_2}}$ are the molar absorptivities of compound B at warelength λ_1 and λ_2, respectively; L is the cell path length in cm, C_B is the solution concentration of compound B in the mixture C solution.

Notice that $\varepsilon_{B_{\lambda_1}}, \varepsilon_{B_{\lambda_2}}$ and L are all constants, which means C_B is a function of $A_{C_{\lambda_1}} - A_{C_{\lambda_2}}$, and that is how the concentration of compound B in the mixture C is obtained.

5.2 Effect of the solvent polarity on ultraviolet characteristic absorption bands

In the ultraviolet spectrometry, the polarity of the solvent is often changed to investigate the changes of absorption bands of some characteristic groups. The increase of the polarity of the solvent can make the fine structure of the absorption spectrum disappear, having an influence both on the wavelength and intensity of absorption peak. But the influence on the wavelength is greater than on the intensity.

In the most of $\pi \rightarrow \pi^*$ transitions, due to solvation in polar solvents, the $\pi \rightarrow \pi^*$ transitional energy (ΔE_2) of molecules decreases compared with the $\pi \rightarrow \pi^*$ transitional energy (ΔE_1) of molecules in non-polar solvents. So absorption peaks of the $\pi \rightarrow \pi^*$ transitions move to higher wavelengths with the polarity increasing (red shift).

Inthe most of $n \rightarrow \pi^*$ transitions, due to the role of hydrogen bonds in polar solvents, the $n \rightarrow \pi^*$ transitional energy (ΔE_2) of molecules increases compared with the $n \rightarrow \pi^*$ transitional energy (ΔE_1) of molecules in non-polar solvents. So absorption peaks of the $n \rightarrow \pi^*$ transitions move to shorter wavelengths with the polarity increasing (blue shift).

6. Discussion

6.1　Give an explanation of the basis of the wavelength selection for the determination of sulfamethoxazole and trimethoprim, respectively.

6.2　Why is the more diluted solution used for the assay of trimethoprim than that for sulfamethoxazole?

6.3　How does the ultraviolet absorption curve of sulfamethoxazole change under alkaline and acidic conditions? Why does this change happen?

（苏梦翔）

实验十三　头孢克洛或头孢克洛胶囊的质量分析

一、目的

（1）掌握抗生素药物质量分析的项目和内容。

（2）掌握 HPLC 梯度法的测定原则。

二、仪器与试药

1. 仪器

水分测定仪（按检定规程中的规定定期检定，应符合规定。按仪器操作说明使用。费休试液，配制和标定见"实验指导"）。

2. 试药

除另有规定外，所有试剂为分析纯级。高效液相色谱实验中应采用色谱纯级的试剂。

三、实验方法

（一）头孢克洛

本品为（6*R*，7*R*）－7－［（*R*）－2－氨基－2－苯乙酰氨基］－3－氯－8－氧代－5－硫杂－1－氮杂双环［4.2.0］辛－2－烯－2－甲酸一水合物。按无水物计算，含头孢克洛（按 $C_{15}H_{14}ClN_3O_4S$ 计）不得少于 95.0%。

1. 头孢克洛的结构式、分子式、相对分子质量

（$C_{15}H_{14}ClN_3O_4S \cdot H_2O$，$M_w = 385.82$）

2. 性状

本品为白色、类白色或微黄色粉末或结晶性粉末；微臭，味苦。

本品在水中微溶，在甲醇、乙醇、三氯甲烷或二氯甲烷中几乎不溶。

比旋度　取本品，精密称定，加水溶解并稀释成每毫升中含 4mg 的溶液，依法测定，比旋度为 +105°至 +120°。

吸收系数　取本品，精密称定，加水溶解并稀释制成每毫升中约含 20μg 的溶液，照紫外－可见分光光度法在 264nm 的波长处测定吸收度，吸收系数（$E_{1cm}^{1\%}$）为 230～255。

3. 鉴别

（1）取本品适量，加水溶解并制成每毫升中约含 2mg 的溶液，滤过，取续滤液作为供试品溶液；另取头孢克洛对照品适量，加水制成每毫升中约含 2mg 的溶液，作为对照溶液；再取对照品和供试品适量，加水制成每毫升中各约含 2mg 的溶液，作为混合溶液。照薄层色谱法试验，吸取上述三种溶液各 2μl，分别点于同一硅胶 H 薄层板［取硅胶 H 2.5g，加 0.1% 羧甲基纤维素钠溶液 8ml，研磨均匀后铺板（10cm×20cm），经 105℃ 活化 1h，放入干燥器中备用］上，以新鲜配制的 0.1mol/L 枸橼酸溶液：0.1mol/L 磷酸氢二钠溶液：6.6% 茚三酮的丙酮溶液（60：40：1.5）为展开剂，展开后晾干，于 110℃ 加热 15min 后检视。供试品溶液所显主斑点的颜色和位置应与对照品溶液的主斑点相同，混合溶液应显一个斑点。

（2）取本品适量，照含量测定项的方法试验，供试品的主峰保留时间应与头孢克洛对照品主峰的保留时间一致。

（3）本品的红外光吸收图谱应与对照的图谱一致。

以上（1）、（2）两项可选做一项。

4. 检查

（1）结晶型　取本品少许，依法检查，应符合规定，为结晶型。

（2）酸度　取本品，加水制成每毫升中含 25mg 的混悬液，依法测定，pH 值应为 3.0～4.5。

（3）有关物质　照高效液相色谱法测定。

色谱条件与系统适用性试验　用十八烷基硅烷键合硅胶为填充剂；以 0.78% 磷酸二氢

钠溶液（取磷酸二氢钠 7.8g，加水溶解并稀释至 1000ml，用磷酸调节 pH 值至 4.0）为流动相 A；以 0.78% 磷酸二氢钠溶液（pH 4.0）：乙腈（55：45）为流动相 B；流速为每分钟 1.0ml，梯度洗脱；检测波长为 220nm。头孢克洛峰和头孢克洛 δ - 3 - 异构体峰的分离度应符合规定，头孢克洛峰的拖尾因子应小于 1.2，理论板数按头孢克洛峰计算应不低于 1500。

测定法　取本品约 50mg，精密称定，置 10ml 量瓶中，用 0.27% 磷酸二氢钠溶液（pH 2.5）溶解，摇匀，作为供试品溶液；精密量取 1ml，置 100ml 量瓶中，加 0.27% 磷酸二氢钠溶液（pH 2.5）至刻度，摇匀，作为对照溶液。取供试品溶液与对照溶液各 20μl，分别注入液相色谱仪，梯度洗脱：0 ~ 30min，流动相 B 的比例从 5% 增加至 25%；45min 时，流动相 B 的比例增加至 100%，维持 10min；56min 时，流动相 A 的比例增加至 95%，维持 15min，记录色谱图。供试品溶液如显杂质峰，单个杂质峰面积（除去主峰和溶剂峰）都应不得大于对照溶液主峰面积的 0.5 倍（0.5%）；各杂质峰面积总和不得超过对照溶液主峰面积的两倍（2.0%）。供试品溶液色谱图中小于对照溶液主峰面积 0.1 倍的峰可忽略不计。

（4）水分　取本品，照水分测定费休法测定，含水分应为 3.0% ~ 6.5%。

（5）重金属　取本品 1.0g，依重金属检查第二法测定，含重金属不得超过百万分之三十。

5. 含量测定

照高效液相色谱法测定。

色谱条件与系统适用性试验　用十八烷基硅烷键合硅胶为填充剂；以磷酸二氢钾溶液（取磷酸二氢钾 6.8g，加水溶解并稀释至 1000ml，用磷酸调节 pH 值至 3.4）：乙腈（92：8）为流动相；流速为每分钟 1ml；检测波长为 254nm。同时，精密称取头孢克洛对照品及头孢克洛 δ - 3 - 异构体对照品适量，加流动相溶解并制成每毫升中分别含头孢克洛及头孢克洛 δ - 3 - 异构体约 0.2mg 的混合溶液，进样测试，头孢克洛峰与头孢克洛 δ - 3 - 异构体峰的分离度应符合规定。理论板数按头孢克洛峰计算应不低于 1500。

测定法　取本品约 20mg，精密称定，置 100ml 量瓶中，加流动相溶解并稀释至刻度，摇匀，取 20μl 注入液相色谱仪；头孢克洛对照品适量，同法测定。按外标法以峰面积计算出供试品中 $C_{15}H_{14}ClN_3O_4S$ 的含量。

（二）头孢克洛胶囊

本品含头孢克洛（按 $C_{15}H_{14}ClN_3O_4S$ 计）应为标示量的 90.0% ~ 110.0%。

1. 性状

本品内容物为类白色或微黄色粉末。

2. 鉴别

取本品内容物适量，加水溶解并制成每毫升中含 2mg 的溶液，滤过，取续滤液作为供试品溶液，照头孢克洛项下的鉴别（1）或（2）项试验，应显相同的结果。

3. 检查

水分　取本品的内容物，照水分测定费休法测定，含水分不得过 8.0%。

溶出度　取本品，照溶出度测定转篮法，以水为溶剂，转速为每分钟 100 转，依法操作，经 30min 时，取溶液适量，滤过，精密量取续滤液适量，用水稀释成每毫升中约含 25μg 的溶液；装量差异项下的内容物，混合均匀，精密称取适量（约相当于一粒的平均装量），按标示量用水制成每毫升中约含 25μg 的溶液。取上述两种溶液，照分光光度法，在 264nm 的波长处分别测定吸收度，按两者吸收度的比值计算每粒的溶出量。限度为 80%，应符合规定。

4. 含量测定

取装量差异项下的内容物，混合均匀，精密称取适量（约相当于头孢克洛 100mg），置量瓶中，加流动相溶解并稀释成每毫升中约含头孢克洛 0.2mg 的溶液（必要时可超声处理），摇匀，滤过，取续滤液 20μl 注入液相色谱仪，照头孢克洛项下的方法测定。

5. 规格

0.25g（按 $C_{15}H_{14}ClN_3O_4S$ 计）。

四、预习提要

（1）头孢克洛属于哪一类抗生素？该类抗生素有哪些结构特点与理化性质？

（2）简述费休水分测定法的原理。

（3）推测头孢克洛水分的上限、下限（6.5% 和 3.0%）制订的依据。

五、实验指导

（一）水分测定法

容量滴定法是根据碘和二氧化硫在吡啶和甲醇溶液中能与水起定量反应的原理以测定水分。所用仪器应干燥，并能避免空气中水分侵入；测定操作宜在干燥处进行。

1. 费休试液的制备与标定

（1）制备 称取碘（置硫酸干燥器内 48h 以上）110g，置干燥的具塞锥形瓶中，加无水吡啶 160ml，注意冷却，振摇至碘全部溶解后加无水甲醇 300ml，称定质量，将锥形瓶置冰浴中冷却，在避免空气中水分侵入的情况下，通入干燥的二氧化硫至质量增加 72g，再加无水甲醇成 1000ml，密塞，摇匀，在暗处放置 24h。本液应遮光，密封，置阴凉干燥处保存，临用前应标定浓度。可以使用稳定的市售卡尔 - 费休试液，市售的试液可以是不含吡啶的其他碱化剂，或不含甲醇的其他醇类等；可以是单一的溶液或由两种溶液混合而成。

（2）标定 精密称取纯化水 10~30mg，用水分测定仪直接标定。精密称取纯化水10~30mg（视费休试液滴定度和滴定管体积而定），置干燥的具塞玻璃瓶中，除另有规定外，加无水甲醇适量，在避免空气水分侵入的情况下，用本液滴定至溶液由浅黄色变为红棕色，或用电化学方法（如永停滴定法等）指示终点。空白试验，按下式计算。

$$F = \frac{W}{A - B}$$

式中，F 为每毫升费休试液相当于水的质量，mg；W 为称取重蒸馏水的质量，mg；A 为滴定所消耗费休试液的体积，ml；B 为空白所消耗费休试液的体积，ml。

2. 测定法

精密称取供试品适量，除另有规定外，溶剂为无水甲醇，用水分测定仪直接测定。精密称取供试品适量（消耗费休试液 1~5ml），置干燥的具塞玻璃瓶中，加溶剂适量，在不断振摇（或搅拌）下用费休试液滴定至溶液由浅黄色至红棕色，或用用电化学方法如（永停滴定法等）指示终点。空白试验，按下式计算。

$$供试品中水分含量（\%）= \frac{(A - B)F}{W} \times 100\%$$

式中，A 为供试品所消耗费休试液的体积，ml；B 为空白所消耗费休试液的体积，ml；F 为每毫升费休试液相当于水的质量，mg；W 为供试品的质量，mg。

称取供试品时，如供试品引湿性较强或毒性较大，可取适量置干燥的容器中，密封（宜在通干燥惰性气体的手套操作箱中操作），精密称定，用干燥的注射器注入适量无水甲醇或其他适宜溶剂，精密称定总质量，振摇使供试品溶解，测定该溶液的水分，洗净并烘干容器，精密称取其质量。同时，测定溶剂的水分，按下式计算。

$$供试品中水分含量（\%）= \frac{(W_1 - W_3)C_1 - (W_1 - W_2)C_2}{(W_2 - W_3)} \times 100\%$$

式中，W_1 为供试品、溶剂和容器的质量，g；W_2 为供试品、容器的质量，g；W_3 为容器的质量，g；C_1 为供试品溶液的水分含量，g/g；C_2 为溶剂的水分含量，g/g。

此外，对热稳定的供试品，亦可将水分测定仪和市售卡氏干燥炉联用测定供试品水分，即将一定量的供试品在干燥炉或样品瓶中加热，并用干燥气体将蒸发出的水分导入水分测定仪中测定。

（二）HPLC 检查有关物质的测定法

1. 内标法

按各品种项的规定，精密称（量）取对照品和内标物质，分别配成溶液，精密量取溶液，混合配成校正因子测定用的对照溶液。取一定量注入仪器，记录色谱图。测量对照品和内标物质的峰面积或峰高，按下式计算校正因子。

$$f = \frac{A_S/C_S}{A_R/C_R}$$

式中，A_S 为内标物质的峰面积或峰高；A_R 为对照品的峰面积或峰高；C_S 为内标物质的浓度；C_R 为对照品的浓度。

再取各品种项含有内标物质的供试品溶液，注入仪器，记录色谱图，测量供试品中待测成分和内标物质的峰面积或峰高，按下式计算含量。

$$C_X = f\frac{A_X}{A_S/C_S}$$

式中，A_X 为供试品的峰面积或峰高；C_X 为供试品的浓度；A_S 为内标物质的峰面积或峰高；C_S 为内标物质的浓度；f 为校正因子。

采用内标法，可避免因样品前处理及进样体积误差对测定结果的影响。

2. 外标法

按各品种项的规定，精密称（量）取对照品和供试品，配制成溶液，分别精密取一定量，注入仪器，记录色谱图，测量对照品溶液和供试溶液中待测成分的峰面积（或峰高），按下式计算含量。

$$C_X = C_R\frac{A_X}{A_R}$$

式中，各符号意义同上。

由于微量注射器不易精确控制进样量，故采用外标法测定供试品中成分或杂质含量时，以定量环或自动进样器进样为好。

3. 加校正因子的主成分自身对照法

测定杂质含量时，可采用加校正因子的主成分自身对照法，在建立方法时，按各品种项的规定精密称（量）取杂质对照品和待测成分对照品各适量，配制测定杂质校正因子的溶液，进样，记录色谱图，按内标法计算杂质的校正因子。此校正因子可直接载入各品种项下，用于校正杂质的实测峰面积。这些须校正计算的杂质通常以主成分为参照，采用相对保留时间定位，其数值一并载入各品种项。

测定杂质含量时，按各品种项规定的杂质限度将供试品溶液稀释成与杂质限度相当的溶液作为对照溶液，进样，调节检测灵敏度（以噪声水平可接受为限）或进样量（以柱子不过载为限），使对照溶液的主成分色谱峰的峰高达满量程的 10% ~ 25% 或其峰面积能准确积分（通常含量低于 0.5% 的杂质，峰面积的相对标准偏差应小于 10%；含量在 0.5% ~ 2% 的杂质，峰面积的 RSD 应小于 5%；含量大于 2% 的杂质，峰面积的 RSD 应小于 2%）。然后，取供试品溶液和对照品溶液适量，分别进样，供试品溶液的记录时间除另有规定外应为主成分色谱峰保留时间的两倍。测量供试品溶液色谱图上各杂质的峰面积，分别乘以相应的校正因子后与对照溶液主成分的峰面积比较，依法计算杂质含量。

4. 不加校正因子的主成分自身对照法

测定杂质含量时，若没有杂质对照品，也可采用不加校正因子的主成分自身对照法。同上述第 3 种法配制对照溶液并调节检测灵敏度后，取供试品溶液和对照品溶液适量，分别进样，前者的记录时间除另有规定外应为主成分色谱峰保留时间的两倍，测量供试品溶液色谱图上各杂质的峰面积并与对照溶液主成分的峰面积比较，计算杂质含量。

若供试品所含的部分杂质未与溶剂峰完全分离，则按规定先记录供试品溶液的色谱图Ⅰ，再记录等体积纯溶剂的色谱图。色谱图Ⅰ上杂质峰的总面积（包括溶剂峰）减去色谱图Ⅱ上的溶剂峰面积即为总杂质峰的校正面积，然后依法计算。

5. 面积归一化法

按各品种项的规定，配制供试品溶液，取一定量注入仪器，记录色谱图。测量各峰的面积和色谱图上除溶剂峰以外的总色谱峰面积，计算各峰面积占总峰面积的百分率。

用杂质检查时，由于峰面积归一化法测定误差大，因此，通常只用于粗略考察供试品中的杂质含量。除另有规定外，一般不宜用于微量杂质的检查。

（三）溶出度测定

溶出度系指活性药物从片剂、胶囊剂或颗粒剂等制剂在规定条件下溶出的速率和程度。凡检查溶出度的制剂，不再进行崩解时限的检查。

1. 篮法仪器装置

（1）转篮　分篮体与篮轴两部分，均为不锈钢或其他惰性材料（所用材料不应有吸附作用或干扰试验中供试品活性药物成分的测定）制成，其形状尺寸如图 4-1 所示。篮体 A 由方孔筛网（丝径为 0.28mm ± 0.03mm，网孔 0.40mm ± 0.04mm）制成，呈圆柱形，转篮内径为 20.2mm ± 1.0mm，上下两端都有封边。篮轴 B 的直径为 9.75mm ± 0.35mm，轴的末端连一圆盘，作为转篮的盖；盖上有一通气孔（孔径 2.0mm ± 0.5mm）；

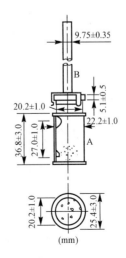

图 4-1　篮法仪器的图示

盖边系两层，上层直径与转篮外径相同，下层直径与转篮内径相同；盖上的 3 个弹簧片与中心呈 120°。

（2）溶出杯 由硬质玻璃或其他惰性材料制成的透明或棕色、底部为半球形的 1000ml 杯状容器，内径为 102mm ± 4mm，高为 185mm ± 25mm；溶出杯可配有适宜的盖子，防止在试验过程中溶出介质的蒸发；盖上有适当的孔，中心孔为篮轴的位置，其他孔供取样或测量温度用，溶出杯置恒温水浴或其他适当的加热装置中。

（3）篮轴 与电动机相连，由速度调节装置控制电动机的转速，使篮轴的转速在各品种规定转速的 ± 4% 范围之内。运转时整套装置应保持平稳，均不能产生明显的晃动或振动（包括装置所处的环境）。转篮旋转时，篮轴与溶出杯的垂直轴在任一点的偏离均不得大于 2mm，转篮下缘的摆动幅度不得偏离轴心 1.0mm。

（4）仪器 一般配有 6 套以上测定装置。

2. 测定法

测定前，应对仪器装置进行必要的调试，使转篮底部距溶出杯的内底部 25mm ± 2mm。分别量取经脱气处理的溶出介质，置各溶出杯内，实际量取的体积与规定体积的偏差应不超过 ±1%，待溶出介质温度恒定在 37℃ ± 0.5℃ 后，取供试品 6 片（粒、袋），分别投入 6 个干燥的转篮内，将转篮降入溶出杯中，注意供试品表面上不要有气泡，按各品种项下规定的转速启动仪器，计时；至规定的取样时间（实际取样时间与规定时间的差异不得过 ±2%），吸取溶出液适量（取样位置应在转篮顶端至液面的中点，距溶出杯内壁不小于 10mm 处；须多次取样时，所量取溶出液的体积之和应在溶出介质的 1% 之内，如超过总体积的 1% 时，应及时补充相同体积的温度为 37℃ ± 0.5℃ 的溶出介质，或在计算时加以校正），立即用适当的微孔滤膜滤过，自取样至滤过应在 30s 内完成。取澄清滤液，照该品种规定的方法测定计算每片（粒、袋）的溶出量。

3. 结果判定

符合下述条件之一者，可判为符合规定。

（1）在 6 片（粒、袋）中，每片（粒、袋）的溶出量按标示量计算，均不低于规定限度（Q）。

（2）在 6 片（粒、袋）中，如有 1 ~ 2 片（粒、袋）低于 Q，但不低于 $Q-10\%$，且其平均溶出量不低于 Q。

（3）在 6 片（粒、袋）中，有 1 ~ 2 片（粒、袋）低于 Q，其中仅有 1 片（粒、袋）低于 $Q-10\%$，但不低于 $Q-20\%$，且其平均溶出量不低于 Q 时，应另取 6 片（粒、袋）复试；初试、复试的 12 片（粒、袋）中有 1 ~ 3 片（粒、袋）低于 Q，其中仅有 1 片（粒、袋）低于 $Q-10\%$，但不低于 $Q-20\%$，且其平均溶出量不低于 Q。

以上结果判断中所示的 10%、20% 是指相对于标示量的百分率（%）。

六、讨论

（1）试述抗生素药物有关物质检查的意义。

（2）试述本品水分测定的意义。

（3）抗生素药物含量或效价测定的方法有哪些？各有什么特点？

（4）有关物质测定的方法有哪些？试述各自的适用范围。

Experiment 13　Analysis of Cefaclor or Cefaclor Capsules

1. Purposes

1. 1　To study the method for the analysis of antibiotics.

1. 2　To experiment on the programmed gradient elution of HPLC method.

2. Instruments and chemical reagents

2. 1　Instruments

Water determination apparatus and dissolution test apparatus　Water determination apparatus and dissolution test apparatus should be checked and calibrated periodically and meet individual appropriate requirements for intended use. The instructions manual should be followed closely.

2. 2　Chemical reagents

All reagents should be of analytical grade unless otherwise stated. HPLC grade reagents must be used in HPLC analysis.

3. Procedures and methods

3. 1　Cefaclor

3. 1. 1　The structure, molecular formula and molecular weight of Cefaclor

$$(C_{15}H_{14}ClN_3O_4S \cdot H_2O, Mw = 385.82)$$

Cefaclor is $(6R, 7R) - 7 - [(R) - 2 - \text{amino} - 2 - \text{phenylacetamido}] - 3 - \text{chloro} - 8 - \text{oxo} - 5 - \text{thia} - 1 - \text{aza} - \text{bicyclo} [4.2.0] \text{oct} - 2 - \text{ene} - 2 - \text{carboxylic acid monohydrate}$. It contains no less than 95.0% $C_{15}H_{14}ClN_3O_4S$, calculated on the anhydrous basis.

3. 1. 2　Description

A white, or almost white or slightly yellow powder or crystalline powder; odour slight; tastes bitter. Slightly soluble in water; practically insoluble in methanol, ethanol, chloroform or methylene chloride.

Specific optical rotation　$+105°$ to $+120°$, in a solution of 4mg per 1ml in water.

Specific absorbance　Measure the absorbance of a solution of 20μg per 1ml in water at 264nm, the value of which(1, 1cm) is 230 ~ 255.

3. 1. 3　Identification

a. Dissolve a quantity in water to produce a solution of about 2mg per 1ml, and filter, using the successive filtrate as solution(1). Dissolve a quantity of cefaclor CRS in water to produce solution(2) of about 2mg per 1ml. Dilute a quantity of solution(1) and(2) with water to produce solution(3) of 2mg per 1ml respectively. Carry out the method for thin-layer chromatography, using

159

a freshly prepared mixture of 0.1mol/L citric acid solution-disodium hydrogen phosphate solution (0.1mol/L)：6.6% solution of ninhydrin in acetone(60：40：1.5)as the mobile phase. Coat the clean plate with homogeneous slurry of 2.5g of silica gel H in 8ml of a 0.1% solution of carboxymethyl-cellulose sodium, dry it in air and activate at 105℃ for 1 hour, and allow it to cool in a desiccator. Apply separately to the plate 2μl each of the three solutions. After developing and removal of the plate, dry it in air and examine. The colour and position of the principal spot in the chromatogram obtained with solution(1)corresponds to that obtained with solution(2), and only a principal spot in the chromatogram obtained with solution(3).

b. The retention time of principal peak of cefaclor in the substance being examined in the chromatogram obtained in the Assay is identical with that of the principal peak of cefaclor CRS solution in the chromatogram.

c. The infrared absorption spectrum is concordant with the reference spectrum of cefaclor.

The obove two methods for identifing may be used alternatively.

3.1.4　Test

a. Crystallinity　Complies with the test for crystallinity. It's crystallographic.

b. Acidity　Dissolve a quantity in water to produce a solution of 25mg per 1ml, pH 3.0~4.5.

c. Related substances　Carry out the method for high performance liquid chromatography.

Chromatographic system　Using a column packed with octadecylsilane bonded silica gel and a 0.78% solution of sodium dihydrogen phosphate(dissolve 2.8g of sodium dihydrogen phosphate in water and dilute to 1000ml, adjust pH value to 4.0 with phosphotic acid)as mobile phase A, a mixture of a 0.78% solution of sodium dihydrogen phosphate(pH 4.0)：acetonitrile(55：45)as mobile phase B. The flow rate is 1.0ml/min and detection wavelength is 220nm. The resolution factor between the peaks of cefaclor and cefaclor δ-3-isomer complies with the related requirements. The tail factor of the column is less than 1.2 and the number of theoretical plates of the column is not less than 1500, calculated with reference to the peak of cefaclor.

Procedure　Dissolve an accurately weighed quantity in a 0.27% solution of sodium dihydrogen phosphate(pH 2.5)to produce solutions(1)containing 5mg per 1ml and(2)containing 50μg per 1ml. Inject separately 20μl into the column, perform a gradient elution program, increase linearly the proportion of mobile phase B from 5% to 25% over a period of 30min, then increase linearly to 100% over a period of 15min, hold for 10min and record the chromatograms for twice the retention time of the principal peak. The sum of the area of all impurity peaks in the chromatogram obtained with solution(1)is not greater than 2 times of area of the principal peak in the chromatogram obtained with solution(2)respectively(2.0%). Any area of impurity peak in the chromatogram obtained with the solution(1)is not greater than 0.5 times of area of the principal peak in the chromatogram obtained with the solution(2)respectively(0.5%). Disregard any peak with an area less than 0.1 times of area of the principal peak in the chromatogram obtained with solution(2).

d. Water　3.0%~6.5%(Karl Fischer's Method).

e. Heavy metals　Carry out the limit test for heavy metals, using 1.0g, not more than 0.00030%.

3. 1. 5 Assay

Carry out the method for high performance liquid chromatography.

Chromatographic system　Using a column packed with octadecylsilane bonded silica gel and a mixture of acetonitrile-phosphate buffer solution(dissolve 6. 8g potassium dihydrogen phosphate in water and dilute to 1000ml, mix well, and adjust pH value to 3. 4 with phosphoric acid)(8 : 92)as the mobile phase. The flow rate is 1ml/min and the detection wavelength is 254nm. Dissolve an accurately weighed quantity of cefaclor $\delta - 3 -$ isomer CRS and cefaclor CRS in bobile phase to produce a mixed solution of 0. 2mg per 1ml. Inject a quantity into the column. The resolution factor between peaks of cefaclor and cefaclor $\delta - 3 -$ isomer complies with the related requirements. The number of the theoretical plates of the column is not less than 1500, calculated with reference to the peak of cefaclor.

Procedure　Dissolve an accurately weighed quantity in mobile phase to produce solution of 0. 2mg per 1ml. Inject 20μl into the column. Repeat the operation, using cefaclor CRS instead of the substance being examined. Calculate the content of $C_{15}H_{14}ClN_3O_4S$ with respect to the peak area obtained in the chromatogram by the external standard method.

3. 2 Cefaclor capsules

Cefaclor capsules conts not less than 90. 0% and not more than 110. 0% of the labelled amount of cefaclor($C_{15}H_{14}ClN_3O_4S$).

3. 2. 1　Description

Capsules contains almost white or slightly yellow powder.

3. 2. 2　Identification

Dissolve a quantity of the contents of the capsules in water to produce a solution of about 2mg of cefaclor per 1ml and filter. The successive filtrate complies with Test(1)and(2)for identification described under cefaclor.

3. 2. 3　Test

Water　Not more than 8. 0%(Karl Fischer's Method), using a quantity of the contents of the capsules.

Dissolution　Carry out the dissolution test, using water as the solvent, adjust the rotational speed of the basket to 100rpm. Withdraw the solution after exact 30 minutes, and filter. Dilute an accurately measured quantity of the successive filtrate with water to produce a solution of 25μg per 1ml. Dissolve an accurately weighed quantity of the mixed contents in the test for weight variation of contents in water to produce a reference solution of 25μg of cefaclor($C_{15}H_{14}ClN_3O_4S$)per 1ml according to the labelled amount. Measure the absorbance of the resulting solutions at 264nm. Calculate the dissolution of $C_{15}H_{14}ClN_3O_4S$ from each capsule. Not less than 80% of the labelled amount is dissolved.

3. 2. 4　Assay

Dissolve an accurately weighed quantity of the mixed contents in the test for weight variation of contents equivalent to about 100mg of cefaclor in mobile phase to produce a solution of 0. 2mg of cefaclor per 1ml, and mix well and filter. Inject 20μl of the successive filtrate into the column, and carry out the Assay under Cefaclor.

3. 2. 5   Strength

0. 25 g(calculated as $C_{15}H_{14}ClN_3O_4S$).

4. Prepare lessons before class

4. 1   Which kind of antibiotics does cefaclor belong to? What are the structure and characteristic of this kind of antibiotics?

4. 2   Explain the principle of Karl Fischer's method for the determination of water.

4. 3   Predict how the upper and lower limits(6. 5% and 3. 0%) of water content for cefaclor are established.

5. Guide for experiment

5. 1   Determination of water

Volumetric titration is based on the quantitative reaction of water with a solution of sulfur dioxide and iodine in pyridine and methanol. The apparatus used should be dry and moisture proof. The determination of water is preferably carried out in a low humidity environment.

5. 1. 1   Preparation and standardization of Karl Fischer reagent

a. Preparation of Karl Fischer reagent   Place 110g of iodine, previously dried in a desiccator over sulfuric acid for more than 48h, in a dry stoppered flask, add 160ml of anhydrous pyridine and cool, and shake to effectively complete dissolution. Add 300ml of anhydrous methanol and weigh the flask. Keep the flask cold in an ice bath, pass dry sulfur dioxide into the flask until the increase of weight is 72g, and add anhydrous methanol to produce 1000ml. Stopper tightly, mix well, and allow to stand for 24h away from light. This reagent should be preserved in tightly closed containers, protected from light and stored in a cool and dry place, and standardized before using. The Karl Fischer reagent is also commercially available.

b. Standardization of Karl Fischer reagent   Standardize with a water determination apparatus directly or place about 30mg of redistilled water, accurately weighed, in a dry stoppered flask, add 2 ~ 5ml of anhydrous methanol. Titrate with Karl Fischer reagent until the colour changes from pale yellow to reddish brown. The end-point may also be determined electrometrically by dead-stop titration. Perform a blank titration and calculate the water equivalent of the reagent in mg of water per 1ml by the formula as follows.

$$F = \frac{W}{A - B}$$

Where F is the weight of water equivalent of the reagent in mg; W is the weight of purified water in mg; A is the volume in ml of the reagent consumed in the titration of water; B is the volume in ml of the reagent consumed in the blank titration.

5. 1. 2   Procedure

Accurately weigh a quantity of the substance being examined and determine with a water determination apparatus directly. The solvent is absolute methanol unless otherwise specified. Or accurately weigh a quantity of the substance being examined which is estimated to consume 1 ~ 5ml of Karl Fischer reagent to a dry flask with stopper, add a quantity of solvent and titrate with Karl

Fischer reagent TS until the colour changes from pale yellow to reddish brown, while shaking or stirring continuously.

The endpoint may also be determined electrometrically by dead-stop titration. Perform a blank titration and calculate the water equivalent of the reagent in mg of water per 1ml by the formula as follows.

$$\text{Content of water} = \frac{(A - B)F}{W} \times 100\%$$

Where A is the volume in ml of Karl Fischer reagent consumed in the titration of water; B is the volume in ml of the reagent consumed in the blank titration; F is the weight of water equivalent of Karl Fischer reagent in mg; W is the of the substance being examined in mg.

If the substance is hygroscopic or poisonous, it can be placed in a dry tared container (for example, a glove box in an atmosphere of dry inert gas) and weighed accurately. Use a dry syringe to add an appropriate volume of accurately measured absolute methanol or other suitable solvent to dissolve the substance, determine the water content, clean and dry the tared container, and weigh it accurately. Determine the water content of the solvent in the same way.

Calculate using the formula as follows.

$$\text{Water content of the substance}(\%) = \frac{(W_1 - W_3)C_1 - (W_1 - W_2)C_2}{(W_2 - W_3)} \times 100\%$$

Where W_1 is the weight of the substance, solvent and dry tared container in g; W_2 is the weight of the substance and tared container in g; W_3 is the weight of the tared container in g; C_1 is the water content of the substance in g/g; C_2 is the water content of the solvent in g/g.

Alternatively, an apparatus, combined with a commercially available Karl Fischer type dry oven can be used to determine the water content. If an oven is used, an appropriate amount of the sample is introduced into the oven and heated, and then the water is evaporated and carried into the apparatus to determine the water content.

5.2 Related substances in HPLC

5.2.1 Corrected internal standard method

Prepare solutions containing an accurately weighed quantity of the reference substance and internal standard respectively as specified in the monograph. Accurately measure each solution and prepare the reference solution for determining the correction factors. Inject a certain amount of solution into the equipment and record the chromatogram. Measure the peak area or height of the reference substance and the internal and calculate the correction factor according to the following equation as follows.

$$f = \frac{A_S/C_S}{A_R/C_R}$$

Where A_S is the peak area or the peak height of the internal standard; A_R is the peak area or the peak height of the reference substance; C_S is the concentration of the internal standard; C_R is the concentration of the reference solution.

Prepare solutions containing the substance being examined and the internal standard as described in the monograph.

Inject the solution into the equipment and record the chromatogram. Measure the peak area or the peak height of the substance being examined and that of the internal standard. Calculate the content as follows.

$$C_X = f\frac{A_X}{A_S/C_S}$$

Where A_x is the peak area or peak height of the substance being examined; C_x is the concentration of the solution of the substance being examined; A_s is the peak area or peak height of the internal standard; C_s is the concentration of the internal standard solution; f is the correction factor.

Using internal standard method can avoid the effect on determination result due to sample pretreatment and injection volume errors.

5.2.2   External standard method

Prepare solutions containing an accurately weighed quantity of the reference substance and substance being examined respectively and inject a certain amount of each solution into the equipment. Record the chromatogram and measure the peak area (or peak height). Calculate the content as follows.

$$C_X = C_R\frac{A_X}{A_R}$$

Where each symbol has the same meaning as that mentioned above.

As the micro syringe is not able to control the amount of solution being injected precisely, the sampling loop or automatic sampler may be used in measuring the content of main components and the impurity in the substance being examined.

5.2.3   Corrected peak areas of impurities compared with that produced by the main peak of a diluted solution of substance being examined

This method could be used to measure the content of the impurity. In the establishment of method, prepare solutions containing an accurately weighed quantity of the reference substances of impurities and the main component as specified in the monograph. Inject a volume and record the chromatogram. Calculate the correction factor of the impurity according to the method described in the 5.2.1. The correction factor could be directly recorded in the individual monograph and used for correction of the measure peak areas of impurities. These impurities, which need correction computation, are generally located by the relative retention time to the main component as reference and all these data are recorded in the individual monograph.

When measuring the content of the impurities, dilute the solution of the substance being examined to a concentration as specified in the individual monograph so that its peak area is around that produced by the impurities in the original concentration. Inject and adjust the attenuation of the detector(limited by the noise level that can be accepted) or vary the injection volume(limited by the load ability of the column) until the peak height of the main component is about $10\% \sim 25\%$ of the full scale or the peak are which could be accurately measured (generally, for the impurity, the content of which is lower than 0.5%, the RSD of the peak area should be less than 10%; for the impurity, the content of which is between $0.5\% \sim 2\%$, the RSD of peak area should be less than 5%; for the impurity whose content is higher than 2%, the RSD of the peak area should be less than 2%). Inject separately an appropriate amount of test solution and reference solution. The recorded time span of the test solution, unless specified otherwise, should be 2 times that of the main component. Measure the peak areas of each impurity on the chromatogram of the main component of the reference solution and calculate the content of the impurities accordingly.

5.2.4 Peak areas of impurities compared with that produced by the main peak of a diluted solution of substance being examined

This method could be used when the impurity reference substance is not available when determining the impurities. Prepare the reference solution according the method 5.2.3 and adjust the attenuation of the detector. Inject separately an appropriate volume of the test solution and reference solution. Record the chromatogram for two times the retention time of the pricipal peak, unless specified otherwise. Measure the peak areas of the impurities on the chromatogram of the test solution and compare them with those of the main component of the reference solution and calculate the content of the impurities.

If there are some impurities in the substance being examined which are not completely separated from the solvent peak, record the chromatogram Ⅰ of the substance being examined according to the specification and then record the chromatogram Ⅱ of the pure solvent of equal volume. The peak area of the solvent solution on the chromatogram Ⅱ is subtracted from the total peak area of the impurities in the chromatogram Ⅰ (including the solvent peak). The result is equal to the correction peak area of the total impurities. Calculate the content of the impurities accordingly.

5.2.5 Peak area normalization method

Prepare test solution as specified in the monograph, inject a certain amount into instrument, and record the chromatogram. In this method, the peak areas of the impurities and total peak on the chromatogram except the solvent peak are measured. Calculate the peak ares of each impurity and he percentage of their sum in the total peak area.

As the deviation of this method is so large that it can be only used to roughly inspect the contents of impurities in the substance being examined. It is not suitable for the determination of minute impurities, unless otherwise specified.

5.3 Dissolution test

Dissolution test is used to determine the dissolution rate and degree of the active pharmaceutical ingredients(APIs) from dosage forms such as tablets, capsules or granules under the specified conditions. When dissolution test is specified in the monograph, disintegration test can be exempted.

5.3.1 Basket apparatus

a. The basket assembly consists of a basket and a shaft made of stainless steel or other inert material(The materials should not be absorptive, or interfere the determination of APIs). The basket (A) is made of stainless steel woven cloth with a nominal aperture of 0.40 mm ± 0.04 mm; the stainless steel wire is 0.28 mm ± 0.03 mm in diameter. The basket is cylindrical, 20.2mm ± 1.0 mm in internal diameter, with a flanged rim at each end. The shaft(B) is 9.75mm ± 0.35mm in diameter and is connected to the lid of the basket. The lid has a vent hole, 2.0 mm ± 0.5mm in diameter and 3 retention springs with 3 tangs on 120°centers. The upper part of the lid has a diameter equal to the outside diameter of the basket and the lower part has a diameter equal to the inside diameter of the basket(Figure 4 – 1).

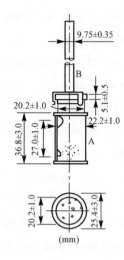

Figure 4 – 1   Basket apparatus

b. The vessel is cylindrical, made of hard glass or other inert, transparent or brown materials, with a hemispherical bottom and a nominal capacity of 1000ml, internal diameter 102 mm ± 4 mm, height 185 mm ± 25 mm. A fitted cover may be used to retard evaporation, the cover has a number of holes, the central one is used for the shaft to pass through, and the others are used for the insertion of thermometer and withdrawal of specimens. The vessel is placed in a constant temperature water bath or other heating device.

c. The shaft is connected with a motor with a speed regulator capable of maintaining the speed of rotation of the basket within ± 4 % of that specified in the individual monograph. When the motor is in operation, no part of the assembly, including the environment in which the assembly is placed, contributes any significant motion or vibration beyond that due to the smoothly rotating element. The shaft is positioned so that its axis is not more than 2mm at any point from the vertical axis of the vessel. The wobbling range is not greater than 1.0 mm during the rotation of the basket.

d. The apparatus with at least six sets of assembly described above.

5.3.2   Procedure

Before testing, adjust the apparatus so that the distance between the inside bottom of the vessel and the bottom of the basket is 25mm ±2mm. Place the stated volume of the degassed medium (+1%) in each of vessels, equilibrate the dissolution medium to 37℃ ± 0.5℃. Place 1 tablet (capsule or packet)in each of 6 dry baskets. Lower the baskets into the vessels. Exclude air bubbles from the surface of the dosage unit, and immediately operate the apparatus under the rotating rate specified in the – monograph and start the counting of time. Withdraw an aliquot of solution from a zone midway between the surface of the dissolution medium and the top of the rotating basket, no less than 10mm apart from the wall of the vessel within the time interval specified, or at each of the times stated(±2%). If two or more sampling times are specified, the sum of the volume of the samples withdrawn should be within 1% of the volume of the dissolution medium. If the sum is greater than 1% , replace the aliquots withdrawn for analysis with equal volumes of fresh – dissolution medium at 37°C immediately, or correct for the volume change in the calculation. Filter immediately through a suitable membrane. Complete taking and filtering a specimen within 30 seconds. Carry out the analysis of active ingredient as directed in the monograph using the successive filtrate and calculate the amount of active ingredient dissolved from each tablet(capsule or packet).

5.3.2   Interpretation

Unless otherwise specified in the monograph, the requirements are met if the quantities of active ingredient dissolved from tablets(capsules or packets)conform to one of the following states.

a. The amount of active ingredient dissolved from each of 6 tablets(capsules or packets) is not less than the specified quantity(Q) calculated on the labeled content.

b. If $1 \sim 2$ of 6 tablets(capsules or packets)fail the requirement, but not less than $Q-10\%$ and the average amount of active ingredient dissolved is not less than Q.

c. If $1 \sim 2$ of 6 tablets(capsules or packets)fail the requirements, and only 1 of tablets(capsules or packets)is less than $Q-10\%$ but not less than $Q-20\%$, and the average amount of active ingredient dissolved is not less than Q, repeat the test on 6 additional tablets(capsules or packets); if $1 \sim 3$ of the total of 12 tablets(capsules or packets)are less than Q, and only 1 of tablets(capsules or packets)is less than $Q-10\%$ but not less than $Q-20\%$, and the average amount of active ingredient dissolved is not less than Q.

The 10% and 20% values stated above interpretation are expressed as percentages of the labeled content.

6. Discussions

6.1　What is the importance of the test of related substances for antibiotics?

6.2　What is the purpose for the test and control of water content for antibiotics?

6.3　What other methods are there for the assay of antibiotics? Give an explanation of the characteristics of each method.

6.4 How many methods are there in related compound test? Explain the scope of application respectively.

（许慧君）

实验十四　石菖蒲的质量检验

一、目的

（1）掌握中药材挥发油的含量测定方法。
（2）熟悉中药材薄层色谱鉴别法中的对照药材法。

二、仪器与试药

1. 仪器
显微镜、紫外光灯（365nm）、坩埚、马弗炉、挥发油测定器、硅胶 G 薄层板。

2. 试药
石菖蒲、石菖蒲对照药材、石油醚（60~90℃）、乙酸乙酯、碘。

三、实验方法

石　菖　蒲

（Acori Tatarinowii Rhizoma）

本品为天南星科植物石菖蒲 *Acorus tatarinowii* Schott. 的干燥根茎。秋、冬二季采挖，除去须根及泥沙，晒干。

1. 性状

本品呈扁圆柱形，多弯曲，常有分枝，长 3～20cm，直径 0.3～1cm；表面棕褐色或灰棕色，粗糙；有疏密不匀的环节，节间长 0.2～0.8cm，具细纵纹，一面残留须根或圆点状根痕；叶痕呈三角形，左右交互排列，有的其上有毛鳞状的叶基残余；质硬，断面纤维性，类白色或微红色，内皮层环明显，可见多数维管束小点及棕色油细胞；气芳香，味苦；微辛。

2. 鉴别

（1）本品横切面。表皮细胞外壁增厚，棕色，有的含红棕色物。皮层宽广，散有纤维束及叶迹维管束；叶迹维管束外韧型，维管束鞘纤维成环，木化；内皮层明显。中柱维管束周木型及外韧型，维管束鞘纤维较少。纤维束及维管束鞘纤维周围细胞中含草酸钙方晶，形成晶纤维。薄壁组织中散有类圆形油细胞；含淀粉粒。

粉末灰棕色。淀粉粒单粒球形、椭圆形或长卵形，直径 2～9μm；复粒由 2～20（或更多）分粒组成。纤维束周围细胞中含草酸钙方晶，形成晶纤维。草酸钙方晶呈多面型、类多角形、双锥形，直径 4～16μm。分泌细胞呈类圆形或长圆形，胞腔内充满黄绿色、橙红色或红色分泌物。石菖蒲横切面图见图 4-2。

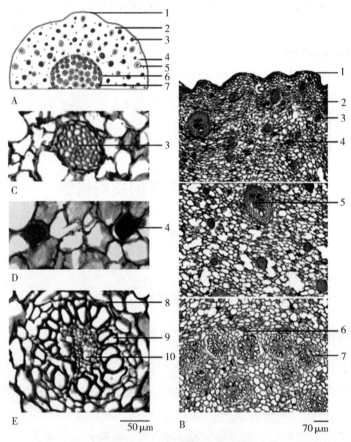

图 4-2 石菖蒲横切面图

A. 简图；B. 切面示意图；C. 纤维束；D. 分泌细胞；E. 中柱维管束

1. 表皮；2. 皮层；3. 纤维束；4. 分泌细胞；5. 叶迹维管束；6. 内皮层；

7. 中柱维管束；8. 维管束鞘；9. 木质部；10. 韧皮部

（2）取本品粉末 0.2g，加石油醚（60～90℃）20ml，加热回流 1h，滤过，滤液蒸干，残渣加石油醚（60～90℃）1ml 溶解，作为供试品溶液。另取石菖蒲对照药材 0.2g，同法制成对照药材溶液。照薄层色谱法试验，吸取上述两种溶液各2μl，分别点于同一硅胶G薄层板上，以石油醚（60~90℃）：乙酸乙酯（4：1）为展开剂，展开，取出，晾干，放置约1h，置紫外光灯（365nm）下检视。在供试品色谱中，在与对照药材色谱相应的位置上，显示相同颜色的荧光斑点；以碘蒸气熏至斑点显色清晰，在供试品色谱中，在与对照药材色谱相应的位置上，显示相同颜色的斑点。

3. 检查

（1）水分　按照烘干法测定，不得过13.0%。

（2）总灰分　不得过10.0%。

（3）浸出物　照醇溶性浸出物测定法项的冷浸法测定，用稀乙醇作溶剂，不得少于12.0%。

4. 含量测定

照挥发油测定法。本品含挥发油不得少于1.0%（ml/g）。

四、预习提要

（1）挥发油测定法的操作及注意事项。

（2）对照药材法鉴别的特点。

五、实验指导

（一）灰分测定法

（1）总灰分测定法　测定用的供试品须粉碎，使能通过二号筛，混合均匀后取供试品2~3g（如需测定酸不溶性灰分，可取供试品3~5g），置炽灼至恒重的坩埚中，称定重量（准确至0.01g），缓缓炽热，注意避免燃烧，至完全炭化时，逐渐升高温度至500~600℃，使完全灰化并至恒重。根据残渣质量，计算供试品中含总灰分的百分数。如供试品不易灰化，可将坩埚放冷，加热水或10%硝酸铵溶液2ml，使残渣湿润，然后置水浴上蒸干，残渣照前法炽灼，至坩埚内容物完全灰化。

（2）酸不溶性灰分测定法　取所得灰分，在坩锅中加入稀盐酸约10ml，用表面皿覆盖坩锅，置水浴上加热10min，表面皿用热水5ml冲洗，洗液并入坩埚中，用无灰滤纸滤过，坩埚内的残渣用水洗于滤纸上，并洗涤至洗液不显氯化物反应为止。滤渣连同滤纸移至同一坩埚中，干燥，炽灼至恒重。根据残渣质量，计算供试品中含酸不溶性灰分的百分数。

（二）浸出物测定法

1. 水溶性浸出物测定法

测定用的供试品须粉碎，使能通过二号筛，并混合均匀。

（1）冷浸法　取供试品约4g，称定质量，置250~300ml的锥形瓶中，精密加入水100ml，塞紧，冷浸，前6h内时时振摇，再静置18h，用干燥滤器迅速滤过。精密量取滤液20ml，置已干燥至恒重的蒸发皿中，在水浴上蒸干，于105℃干燥3h，移置干燥器中，冷却30min，迅速精密称定质量。除另有规定外，以干燥品计算供试品中水溶性浸出物的含量（%）。

（2）热浸法　取供试品约2~4g，称定质量，置100~250ml的锥形瓶中，精密加入水50~100ml，塞紧，称定质量，静置1h后，连接回流冷凝管，加热至沸腾，并保持微沸1h。放冷后，取下锥形瓶，密塞，称定质量，用水补足减失的质量，摇匀，用干燥滤器滤过。

精密量取滤液 25ml，置已干燥至恒重的蒸发皿中，在水浴上蒸干，于 105℃ 干燥 3h，移置干燥器中，冷却 30min，迅速精密称定质量。除另有规定外，以干燥品计算供试品中水溶性浸出物的含量（%）。

2. 醇溶性浸出物测定法

照水溶性浸出物测定法测定。除另有规定外，以各品种项下规定浓度的乙醇代替水为溶剂。

3. 挥发性醚浸出物测定法

取供试品（过四号筛）2~5g，精密称定，置五氧化二磷干燥器中干燥 12h，置索氏提取器中，加乙醚适量。除另有规定外，加热回流 8h，取乙醚液，置干燥至恒重的蒸发皿中，放置，挥去乙醚，残渣置五氧化二磷干燥器中干燥 18h，精密称定，缓缓加热至 105℃，并于 105℃ 干燥至恒重，其减失质量即为挥发性醚浸出物的质量。

（三）挥发油测定法

1. 原理

挥发油测定法利用供试品用水蒸馏，挥发油和水能一起蒸馏出，经回流冷凝管冷却并滴入挥发油测定器中，由于两者互不混溶，且相对密度不同而分层，水经挥发油测定器下端的联通装置不断溢流入烧瓶中，而挥发油则留在测定器中。如此连续反复蒸馏，直至供试品中挥发油全部馏出。根据供试品中所含挥发油的相对密度分别选用甲法或乙法：甲法适用于相对密度 1.0 以下的挥发油测定；乙法适用于相对密度 1.0 以上的挥发油测定。采用二甲苯与挥发油混溶使相对密度降至 1.0 以下。

2. 仪器装置

如图 4-3 所示，A 为 1000ml（或 500ml、2000ml）的硬质圆底烧瓶，上接挥发油测定器 B，B 的上端连接回流冷凝管 C。以上各部均用玻璃磨口连接。测定器 B 应具有 0.1ml 的刻度。全部仪器应充分洗净，并检查接合部分是否严密，以防挥发油逸出。

3. 测定法

测定用的供试品，除另有规定外，须粉碎使能通过二号至三号筛，并混合均匀。

甲法：本法适用于测定相对密度在 1.0 以下的挥发油。取供试品适量（相当于含挥发油 0.5~1.0ml），称定质量（准确至 0.01g），置烧瓶中，加水 300~500ml（或适量）与玻璃珠数粒，振摇混合，连接挥发油测定器与回流冷凝管。自冷凝管上端加水使充满挥发油测定器的刻度部分，并溢流入烧瓶时为止。置电热套中或用其他适宜方法缓缓加热至沸，并保持微沸约 5h，至测定器中油量不再增加，停止加热，放置片刻，开启测定器下端的活塞，将水缓缓放出，至油层上端到达刻

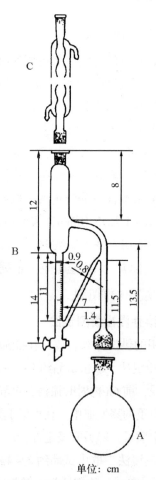

单位：cm

图 4-3 挥发油测定法的装置示意图

注：装置中挥发油测定器的支管分岔处应与基准线平行

170

度 0 线上面 5mm 处为止。放置 1h 以上，再开启活塞，使油层下降至其上端恰与刻度 0 线平齐，读取挥发油量，并计算供试品中挥发油的含量（%）。

乙法：本法适用于测定相对密度在 1.0 以上的挥发油。取水约 300ml 与玻璃珠数粒，置烧瓶中，连接挥发油测定器。自测定器上端加水使充满刻度部分，并溢流入烧瓶时为止，再用移液管加入二甲苯 1ml，然后连接回流冷凝管。将烧瓶内容物加热至沸腾，并继续蒸馏，其速度以保持冷凝管的中部呈冷却状态为度。30min 后，停止加热，放置 15min 以上，读取二甲苯的容积。然后照甲法自"取供试品适量"起，依法测定，自油层量中减去二甲苯量，即为挥发油量，再计算供试品中挥发油的含量（%）。

4. 注意事项

（1）挥发油测定采用水蒸气蒸馏法提取测定，采用的回流冷凝管必须有足够长度，以保证冷凝效率。

（2）应按照各品种项规定的条件取样测定，否则由于水溶液饱和的影响，结果会有偏差。

（3）乙法由于二甲苯的溶剂提取作用，测定结果通常更稳定。乙法也适用于相对密度在 1.0 以下样品的测定。

（4）乙法进行挥发油测定时，也可采用其他与水不混溶且密度比水小的有机溶剂替代二甲苯。为了准确测定，使用乙法进行空白蒸馏的时间应与样品测定的蒸馏时间相同，以免逸失不同而导致误差。

六、讨论

（1）石菖蒲的主要化学成分有哪些？

（2）本品挥发油用甲法进行测定。若用乙法测定须加入二甲苯 1.0ml，其目的是什么？

（3）供挥发油测定用的供试品须如何进行预处理？

Experiment 14　Analysis of Acori Talarinowii Rhizoma

1. Purposes

1.1　To master the method for the determination of volatile oil in the traditional Chinese materia medica.

1.2　To experiment on the identification of the traditional Chinese materia medica by TLC using reference crude herb.

2. Instruments and chemical reagents

2.1　Instruments

Microscope, ultra-violet light (365nm), crucible, Muffle furnace, volatile oil extractor, silica gel G TLC plate.

2.2　Chemical reagents

Acori Talarinowii Rhizoma and its reference crude herb, petroleum ether (60 ~ 90℃), ethyl acetate, iodine.

3. Procedures and methods

Acori Talarinowii Rhizoma(Shichangpu)

Acori Tatarinowii Rhizoma is the dried rhizome of *Acorus tatarinowii* Schott. (Araceae). The rhizome is collected in autumn and winter, fibrous roots and soil removed, and then dried under the sun to obtain Acori Tatarinowii Rhizoma.

3.1 Description

Compressed-cylindrical, frequently tortuous, normally branched, 3 ~ 20cm long, 0.3 ~ 1cm in diameter. Externally brown or greyish-brown, rough, with uneven annulations, internodes 0.2 ~ 0.8cm long, with fine longitudinal wrinkles, one surface with remains of fibrous roots or rounded root scars; leaf scars triangular, arranged alternately, some with hairy and scaly remains of leaf bases. Texture hard. Fracture fibrous, white or pale red, an endodermis ring distinct, numerous dotted vascular bundles and brown oil cells visible. Odor aromatic; tastes bitter and slightly pungent.

3.2 Identification

3.2.1 Transverse section. Epidermis consists of 1 layer of brown cells with thickened outer wall, some of which contain reddish-brown contents. Cortex broad, scattered with fibre bundles and leaf-trace vascular bundles, and each surrounded by a vascular bundle sheath of lignified fibres. Endodermis distinct. Amphivasal or collateral vascular bundles scattered throughout the stele, with less fibrous bundle sheath. Fibre bundles and bundle sheaths surrounded by cells containing prisms of calcium oxalate, forming crystal fibres. Parenchyma scattered with surrounded oil cells, containing starch granules.

Powder: Colour yellowish-brown. Simple starch granules ellipsoid, spheroidal or long-ovoid, 2 ~ 9μm in diameter, compound starch granules composed of 2 ~ 20(even more)units. Fibre bundles surrounded by cells containing prisms of calcium oxalate, forming crystal fibres. Prisms of calcium oxalate polyhedral, subpolygonal or polyconelike, 4 ~ 16μm in diameter. Secretory cells subrounded or elongated-rounded, filled with yellow-green, orange or red secretions(Figure 4 − 2).

3.2.2 Weigh 0.2g of the powdered sample, then add 20ml of petroleum ether(60 ~ 90℃) followed by heating under reflux for 1h. Filter, evaporate the filtrate to dryness and dissolve the residue in 1ml of petroleum ether(60 ~ 90℃) as the test solution. Produce a reference herb solution of Acori Rhizoma Talarinowii reference crude herb in the same manner. Carry out the method for thin layer chromatography, using silica gel G as the coating substance and petroleum ether(60 ~ 90℃) : ethyl acetate(4 : 1)as the developing solvent system. Apply separately the test solution and reference herb solution(2μl each)to the plate. After the development, remove the plate from the chamber, dry it in air, allow to stand for 1 hour and examine under ultraviolet light(365nm). The fluorescent spots in the chromatogram obtained with the test solution correspond in position and color to the spots in the chromatogram obtained with the reference herb solution. Expose to iodine vapour to visualize clearly under daylight. The spots in the chromatogram obtained with the test solution correspond in position and colour to the spots in the chromatogram obtained with the reference herb solution.

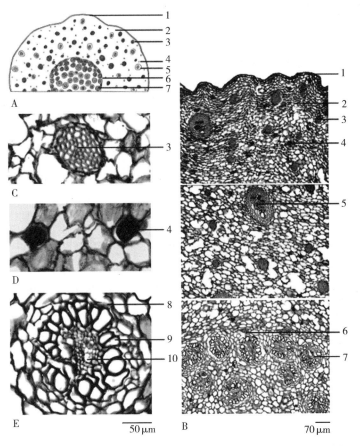

Figure 4 − 2 Microscopic features of transverse section of Acori Tatarinowii Rhizoma

A. Sketch,B. Section illustration,C. Fibre bundle,D. Secretory cell,E. Stele vascular bundle

1. Epidermis,2. Cortex,3. Fibre bundle,4. Secretory cell,5. Leaf – trace vascular,6. Endodermis,

7. Stele vascular bundle,8. Vascular bundle sheath,9. Xylem,10. Phloem

3. 3   Test

Water Content   Not more than 13. 0% .

Total ash   Not more than 10. 0% .

Extractives   Ethanol-soluble extractives(cold extraction method with dilute ethanol): not less than 12. 0% (Chinese Pharmacopeia 2010,Volume 1).

3. 4   Assay

Carry out the method for the determination of volatile oil(Chinese Pharmacopeia 2010,Volume 1). It contains not less than 1. 0% (ml/g)of volatile oil.

4. Prepare lessons before class

4. 1   Describe the procedures and key points for the determination of volatile oil.

4. 2   Describe the features of the identification by comparing with reference crude herb.

5. Guide for experiment

5. 1   Determination of ash

5. 1. 1   Total ash

a. Pulverize CMM sample,pass through No. 2 sieve and mix well. Accurately weigh 2 ~ 3g

(3 ~ 5g for the determination of acid-insoluble ash) of the powdered sample in a tared crucible(to the nearest 0. 01g). Ignite the sample gently until completely carbonized, keep it from burning, and then gradually increase the temperature to 500 ~ 600℃. Continue the ignition until a constant weight of carbon-free ash is obtained. Calculate the percentage of total ash in the weight of CMM sample.

b. If a carbon-free ash cannot be obtained in this way, cool the crucible, and moisten the residue with hot water or 2ml of aqueous ammonium nitrate solution(10% , V/V) , and then dry the residue on a water bath. Ignite the residue again as directed above until a carbon-free ash is obtained.

5. 1. 2　Acid-insoluble ash

To a crucible containing the total ash, add 10ml of dilute hydrochloric acid(10% , V/V) , cover with a watch glass and gently heat for 10min on a water bath. Rinse the watch glass with 5ml of hot water and add the rinsing to the crucible. Transfer the insoluble matter and rinse the remaining residues from the crucible onto an ashless filter paper, and wash with hot water until the filtrate is free of chlorides. Transfer the ashless filter paper containing the insoluble matter to the original crucible, dry and ignite to constant weight. Calculate the percentage of acid-insoluble ash in the weight of CMM sample.

The amount of total ash and acid-insoluble ash in CMM samples should be not more than the percentages specified in the individual monograph.

5. 2　Determination of extractives

5. 2. 1　Determination of water-soluble extractives.

Pulverize CMM sample, pass through a No. 2 sieve and mix well.

a. Cold extraction method　Place 4. 0g of the powdered sample, accurately weighed, in a 250 ~ 300ml conical flask with a stopper. Accurately add 100ml of water, insert the stopper and extract for 24h. Shake frequently during the first 6h, then allow to stand for 18h. Filter rapidly through a dry filter. Accurately transfer 20ml of the filtrate to an evaporating dish, previously dried to constant weight, and evaporate to almost dryness on a water bath, then dry at 105 °C for 3h. Cool in a desiccator for 30min, and then weigh immediately and accurately. Calculate the percentage of water-soluble extractives with reference to the dried CMM sample.

b. Hot extraction method　Place 2 ~ 4g of the powdered sample, accurately weighed, in a 100 ~ 250ml conical flask with a stopper. Accurately add 50 ~ 100ml of water, insert the stopper and weigh. Allow to stan d for 1h. Attach a reflux condenser to the flask and boil gently for 1h, then cool to room temperature and weigh, readjust to the original weight with water. Shake and filter through a dry filter. Accurately transfer 25ml of the filtrate to an evaporating dish, previously dried to constant weight, and evaporate to dryness on a water bath, then dry at 105℃ for 3h. Cool in a desiccator for 30min, and then weigh immediately and accurately. Calculate the percentage of water-soluble extractives with reference to the dried CMM sample.

5. 2. 2　Determination of ethanol-soluble extractives.

Proceed as directed under determination of water-soluble extractives using ethanol of a concentration specified in individual monograph as the solvent instead of water.

5.2.3 Determination of volatile ether extractives.

Place 2~5g of the powdered material(through No. 4 sieve), accurately weighed, dry for 12h in a desiccator with P_2O_5. Place in a Soxhlet's extractor, add a quantity of ether, and heat under reflux for 8h, unless otherwise specified in the monography. Place in an evaporating dish, previously dried to constant weight, and evaporate to dryness. Dry for 18h in a desiccator with P_2O_5, weigh accurately, heat to 105℃ slowly, dry at 105℃ to constant weight. The weight loss is the weight of volatile ether extractives.

5.3 Determination of volatile oil

5.3.1 Theory

The determination of volatile oils in the drug is performed by distillation with water, collecting the distillate in a graduated tube with a structure such as allows that the aqueous phase get separated from the oil phase and is returned to the distillation flask. When the essential oil has a density near to the density of water or when the separation phase is difficult, it is added into the graduated tube a premeasured amount of low density solvent with appropriate boiling point (for example, xylene), which allows to dissolve the essential oil and facilitate the separation.

5.3.2 Apparatus

The apparatus consists of a 1000ml(500ml or 2000ml) round-bottomed flask(A), a volatile oil determination tube (B) and a reflux condenser(C). All parts are connected via ground glass joints. The measuring tube of B is graduated in 0.1ml. The apparatus should be cleaned before use and all parts of apparatus should be tightly connected to avoid the loss of volatile oil(Figure 4-3).

Note: The volatile oil determination tube should be set vertically. The connecting point between the side tube and the graduated tube is at a horizontal level.

5.3.3 Method

Preparation of test sample. Pulverize the sample, pass through No. 2 or No. 3 sieves and mix well, unless otherwise specified.

Method A   This method is used to determine the volatile oils with relative density less than 1.0. Take a quantity of the powdered sample which is expected to give 0.5~1.0ml of volatile oil, weigh accurately to closest to 0.01g, and put into a round-bottomed flask. Add 300~500ml of water(or appropriate amount) and a few glass beads, shake and mix well. Connect the round-bottomed flask to a volatile oil determination tube and then connect the volatile oil determination tube to a reflux condenser. Add

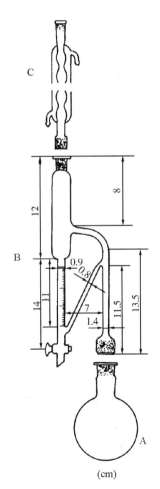

(cm)

Figure 4-3 Apparatus for the determinationof volatile oil

water through the top of reflux condenser until the graduated tube of volatile oil determination tube is filled and overflows to the round-bottomed flask. Heat the flask gently until boiling by using an electric heating jacket or other appropriate means. Continue the gentle boiling for about 5h until the volume of oil does not increase. Stop heating, allow it to stand for a while. Open the stopcock at the lower part of volatile oil determination tube and run off the water layer slowly until the oily layer is 5mm above the zero mark. Allow to stand for at least 1h, open the stopcock again, run off the remaining water layer carefully until the oily layer is just on the zero mark. Record the volume of oil in the graduated tube of volatile oil determination tube and calculate the percentage of volatile oil in the sample.

Method B   This method is used to determine the volatile oils with relative density more than 1. 0. Add 300ml of water and a few pieces of glass beads into a round-bottomed flask. Connect the round-bottomed flask to volatile oil determination tube. Add water through the top of volatile oil determination tube until the graduated tube is filled and overflows to the round-bottomed flask. Add 1ml of xylene by using a pipette and then connect the reflux condenser to volatile oil determination tube. Heat the flask until boiling, continue the heating to allow the distillation proceed at a rate that will keep the middle part of the condenser cold. Stop heating after 30min, and allow it to stand for at least 15min. Record the volume of xylene in the graduated tube of volatile oil determination tube. Carry out the procedure as described in Method A beginning with the words "Take a quantity of the powdered sample". Subtract the volume of xylene previously observed from the volume of oily layer, the difference in volume is taken to be the content of volatile oil, and calculate the percentage of volatile oil in the sample.

5. 4   Key points

5. 4. 1   The reflux condenser should be long enough to ensure the efficacy of condensation.

5. 4. 2   Assay should be performed under the required conditions specified in the pharmacopoeia monograph of each sample to decrease the error.

5. 4. 3   Due to the addition of xylene, Method B usually provides more stable results and can be also used to determine the volatile oils with relative density less than 1. 0.

5. 4. 4   In Method B for the determination of volatile oil, xylene can be replaced with other organic solvents which are insoluble in water and with lower density less than water.

6. Discussion

6. 1   Describe the main components found in Acori Tatarinowii Rhizoma.

6. 2   Method A is adopted for the determination of volatile oil in Acori Tatarinowii Rhizoma. Describe the purpose for adding 1. 0ml of xylene.

6. 3   What should be done to the sample before the determination of volatile oil?

（许慧君）

实验十五 六味地黄丸的质量检验

一、目的

（1）掌握中成药鉴别试验及含量测定中检测对象的选择原则。

（2）掌握蜜丸类中成药在样品处理过程中的脱蜜方法。

（3）熟悉中成药中有效成分含量测定的高效液相色谱法。

（4）熟悉中成药中各药材粉末的显微鉴别法。

二、仪器与试药

1. 仪器

显微镜、万分之一天平、超声波震荡仪、具塞锥形瓶、高效液相色谱仪、C_{18}色谱柱。

2. 试药

小蜜丸、大蜜丸、水蜜丸、丹皮酚对照品、马钱苷对照品、中性氧化铝、硅胶 G 薄层板、环己烷、乙酸乙酯、盐酸酸性 5% 三氯化铁乙醇溶液、10% 硫酸乙醇溶液、四氢呋喃、乙腈、甲醇、乙醚、丙酮、磷酸。

三、实验方法

1. 处方

熟地黄 160g、酒萸肉 80g、牡丹皮 60g、山药 80g、茯苓 60g、泽泻 60g。

2. 制法

以上六味粉碎成细粉，过筛，混匀。每 100g 粉末加炼蜜 35～50g 与适量的水，制丸，干燥，制成水蜜丸，或加炼蜜 80～110g 制成小蜜丸或大蜜丸，即得。

3. 性状

本品为棕黑色的水蜜丸、棕褐色至黑褐色的小蜜丸或大蜜丸，味甜而酸。

4. 鉴别

（1）取本品，置显微镜下观察。淀粉粒三角状卵形或矩圆形，直径 24～40μm，脐点短缝状或"人"字状（山药）。不规则分枝状团块无色，遇水合氯醛试液溶化；菌丝无色，直径 4～6μm（茯苓）。薄壁组织灰棕色至黑棕色，细胞多皱缩，内含棕色核状物（熟地黄）。草酸钙簇晶存在于无色薄壁细胞中，有时数个排列成行（牡丹皮）。果皮表皮细胞橙黄色，表面观类多角形，垂周壁连珠状增厚（酒萸肉）。薄壁细胞类圆形，有椭圆形纹孔，集成纹孔群；内皮层细胞垂周壁波状弯曲，较厚，木化，有稀疏细孔沟（泽泻）。

（2）取本品水蜜丸 6g，研碎，或取小蜜丸或大蜜丸 9g，剪碎，加硅藻土 4g，研匀。加乙醚 40ml，回流 1h，滤过，滤液挥去乙醚，残渣加丙酮 1ml 溶解，作为供试品溶液。另取丹皮酚对照品，加丙酮制成每毫升含 1mg 的溶液，作为对照品溶液。照薄层色谱法（《中国药典》一部）试验，吸取上述两种溶液各 10μl，分别点于同一硅胶 G 薄层板上，以环己烷－乙酸乙酯（3∶1）为展开剂，展开，取出，晾干，喷以盐酸酸性 5% 三氯化铁乙醇溶液，加热至斑点显色清晰。在供试品色谱中，在与对照品色谱相应的位置上显示相同颜色的斑点。

（3）取本品水蜜丸6g，研细，或取小蜜丸或大蜜丸9g，剪碎，加硅藻土4g，研匀。加乙酸乙酯40ml，加热回流20min，放冷，滤过，滤液浓缩至约0.5ml，作为供试品溶液。另取泽泻对照药材0.5g，加乙酸乙酯40ml，同法制成对照药材溶液。照薄层色谱法（《中国药典》一部）试验，吸取上述两种溶液各5～10μl，分别点于同一硅胶G薄层板上，以三氯甲烷：乙酸乙酯：甲酸（12：7：1）为展开剂，展开，取出，晾干，喷以10%硫酸乙醇溶液，在105℃加热至斑点显色清晰。在供试品色谱中，在与对照药材色谱相应的位置上显示相同颜色的斑点。

六味地黄丸显微结构图见图4-4。

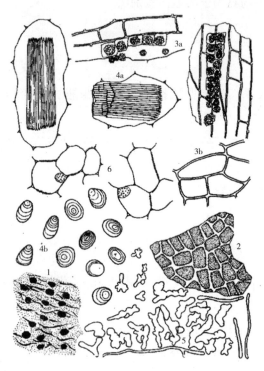

图4-4 六味地黄丸显微结构图

1. 熟地黄；2. 酒萸肉；3. 牡丹皮；4. 山药；5. 茯苓；6. 泽泻

5. 检查

应符合丸剂项有关的各项规定。

6. 含量测定

（1）酒萸肉 照高效液相色谱法测定。

色谱条件与系统适用性试验 以十八烷基硅烷键合硅胶为填充剂，以四氢呋喃：乙腈：甲醇：0.05%磷酸溶液（1：8：4：87）为流动相，检测波长为236nm，柱温40℃。理论板数按马钱苷峰计算应不低于4000。

对照品溶液的制备 取马钱苷对照品适量，精密称定，加50%甲醇制成每毫升含20μg的溶液，即得。

供试品溶液的制备 取本品水蜜丸或小蜜丸，切碎，取约0.7g，精密称定，或取质量差异项下的大蜜丸，剪碎，取约1g，精密称定，置具塞锥形瓶中，精密加入50%甲醇25ml，密塞，称定质量，超声处理（功率250W，频率33kHz）15min溶散，加热回流1h，放冷，再称定质量，用50%甲醇补足减失的质量，摇匀，滤过。精密量取续滤液10ml，置中性氧化铝柱（100～200目，4g，内径1cm）上，用40%甲醇50ml洗脱，收集流出液及洗脱液，蒸干，残渣加50%甲醇适量溶解，并转移至10ml量瓶中，加50%甲醇稀释至刻度，摇匀，即得。

测定法 分别精密吸取供试品溶液与对照品溶液各10μl，注入液相色谱仪，测定，即得。

本品含酒萸肉以马钱苷（$C_{17}H_{26}O_{10}$）计，水蜜丸每克不得少于0.70mg，小蜜丸每克不得少于0.50mg，大蜜丸每丸不得少于4.5mg。

（2）牡丹皮 照高效液相色谱法测定。

色谱条件与系统适用性试验 以十八烷基硅烷键合硅胶为填充剂，以甲醇–水（70∶30）为流动相，检测波长为274nm。理论板数按丹皮酚峰计算应不低于3500。

对照品溶液的制备 取丹皮酚对照品适量，精密称定，加甲醇制成每毫升含20μg的溶液，即得。

供试品溶液的制备 取本品水蜜丸或小蜜丸，切碎，取约0.3g，精密称定，或取质量差异项下的大蜜丸，剪碎，取约0.4g，精密称定，置具塞锥形瓶中，精密加入50%甲醇50ml，密塞，称定质量，超声处理（功率250W，频率33kHz）45min，放冷，再称定质量，用50%甲醇补足减失的质量，摇匀，滤过，取续滤液，即得。

测定法 分别精密吸取供试品溶液20μl与对照品溶液10μl，注入液相色谱仪，测定，即得。

本品含牡丹皮按丹皮酚（$C_9H_{10}O_3$）计，水蜜丸每克不得少于0.9mg；小蜜丸每克不得少于0.70mg；大蜜丸每丸不得少于6.3mg。

四、预习提要

（1）中药丸剂的常规检查项目有哪些？
（2）中药分析时样品的预处理方法有哪些？
（3）高效液相色谱仪使用时应注意什么？

五、实验指导

（一）中药丸剂的分类与检查

1. 丸剂分类

丸剂系指药材细粉或药材提取物加适宜的黏合剂或其他辅料制成的球形或类球形制剂，分为蜜丸、水蜜丸、水丸、糊丸、蜡丸和浓缩丸等类型。

蜜丸系指饮片细粉以蜂蜜为黏合剂制成的丸剂。其中，每丸质量在0.5g（含0.5g）以上称大蜜丸，每丸质量在0.5以下称小蜜丸。

水蜜丸系指饮片细粉以蜂蜜和水为黏合剂制成的丸剂。

水丸系指饮片细粉以水（或根据制法用黄酒、醋、稀药汁、糖液等）为黏合剂制成的丸剂。

糊丸系指饮片细粉以米粉、米糊或面糊等为黏合剂制成的丸剂。

蜡丸系指饮片细粉以蜂蜡为黏合剂制成的丸剂。

浓缩丸系指药材或部分药材提取浓缩，与适宜的辅料或其余药材细粉，以水、蜂蜜或蜂蜜和水为黏合剂制成的丸剂。根据所用的黏合剂，分为浓缩水丸、浓缩蜜丸和浓缩水蜜丸。

2. 丸剂检查项目

除另有规定外，丸剂应进行以下相应的检查。

（1）水分　照水分测定法测定。除另有规定外，蜜丸和浓缩蜜丸中所含水分不得过15.0%；水蜜丸和浓缩水蜜丸不得过12.0%；水丸、糊丸和浓缩水丸不得过9.0%。蜡丸不检查水分。

（2）重量差异　除另有规定外，丸剂照下述方法检查，应符合规定。

检查法　以10丸为1份（丸重1.5g及1.5g以上的丸剂以1丸为1份），取供试品10份，分别称定质量，再与每份标示质量（每丸标示量×称取丸数）相比较（无标示质量的丸剂，与平均质量比较），按表4-1的规定，超出质量差异限度的不得多于2份，并不得有1份超出限度1倍。

表4-1　标示重量及其差异限度

标示质量（或平均质量）	质量差异限度
0.05g及0.05g以下	±12%
0.05g以上至0.1g	±11%
0.1g以上至0.3g	±10%
0.3g以上至1.5g	±9%
1.5g以上至3g	±8%
3g以上至6g	±7%
6g以上至9g	±6%
9g以上	±5%

包糖衣丸剂应检查丸芯的质量差异并符合规定，包糖衣后不再检查质量差异，其他包衣丸剂应在包糖衣后检查重量差异并符合规定。凡进行装量差异检查的单剂量包装丸剂，不再进行质量差异检查。

装量差异　单剂量包装的丸剂照下述方法检查，应符合规定。

检查法　取供试品10袋（瓶），分别称定每袋（瓶）内容物的质量，每袋（瓶）装量与标示装量相比较，按表4-2的规定，超出装量差异限度的不得多于2袋（瓶），并不得有1袋（瓶）超出限度1倍。

表4-2　标示装量及其差异限度

标示装量	装量差异限度
0.5g及0.5g以下	±12%
0.5g以上至1g	±11%
1g以上至2g	±10%
2g以上至3g	±8%
3g以上至6g	±6%
6g以上至9g	±5%
9g以上	±4%

（3）装量　装量以质量标示的多剂量包装丸剂，照最低装量检查法检查，应符合规定。以丸数标识的多剂量包装丸剂，不检查装量。

（4）溶散时限　除另有规定外，取供试品6丸，选择适当孔径筛网的吊篮（丸剂直径在2.5mm以下的用孔径约0.42mm的筛网；在2.5~3.5mm之间的用孔径约1.0mm的筛网；在3.5mm以上的用孔径约2.0mm的筛网），照崩解时限检查法（《中国药典》四部通则）片剂项下的方法加挡板进行检查。除另有规定外，小蜜丸、水蜜丸和水丸应在1h内全部溶散；浓缩丸和糊丸应在2h内全部溶散。操作过程中如供试品黏附挡板妨碍检查时，应另取供试品6丸，以不加挡板进行检查。

上述检查时，应在规定时间内全部通过筛网。如有细小颗粒状物未通过筛网，但已软化且无硬芯者可按符合规定论。

蜡丸照崩解时限检查法片剂项下的肠溶衣片检查法检查，应符合规定。

除另有规定外，大蜜丸不检查溶散时限。

微生物限度　照微生物限度检查法检查，应符合规定。

（二）中药材及其制剂的前处理

1. 中药材及其制剂样品预处理的目的

中药材成分复杂，干扰因素多，且这些成分存在于中药材组织和细胞中，不易提取，因此，进行中药材含量测定时，应综合考虑待测成分的理化性质、存在状态及各成分之间的相互干扰程度，选择适宜的预处理技术对其进行提取分离和纯化。

2. 常见的提取方法

为使待测成分易于提取，同时保证取样均一，应将中药材粉碎、过筛后再行提取。常见的提取方法有冷浸法、回流提取法、连续回流提取法、超声提取法和水蒸气蒸馏法，特点比较列于表4-3。

表4-3　中药材含量测定常用的提取方法特点比较

提取方法	适用范围	优点	缺点
冷浸法	遇热不稳定成分	操作简便	时间较长
回流提取法	对热稳定或无挥发性的组分	提取速度快	操作繁琐
连续回流提取法	对热应稳定，应选用低沸点的溶剂	节省溶剂，提取效率高	时间较长
超声提取法	范围广	简便，提取时间短	某些成分易破坏
水蒸气蒸馏法	具有挥发性，可随水蒸气流出而不被破坏的难溶于水的成分	有一定纯化作用	操作繁琐

除选择合适的提取方法外，提取溶剂和提取时间也是确保待测成分提取完全的重要因素。根据组分的物理性质和溶解行为选择合适的溶剂提取，提取时间经实验比较方能确定。一些样品经提取后还不能直接进行测定，有时须进一步纯化并去除杂质。常用的净化方法有液-液萃取法、沉淀法和各种色谱法等。采用这些预处理技术时，一定要注意保证方法的准确度和重复率。

总之，对于不同药材不同成分，应具体问题具体分析，选择合适的预处理方法，使制得的供试品溶液纯净且提取完全。

六、讨论

（1）中成药鉴别试验及含量测定中检测对象的选择原则有哪些？本品为什么选择马钱苷和丹皮酚进行含量测定？

（2）中药制剂的含量测定为何往往选用置具塞锥形瓶而非量瓶进行定量操作？

（3）中药与化学药的质量分析有何不同？

（4）目前，中药质量评价的方法有哪些？如何有效地控制中药质量？

Experiment 15　Analysis of Liuwei Dihuang Wan

1. Purposes

1.1　To master the principles for the selection of components for the identification and assay of traditional Chinese materia medica.

1.2　To master the sample pretreatment method for the honeyed pills.

1.3　To study the high performance liquid chromatography method for the assay of the traditional Chinese materia medica.

1.4　To experiment on the microscopic identification method for the traditional Chinese materia medica.

2. Instruments and chemical reagents

2.1　Instruments

Microscope, weight, ultrasonic vibration instrument, conical flask with stopper, HPLC, C_{18} column.

2.2　Chemical reagents

Small honeyed pills, big honeyed pills, water-honeyed pills, paeonol CRS, loganin CRS, neutral aluminum oxide, silica G TLC plate, cyclohexane, ethyl acetate, 5% solution of ferric chloride in ethanol acidified with hydrochloric acid, 10% solution of sulphuric acid in ethanol, tetrahydrofuran, acetonitrile, methanol, ether, acetone, phosphoric acid.

3. Procedures and methods

3.1　Ingredients

Radix Rehmanniae preparata 160g, Liquor Cornus 80g, Cortex Moutan 60g, Rhizoma Dioscoreae 80g, Poria 60g, Rhizoma Alismatis 60g.

3.2　Procedures

Pulverize the above six ingredients to fine powder, sift and mix well. To each 100g of the powder add 35 ~ 50g of refined honey and a quantity of water to make water-honeyed pills and dry. Alternatively add 80 ~ 110g of refined honey to make small honeyed pills or big honeyed pills.

3.3　Description

Brown-black water-honeyed pills, black-brown small honeyed pills or big honeyed pills; tastes sweet and sour.

3.4　Identification

3.4.1　Starch granules triangular-ovoid or oblong (Figure 4 - 4), 24 ~ 40μm in diameter, hilum short cleft or V-shaped(Rhizoma Dioscoreae). Irregular branched masses colorless,dissolved in chloral hydrate solution; hyphae colorless,4 ~ 6μm in diameter(Poria). Parenchyma greyish-brown to black-brown,cells mostly shrunken,and each containing a brown nucleus-like mass(Radix Rehmanniae preparata). Clusters of calcium oxalate occurring in colorless parenchymatous cells, sometimes several clusters arranged in rows(Cortex Moutan). Epidermal cells of pericarp orange-yellow, polygonal in surface view, with somewhat beaded anticlinal walls (Liquor Cornus). Parenchymatous cells subrounded,with elliptical pits,gathered into pit groups(Rhizoma Alismatis), see the supplementary figure.

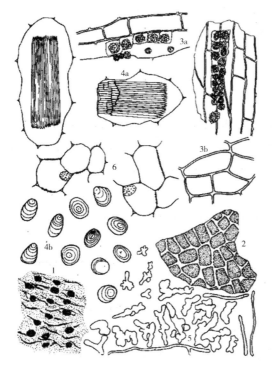

图 4 – 4　Microscopic features of Liuwei Dihuang Wan

1. Radix Rehmanniae preparata;2. Liquor Cornus;3. Cortex Moutan;

4. Rhizoma Dioscoreae;5. Poria;6. Rhizoma Alismatis

3.4.2　Pulverize 6g of water-honeyed pills,or take 9g of small honeyed pills or big honeyed pills,in powder,add 4g of kieselguhr and triturate well. Heat under reflux with 40ml of ether for 1 hour,filter and evaporate to remove ether. Dissolve the residue in 1ml of acetone as the test solution. Dissolve paeonol CRS in acetone to produce a solution containing 1mg per 1ml,as the reference solution. Carry out the method for thin layer chromatography,using silica gel G as the coating substance and cyclohexane：ethyl acetate(3：1) as the developing solvent solution. Apply separately two solutions(each 10μl) to the plate. After the development,remove the plate from the chamber,and dry it in air. Spray with 5% solution of ferric chloride in ethanol acidified with hydrochloric acid and visualize under a current of hot air. The spot in the chromatogram obtained with the test solution corresponds in position and color to the spot in the chromatogram obtained with the reference solution.

3.4.3　Pulverize 6g of water-honeyed pills,or take 9g of small honeyed pills or big honeyed pills, in powder, add 4g of kieselguhr and triturate well. Heat under reflux with 40ml of ethyl acetate for 20 minutes, filter, and concentrate the filtrate to approximate 0. 5ml as the test solution. Produce a reference herb solution of Rhizoma Alismatis reference crude herb in the same manner. Carry out the method for thin layer chromatography, using silica gel G as the coating substance and chloroform : ethyl acetate : formic acid (12 : 7 : 1) as the developing solvent solution. Apply separately two solutions (each 5 ~ 10μl) to the plate. After the development, remove the plate from the chamber, and dry it in air. Spray with 10% solution of of sulphuric acid in ethanol and visualize under 105℃. The spot in the chromatogram obtained with the test solution corresponds in position and color to the spot in the chromatogram obtained with the reference herb solution.

3. 5 Other requirements

Comply with the general requirements for pills.

3. 6 Assay

3. 6. 1 Liquor Cornus

Carry out the method for high performance liquid chromatography.

Chromatographic system and system suitability Use octadecylsilane bonded silica gel as the stationary phase and a mixture of tetrahydrofuran, acetonitrile, methanol and 0. 05% solution of phosphoric acid (1 : 8 : 4 : 87) as the mobile phase. As detector a spectrophotometer set at 236nm, maintain the column temperature at 40℃. The number of theoretical plates of the column is not less than 4000, calculated with reference to the peak of loganin.

Reference solution Dissolve a quantity of loganin CRS, accurately weighed, in 50% methanol to prepare a solution containing 20μg per 1ml.

Test solution Take 0. 7g of the powered water-honeyed pills or small honeyed pills, or 1g of big honeyed pills used for weigh variance test, accurately weighed, place to a stopper conical flask, add accurately 25ml of 50% methanol, stopper tightly and weigh. Ultrasonicate (power 250W, frequency 33kHz) for 15 minutes, heat under reflux for 1 hour and cool. Weigh again and replenish the lost weight with 50% methanol, mix well and filter. Measure accurately 10ml of the successive filtrate, apply to a column (1cm in internal diameter) packed with neutral aluminium oxide (100 ~ 200 mesh, 4g). Elute with 50ml of 40% methanol, collect the eluate, evaporate to dryness and dissolve the residue with 50% methanol, transfer to a 10ml volumetric flask, dilute with 50% methanol to volume, and mix well.

Procedure Inject accurately 10μl of the reference solution and 10μl of the test solution into the column, and calculate the content.

It contains not less than 0. 70mg, 0. 50mg and 4. 5mg of loganin ($C_{17}H_{26}O_{10}$) every 1g of water-honeyed pills, small honeyed pill and big honeyed pills respectively, referred to Liquor Cornus.

3. 6. 2 Cortex Moutan

Carry out the method for high performance liquid chromatography

Chromatographic system and system suitability Use octadecylsilane bonded silica gel as the stationary phase and mixture of methanol and water (70 : 30) as the mobile phase. As detector a spectrophotometer set at 247nm. The number of theoretical plated of the column is not less than 3500, calculated with the reference to the peak of paeonol.

Reference solution　　Dissolve a quantity of paeonol CRS, accurately weighed, in methanol to prepare a solution containing $20\mu g$ per 1ml.

Test solution　　Take 0.3g of the powered water-honeyed pills or small honeyed pills, or 0.4g of the powered big honeyed pills used for weigh variance test, weigh accurately, place to a stopper conical flask, add exactly 50ml of 50% methanol, stopper tightly, and weigh. Ultrasonicate (power 250W, frequency 33kHz) for 45 minutes, allow to cool, and weigh again. Replenish the lost weight with 50% methanol, mix well and filter. Use the successive filtrate as the test solution.

Procedure　　Inject accurately $10\mu l$ of the reference of solution and $20\mu l$ the test solution into column, and calculated the content.

It contains not less than 1.8mg every 1g of concentrated pills of paeonol ($C_9H_{10}O_3$), referred to Cortex Moutan.

It contains not less than 0.9mg, 0.70mg and 6.3mg of paeonol ($C_9H_{10}O_3$) every 1g of water-honeyed pills, small honeyed pill and big honeyed pills respectively, referred to Cortex Moutan.

4. Prepare lessons before class

4.1　Describe the general tests for pills.

4.2　Which methods can be used to pretreat TCM samples?

4.3　What should we take care of when using HPLC?

5. Guide for experiment

5.1　Classification and tests of pills

5.1.1　Classification of pills

Pills are spherical or spherical-like solid dosage forms made of finely powdered crude drugs or crude drug extracts, proper binders or other excipients. They are classified into honeyed pills, water-honeyed pills, watered pills, pasted pills, waxed pills and concentrated pills etc.

Honeyed pills are made of fine powder of crude drugs, using honey as binder. Among them, pills weighing more than 0.5g (including 0.5g) per pill are big honeyed pills, pills weighing less than 0.5g per pill are small honeyed pills.

Water-honeyed pills are made of fine powder of crude drugs, using honey and water as binders.

Watered pills are made of fine powder of crude drugs, using water (or yellow rice wine, vinegar, dilute medicinal juice, dilute syrup) as binder.

Pasted pills are made of fine powder of crude drugs, using rice powder rice-paste or flour-paste as binder.

Waxed pills are made of fine powder of crude drugs, using beeswax as binder.

Concentrated pills are made of condensed extract of crude drugs or partial crude drugs, mixing with appropriate excipients or fine powder of other crude drugs, using water, honey or honey and water as binders. They may be classified into concentrated watered pills, concentrated honeyed pills and concentrated water-honeyed pills based upon the different binders used in the production.

5.1.2　General requirements for pills

Following relevant tests should be carried out for pills.

Determination of water　Carry out the method for the determination of water in general. Unless specified otherwise, honeyed pills and concentrated honeyed pills contain not more than 15.0% of water, water-honeyed pills and concentrated water-honeyed pills not more than 12.0% of water, watered pills, pasted pills and concentrated watered pills not more than 9.0%. No determination of water is required for waxed pills.

Weight variation　Unless specified otherwise, pills examined by the following method should comply with the requirement.

Method　Take 10 pills as one part(1 pill as one part for pills weighing 1.5g or more than 1.5g per pill). Weigh separately 10 parts and compare with the labeled total weight(labeled weight per pill × the number of pills weighed. If no labeled weight per pill is stated, compare with the average weight calculated. According to the requirements stated in Table 4 – 1, not more than 2 parts exceed the limit of weight variation and none doubles the limit of weight variation.

Table 4 – 1　Labeled total weight and weight variation limit

Labeled total weight(or average weight)	Weight variation limit
0.05g or less	±12%
0.05g to 0.1g	±11%
0.1g to 0.3g	±10%
0.3g to 1.5g	±9%
1.5g to 3g	±8%
3g to 6g	±7%
6g to 9g	±6%
more than 9g	±5%

Weight variation of sugar-coated pills should be examined before coating, pills are not to be coated until the weight variation of the pill cores complies with the requirements. The weight variation of pills is no longer examined after sugar-coating, Other coated pills should be examined the weight variation after coating and comply with the requirements. The weight variation is no longer examined for the single dose packed pills, which have been examined according to the filling variation standards.

Filling variation　The filling variation of pills presented in single dose pack should comply with the following requirements.

Procedure　Take ten packs(or vials) of pills, weigh separately the content of each pack(or vial), and compare with the labeled weight. According to the requirement stated in Table 4 – 2, not more than 2 packs exceed the filling variation limit and none doubles the limit.

Table 4 – 2　Labeled filling and filling vasiation limit

Labeled filling	Filling variation limit
0.5g or less	±12%
0.5g to 1g	±11%

continued

Labeled filling	Filling variation limit
1g to 2g	±10%
2g to 3g	±8%
3g to 6g	±6%
6g to 9g	±5%
more than 9g	±4%

Filling   The filling of multiple doses packed pills of which filling is labeled in weight should comply with the test for minimum filling.

No filling test is required for multiple doses packed pills of which filling is labeled by the number of pills.

Disintegration test   Unless specified otherwise, take 6 pills, select a basket with proper porosity of sieve (for pills with the diameter of less than 2.5mm, 2.5 ~ 3.5mm and more than 3.5mm, using sieves with pores of 0.42mm, 1.0mm and 2.0mm in diameter respectively). Carry out the test as described under the disintegration test for tablets, using disk. Unless specified otherwise, small honeyed pills, water-honeyed pills and watered pills should be completely disintegrated within 1 hour, concentrated pills and pasted pills should be within 2 hours. During the procedure, if pills adhere to the disk, thus hindering the determination, take another 6 pills and carry out the test without disk.

Disintegration is considered to be achieved when no residue remains on the screen within the specified time, or if there is a residue, it consists of a soft mass having no palpably firm, unmoistened core.

Waxed pills should comply with the requirements stated in Determination of Disintegration   for enteric-coated tablets.

No disintegration test is required for big honeyed pills.

Microbial limit test   Comply with the requirements stated under Microbial limit test.

5.2   Common pretreatment methods in TCM analysis

5.2.1   Aim of the pretreatment

The constituents in Chinese drug are complicated, and they influence each other when being determined. Moreover, these constituents are in the tissues or cells of crud drugs, which make it difficult to be extracted. Therefore, physico chemical properties, existing style and interfering degree of the analytes should be considered. Correspondingly, pretreating technologies should be optimized to extract, isolate and purify the analytes from the drug samples.

5.2.2   Common methods

In order to extract the analytes easily and ensure the homogenicity of sampling, the crude drug samples should be powdered to a homogeneous size and sieved before being extracted. There are some extraction methods such as soaking, refluxing, continuous refluxing, ultrasonic extraction and steam distillation. These methods are listed in the Table 4 – 3.

Table 4 – 3　The extraction methods used for the assay of Chinese drug

Methods	Application	Advantages	Disadvantages
Soaking	Heat labile components	Simple	Consume time
Refluxing	Thermostable and nonvolatile components	Rapid	Tedious operation
Continuous refluxing	Thermostable components, using lower boiling point solvent	Save solvent, high extraction of efficiency	Consume time
Ultrasonic extraction	Widely used	Simple, save time	Some components are demolished
Steam distillation	The components are volatile, able to outflow following steam, stable and indissolvable in water	The extract is relatively pure	Tedious operation

Except for extraction method, extraction solvent and time are important factors to ensure thorough extraction of the analytes. The solvent is chosen according to the physico chemical properties and solubility of the analytes. The extraction time also needs to be optimized.

Some extraction solution can't be directly analyzed and then the purification procedure to remove interference is required. There are many commonly used purification methods such as liquid-liquid extraction, precipitation and chromatography. The accuracy and repeatability of the method should be taken care of when these methods are used. In a word, proper pretreatment methods are needed to ensure purification and thorough extraction of the analytes for different materials.

6. Discussions

6. 1　Describe the principle for the assay and identification of traditional Chinese materia medica. Explain why loganin and paeonol are selected for the assay of Liuwei Dihuang Wan.

6. 2　Why stopper conical flask rather than volumetric flask is generally adopted for the quantitative analysis of Chinese materia medica preparations?

6. 3　What are the differences between the analysis of TCM and pharmaceutical chemicals?

6. 4　Which methods can be used to evaluate the quality of TCM? How to efficiently control the quality of TCM?

（许慧君）

实验十六　双黄连口服液的质量检验

一、目的

（1）掌握中成药特征成分的薄层对照品法及对照药材法的鉴别。

（2）掌握高效液相色谱外标法测定中药制剂中指标成分的原理与方法。

二、仪器与试药

1. 仪器

万分之一天平，比重瓶，酸度计，聚酰胺薄膜，硅胶 G 薄层板，紫外光灯（365nm），中性氧化铝（100～120 目、6g、内径为 1cm），棕色量瓶，超声震荡仪，具塞锥形瓶，高效液相色谱仪，C_{18} 色谱柱。

2. 试药

黄芩苷对照品、绿原酸对照品、连翘苷对照品、连翘对照药材、乙酸、甲醇、三氯甲烷、10% 硫酸乙醇溶液、水、冰乙酸、乙腈。

三、实验方法

1. 处方

金银花 375g、黄芩 375g、连翘 750g。

2. 制法

以上三味，黄芩加水煎煮 3 次，第一次 2h，第二、三次各 1h，合并煎液，滤过，滤液浓缩并在 80℃时加入 2mol/L 盐酸溶液适量调节 pH 值至 1.0～2.0，保温 1h，静置 12h，滤过，沉淀加 6～8 倍量水，用 40% 氢氧化钠溶液调节 pH 值至 7.0，再加等量乙醇，搅拌溶解，滤过，滤液用 2mol/L 盐酸溶液调节 pH 值至 2.0，60℃保温 30min，静置 12h，滤过，沉淀用乙醇洗至 pH 值为 7.0，回收乙醇备用；金银花、连翘加水温浸 30min 后，煎煮两次，每次 1.5h，合并煎液，滤过，滤液浓缩至相对密度为 1.20～1.25（70～80℃）的清膏，冷至 40℃时缓缓加入乙醇，使含醇量达 75%，充分搅拌，静置 12h，取上清液，残渣加 75% 乙醇适量，搅匀，静置 12h，滤过，合并乙醇液，回收乙醇至无醇味，加入上述黄芩提取物，并加水适量，以 40% 氢氧化钠溶液调节 pH 值至 7.0，搅匀，冷藏（4～8℃）72h，滤过，滤液加入蔗糖 300g，搅拌使溶解，或再加入香精适量并调节 pH 值至 7.0，加水制成 1000ml，搅匀，静置 12h，滤过，灌装，灭菌，即得。

3. 性状

本品为棕红色的澄清液体；味甜，微苦。

4. 鉴别

（1）黄芩苷和绿原酸：取本品 1ml，加 75% 乙醇 5ml，摇匀，作为供试品溶液。另取黄芩苷对照品、绿原酸对照品，分别加 75% 乙醇制成每毫升含 0.1mg 的溶液，作为对照品溶液。照薄层色谱法试验，吸取上述三种溶液各 1～2μl，分别点于同一聚酰胺薄膜上，以乙酸为展开剂，展开，取出，晾干，置紫外光灯（365nm）下检视。在供试品色谱中，在与黄芩苷对照品色谱相应的位置上，显示相同颜色的荧光斑点；在与绿原酸对照品色谱相应的位置上，显示相同颜色的荧光斑点。

（2）连翘对照药材：取本品 1ml，加甲醇 5ml，振摇溶解，静置，取上清液，作为供试品溶液。另取连翘对照药材 0.5g，加甲醇 10ml，加热回流 20min，滤过，滤液作为对照药材溶液。照薄层色谱法试验，吸取上述两种溶液各 5μl，分别点于同一硅胶 G 薄层板上，以三氯甲烷:甲醇（5:1）为展开剂，展开，取出，晾干，喷以 10% 硫酸乙醇溶液，在 105℃加热至斑点显色清晰。在供试品色谱中，在与对照药材色谱相应的位置上，显示相同颜色的斑点。

5. 检查

（1）相对密度：应不低于 1.12。

（2）pH 值：应为 5.0～7.0。

（3）其他：应符合合剂项下有关的各项规定。

6. 含量测定

（1）黄芩

色谱条件与系统适用性试验：以十八烷基硅烷键合硅胶为填充剂；以甲醇：水：冰乙酸（50：50：1）为流动相；检测波长为274nm。理论板数按黄芩苷峰计算应不低于1500。

对照品溶液的制备：取黄芩苷对照品适量，精密称定，加50%甲醇制成每毫升含0.1mg的溶液，即得。

供试品溶液的制备：精密量取本品1ml，置50ml量瓶中，加50%甲醇适量，超声处理20min，放置至室温，加50%甲醇稀释至刻度，摇匀，即得。

测定法：分别精密吸取对照品溶液和供试品溶液各5μl，注入液相色谱仪，测定，即得。

本品每毫升含黄芩以黄芩苷（$C_{21}H_{18}O_{11}$）计，不得少于10.0mg。

（2）金银花

色谱条件与系统适用性试验：以十八烷基硅烷键合硅胶为填充剂；以甲醇：水：冰乙酸（20：80：1）为流动相；检测波长为324nm。理论板数按绿原酸峰计算应不低于6000。

对照品溶液的制备：取绿原酸对照品适量，精密称定，置棕色量瓶中，加水制成每毫升含40μg的溶液，即得。

供试品溶液的制备：精密量取本品2ml，置50ml棕色量瓶中，加水稀释至刻度，摇匀，即得。

测定法：分别精密吸取对照品溶液10μl与供试品溶液10～20μl，注入液相色谱仪，测定，即得。

本品每毫升含金银花以绿原酸（$C_{16}H_{18}O_9$）计，不得少于0.60mg。

（3）连翘

色谱条件与系统适用性试验：以十八烷基硅烷键合硅胶为填充剂；以乙腈：水（25：75）为流动相；检测波长为278nm。理论板数按连翘苷峰计算应不低于6000。

对照品溶液的制备：取连翘苷对照品适量，精密称定，加50%甲醇制成每毫升含60μg的溶液，即得。

供试品溶液的制备：精密量取本品1ml，加在中性氧化铝柱（100～120目，6g，内径为1cm）上，用70%乙醇40ml洗脱，收集洗脱液，浓缩至干，残渣加50%甲醇适量，温热使溶解，转移至5ml量瓶中，并稀释至刻度，摇匀，即得。

测定法：分别精密吸取对照品溶液与供试品溶液各10μl，注入液相色谱仪，测定，即得。

本品每毫升含连翘以连翘苷（$C_{27}H_{34}O_{11}$）计，不得少于0.30mg。

四、预习提要

（1）高效液相色谱法中如何优化色谱条件？

（2）中药制剂的含量测定可选择的方法有哪些？

（3）口服液常规检查有哪些？

五、实验指导

1. 聚酰胺薄膜层析常用于黄酮类、酚类、生物碱类、磺胺类、解热镇痛类药物及复方制剂的分析。聚酰胺是一种吸附剂，其对极性物质的吸附作用是由于其分子内存在酰胺键，可与酚类、酸类、醌类及硝基化合物等形成氢键。各化合物与聚酰胺形成氢键的能力不同，决定吸附力也不同。影响吸附力强弱的因素主要有化合物结构、展开剂的种类和聚酰胺的性质。一般来讲，在水中形成氢键的能力最强，在有机溶剂中形成氢键的能力较弱，在碱性溶剂中形成氢键能力最弱。在下列溶剂中形成氢键能力的强弱次序是：水 > 甲醇或乙醇 > 丙酮 > 稀氨水 > 二甲基甲酰胺。

聚酰胺薄膜的制备是将聚酰胺溶于甲酸或乙酸与乙醇的混合液中，涂于涤纶片基上使成一层薄膜，也可涂于清洁的玻璃片上，但涂于涤纶片基上便于保存。

2. 合剂系指饮片用水或其他溶剂，采用适宜方法提取制成的口服液体制剂（单剂量灌装者也可称口服液）。

（1）合剂在生产与贮藏期间应符合下列有关规定：

①饮片应按个品种项规定的方法提取、纯化、浓缩至一定体积。除另有规定外，含有挥发性成分的药材宜先提取挥发性成分，再与余药共同煎煮。

②根据需要可加入适宜的附加剂。在确定制剂处方时，抑菌剂的抑菌效力应符合抑菌效力检查法的规定。如需加入防腐剂，山梨酸和苯甲酸的用量不得超过 0.3%（其钾盐、钠盐的用量分别用酸计），羟苯酯类的用量不得超过 0.05%，如须加入其他附加剂，其品种与用量应符合国家标准的有关规定，不影响成品的稳定性，并应避免对检验产生干扰。必要时可加入适量的乙醇。

③合剂若加蔗糖作为附加剂，除另有规定外，含蔗糖量应不高于 20%（g/ml）。

④除另有规定外，合剂应澄清。在贮存期间不得有发霉、酸败、变色、产生气体或其他变质现象，允许有少量摇之易散的沉淀。

⑤一般应检查相对密度、pH 值等。

⑥除另有规定外，合剂应密封，于 30℃ 以下避光置干燥处贮存。

（2）除另有规定外，合剂应进行以下相应的检查程序：

①装量 单剂量灌装的合剂，照下述方法检查应符合规定。

检查法 取供试品 5 支，将内容物分别倒入经标化的干燥量入式量筒内，在室温下检视，每支装量与标示装量相比较，少于标示装量的不得多于 1 支，并不得少于标示装量的 95%。

②多剂量灌装的合剂，照最低装量检查法检查，应符合规定。

③微生物限度照非无菌产品微生物限度检查法检查，应符合规定。

六、讨论

（1）中药及其制剂的鉴别方法主要包括哪些？

（2）在中成药及中药材的薄层色谱鉴别中何时采用对照药材法？

（3）中药及其制剂含量测定项目的选定原则是什么？

（4）中药及其制剂高效液相色谱法测定的注意事项有哪些？

（5）在黄芩苷高效液相色谱含量测定中，流动相中的冰乙酸有何作用？

Experiment 16   Analysis of Shuanghuanglian Koufuye

1. Purposes

1. 1   To study the method for the identification of traditional Chinese materia medica with reference to CRS or reference drug.

1. 2   To experiment on the assay of traditional Chinese materia medica by HPLC using CRS.

2. Instruments and chemical reagents

2. 1   Instruments

Analytical balance(with an accuracy of 0. 1mg), specific gravity bottle, pH-meter, polyamide thin film, silica gel G thin layer plate, ultraviolet lamp(365nm), neutro-alumina column(100 ~ 200mesh, 6g, 1cm in internal diameter), brown volumetric flask, ultrasonic vibration instrument, erlenmeyer flask with stopper, HPLC, C_{18} column.

2. 2   Chemical reagents

Baicalin CRS, chlorogenic acid CRS, forsythin CRS, forsythin contrast drug, ethanoic acid, methanol, trichlormethane, ethanol solution with 10% sulphuric acid, water, glacial acid, acetonitrile.

3. Procedures and methods

3. 1   Ingredients

Flos Lonicerae 375g, Radix Scutellariae 375g, Fructus Forsythiae 750g.

3. 2   Procedures

Cut Radix Scutellariae into slices, decoct with water for 3 times, 2h for the first time, 1h for the second and third time respectively, combine the decoction, filter, concentrate the filtrate, adjust pH to 1. 0 ~ 2. 0 with a quantity of 2mol/L solution of hydrochloric acid at a temperature of 80℃, keep the temperature for 1h, and allow to stand for 12h, filter. Stir the precipitate in 6 ~ 8 times amount of water, adjust the pH value to 7. 0 with 40% solution of sodium hydroxide and add an equal quantity of ethanol to dissolve by stirring, filter, adjust the pH value to 2. 0 with a quantity of 2mol/L solution of hydrochloric acid at a temperature of 60℃, keep the temperature for 30min, allow to stand for 12h, filter, wash the precipitate with ethanol to pH 7. 0, and completely expel ethanol to obtain reserved extract. Macerate warmly Flos Lonicerae and Fructus Forsythiae in water for half an hour, decoct for 2 times, 1. 5h for each, combine the decoctions, filter, concentrate the filtrate to a thick extract with a relative density of 1. 20 ~ 1. 25(70 ~ 80℃), allow to cool to 40℃, gently add ethanol, stir constantly, to a content of 75% ethanol, stir thoroughly, allow to stand for 12h, filter to obtain the supernatant liquid, stir well the residue in a quantity of 75% ethanol solution, allow to stand for 12h, filter, combine the ethanol liquid, completely recover ethanol, add the above reserved extract and a quantity of water, adjust pH to 7. 0 with 40% solution of sodium hydroxide, stir well, refrigerate for 72h under 4 ~ 8℃, filter, dissolve 300g of sucrose in the filtrate by stirring, add a quantity of essence and adjust pH to 7.0, and water to produce 1000ml, stir well, allow to stand for 12h, filter, pack and sterilize.

3.3　Description

A clear, brownish-red liquid; taste, sweet and slightly bitter.

3.4　Identification

3.4.1　Mix well 1ml of the mixture with 5ml of 75% ethanol as the test solution. Dissolve respectively chlorogenic acid CRS and baicalin CRS in 75% ethanol to produce two solutions containing 0.1mg/ml as the reference solution. Carry out the method for thin layer chromatography, using polyamide film as the coating substance and acetic acid as the mobile phase. Apply separately to the film 1~2μl each of above the three solutions. After developing and removing of the film, dry it in air, and examine under ultraviolet light(365nm). The spots in the chromatogram obtained with the test solution correspond in position and color to the spots in the chromatogram obtained with the chlorogenic acid CRS. The fluorescence spots in the chromatogram obtained with the test solution correspond in position and color to those in the chromatogram obtained with the baicalin CRS.

3.4.2　Dissolve 1ml of the mixture in 5ml of methanol with shaking, and allow to stand, using the supernatant liquid as the test solution. Heat under reflux 0.5g of Fructus Forsythiae reference drug with 10ml of methanol for 20min on a water bath, filter, using the filtrate as the reference drug solution. Carry out the method for thin layer chromatography, using silica gel G containing sodium carboxymethylcellulose as the coating substance and a mixture of chloroform-methanol(5:1) as the mobile phase. Apply separately to the plate 5μl each of the above two solutions. After developing and removing of the plate, dry it in air. Spray with 10% solution of sulfuric acid in ethanol, heat at 105℃ until the spots are clear. The spots in the chromatogram obtained with the test solution correspond in position and color to those in the chromatogram obtained with the reference drug solution.

3.5　Test

Relative density　Not less than 1.12.

pH Value　5.0~7.0.

Other requirements　Comply with the general requirements for mixtures.

3.6　Assay

3.6.1　Radix Scutellariae

Carry out the method for high performance liquid chromatography.

Chromatographic system and system suitability　Use notadecylsilane bonded silica gel as the stationary phase and a mixture of methanol : water : acetic acid(50:50:1) as the mobile phase. The wavelength of detector is 274nm. The number of theoretical plates of the column is not less than 1500, calculated with reference to the peak of baicalin.

Preparation of reference solution　Weigh accurately a quantity of baicalin CRS, add a quantity of 50% methanol to obtain the solution containing 0.1mg/ml of baicalin.

Preparation of test solution　Measure accurately 1ml of the mixture, in a 50ml volumetric flask, add a quantity of 50% methanol, ultrasonic for 20min, stand to room temperature, dilute with 50% methanol to the volume and mix well.

Procedure   Inject accurately $5\mu l$ each of the reference solution and test solution into the column and measure.

It contains not less than 10. 0mg/ml of baicalin($C_{21}H_{18}O_{11}$), referring to Radix Scutellariae.

3. 6. 2   Flos Lonicerae

Carry out for the method for high performance liquid chromatography

Chromatographic system and system suitability   Use octadecylsilane bonded silica gel as the stationary phase and a mixture of methanol : water : glacial acetic acid (20: 80 : 1) as the mobile phase. The wavelength of detector is 324nm. The number of theoretical plates of the column is not less than 6000, calculated with reference to the peak of the chlorogenic acid.

Preparation of reference solution   Weigh accurately chlorogenic acid. In a 50ml brown volumetric flask, add water to obtain a solution containing $40\mu g/ml$ of chlorogenic acid.

Preparation of test solution   Measure accurately 2ml of the mixture, in a 50ml brown volumetric flask, add a quantity of water to the volume and mix well.

Procedure   Inject accurately $10\mu l$ of the reference solution and $10 \sim 20\mu l$ of the test solution into the column and measure.

It contains not less than 0. 6mg/ml of chlorgenic acid($C_{16}H_{18}O_{9}$), referring to Flos Lonicerae.

3. 6. 3   Fructus Forsythiae

Chromatographic system and system suitability   Use octadecylsilane bonded silica gel as the stationary phase and a mixture of acetonitrile : water (75 : 25) as the mobile phase. The wavelength of detector is 278nm. The number of theoretical plates of the column is not less than 6000, calculated with reference to the peak of forsythin.

Preparation of reference solution   Weigh accurately 10mg of forsythin CRS, add a quantity of 50% methanol to obtain reference solution containing $60\mu g/ml$ of forsythin.

Preparation of test solution   Measure accurately 1ml of the mixture, set it in the neutral aluminium oxide column($100 \sim 200$mesh, 6g, 1cm in interval diameter). Wash with 40ml of 70% methanol, collect eluent. Concentrate to dryness. Add a quantity of 50% methyl alcohol and warm to dissolve the residual. Transfer it to a 5ml of volumetric flask, dilute to the volume and mix well.

Procedure   Inject accurately $10\mu l$ each of the reference solution and the test solution into the column and measure.

It contains not less than 0. 30mg/ml of forsythin($C_{27}H_{34}O_{11}$), referring to Fructus Forsythise.

4. Prepare lessons before class

4. 1   How to optimize chromatographic conditions by HPLC?

4. 2   What methods can be applied to TCM assay?

4. 3   What are general tests of oral liquid?

5. Guide for experiment

5. 1   Polyamide thin film chromatography is extensively applied to the analysis of flavonoid, phenol, alkaloid, sulfanilamide, antipyretic analgesic drugs and compound preparations. Polyamide is a kind of absorbent, which can selectively absorb polarity substance, this role is attributed to amide

bonds in its molecule, and it forms hydrogen bonds with phenol, acids, quinine, and nitro compounds. It is obvious that the ability of all kinds of compounds forming hydrogen bonds with polyamide is different, and it contributes to the difference of absorption. The factors influencing absorption include the structure of compounds, different kinds of solvents and properties of polyamide. Generally speaking, the ability of forming hydrogen bonds is strongest in water, the ability of forming hydrogen bonds is relatively weaker in organic solvents and is weakest in alkaline. The ability of forming hydrogen bonds in following solvent is in a descending order: water > carbinol or ethanol > acetone > low concentration ammonia water > dimethyl formamide.

Polyamide thin film can be prepared in this way: solve polyamide to the mixture of formic acid and ethanol or the mixture of acetic acid and ethanol, and then smear it on dacron slice or clean glass. However, the latter is more likely to store.

5.2 Mixtures are liquid preparations intended for oral administration, prepared by extracting the crude drugs with water or other solvents in suitable ways(package of a single dose is also known as oral liquids).

5.2.1 The production and storage of mixtures should comply with following requirements.

a. The drugs should be extracted, purified and concentrated to a certain volume by the methods as described under individual monograph. Unless otherwise specified, the volatile ingredients in crude drugs should be extracted first, and then the remaining crude drugs are decocted with other drugs together.

b. Suitable additives may be added to mixtures. If preservatives are needed, the amount of sorbic acid and benzoic acid should not be more than 0.3% (its potassium or sodium salt should be taken by the acid amount) or the amount of p-hydroxybenzoic acid esters, not more than 0.05%. If other additives are added, the variety and quantity to be used should comply with the requirements of the national standard, without affecting the stability and interfere with the tests for mixtures. If necessary, mixtures should also contain a proper quantity of alcohol.

c. If sucrose is used as an additive in mixture, unless specified otherwise the content of it is not more than 20% (g/ml).

d. Unless otherwise specified, mixtures should be clear, with no evidence of mold contamination, rancidity, foreign matters, color changing, gas or other deterioration during storage, but a small amount of dispersible precipitates are allowed.

e. In general, relative density and pH value etc. should be determined.

f. Mixtures should be preserved in tightly closed containers and stored in a cool place under 30℃, unless specified otherwise.

5.2.2 The following relevant test should be carried out for mixture.

a. Filling variation for mixtures packed in a single dose should comply with following test.

Assay　Take 5 bottles of mixture, pour the content separately to the calibrated dry graduated cylinders, and examine at room temperature. Compare the filling volume of each pack with the labeled amount, not more than 1 bottle is less than the labeled amount, none is less than 95% of the labeled amount.

b. Mixtures filled in multiple doses should comply with the requirements stated in Minimum

Filling.

c. Microbial limit test Comply with the requirements stated under Microbial Limit Tests.

6. Discussions

6. 1　Which methods can be used to identify traditional Chinese materia medica?

6. 2　When should the reference drug be used for the thin layer chromatography identification of traditional Chinese materia medica?

6. 3　What is the principle for the assay of traditional Chinese materia medica.

6. 4　What precautions should be taken for the assay of traditional Chinese materia medica in HPLC?

6. 5　What is the effect of the acetic acid in the mobile phase in the HPLC assay of baicalin?

（许慧君）

第五章　生物样本中药物的分析

Chapter 5　Quantitation of Drugs in Biological Matrix

实验十七　兔血清中茶碱的高效液相色谱法测定

一、目的

（1）掌握血清样品的一般处理方法，熟悉血样收集方法。

（2）掌握高效液相色谱测定血清中茶碱含量的方法和步骤。

二、仪器与试药

1. 仪器

高效液相色谱仪 – 紫外检测器，微量注射器（10μl），分析天平，离心机，超声波清洗器，氮吹仪，微量移液器（1000μl、100μl），涡旋混合振荡器，量瓶（100ml、10ml），量筒（500ml），离心管（5ml、1.5ml），吸液头（1000μl、100μl），移液管（5ml、1ml）。

2. 试药

茶碱水溶液（17.5mg/ml）、茶碱对照品、1,3 – 二硝基苯对照品、乙酸乙酯（AR.）、磷酸氢二钠（AR.）、盐酸（AR.）、三氯甲烷（AR.）、甲醇（HPLC）、二次重蒸水。

三、实验方法

1. 药物简介

茶碱，即1,3 – 二甲基 – 3,7 – 二氢 – 1H – 嘌呤 – 2,6 – 二酮一水合物，分子式为$C_7H_8N_4O_2 \cdot H_2O$，相对分子质量为198.18。白色结晶性粉末，易溶于氢氧化钾溶液或氨溶液，微溶于乙醇或三氯甲烷；几乎不溶于乙醚。

1,3 – 二硝基苯（内标），分子式为$C_6H_4N_2O_4$，相对分子质量为168.11。

2. 样本来源及取样方法

取体重约为2.5 kg的健康家兔，从颈静脉（或耳静脉）取血约2ml，放置，待凝固后离心，分取空白血清。然后从耳静脉快速注射茶碱水溶液（17.5mg/ml）1ml，分别于给药后5、15、30 min 及1、2、3、4、6、8、10、12h 采集颈静脉（或耳静脉）血2ml，放置，离心（3500 rpm）10 min，分离血清，于 −20℃ 冷冻保存、待测。

3. 标准溶液的制备

（1）茶碱对照品溶液　精密称取茶碱对照品100mg，置100ml 量瓶中，用水溶解，并稀释制成每毫升含1000μg 的标准储备液，精密量取茶碱标准储备液适量，用水稀释制成浓度分别为2.0、5.0、10.0、20.0、30.0、40.0、50.0 和 100.0μg/ml 的茶碱标准系列溶液，4℃冷藏。

（2）1，3−二硝基苯内标溶液　精密称取1，3−二硝基苯对照品10mg，置100ml 量瓶中，用乙酸乙酯溶解，并定量稀释制成每毫升含100μg 的储备溶液；精密量取该溶液1ml，置100ml 量瓶中，用乙酸乙酯稀释至刻度配成1μg/ml 的标准溶液，4℃冷藏。

4. 茶碱血清样品处理

取冷冻的血清样品，在37℃水浴下解冻，精密吸取100μl，置10ml 具塞离心管中，加水100μl，混匀，在38℃的水浴中保温30min，精密加入1，3−二硝基苯内标溶液1ml，涡旋混合3min，离心，分取上层有机相0.8ml，置于另一干燥塑料离心管中，于50℃水浴中氮气流吹干，残渣加100μl 流动相涡旋溶解，离心，取上清液5μl 进样。

5. 方法学验证

（1）标准曲线　取空白血清100μl，分别置10ml 离心管中，精密加入每毫升含茶碱2、5、10、20、30、40、50 与100μg 的标准溶液各0.1ml，旋涡混合3s，在38℃水浴中保温30min，按"茶碱血清样品处理"项自"精密加入1，3−二硝基苯内标溶液1ml"起，同法处理，进样5μl，记录色谱图。以茶碱血清浓度为横坐标，茶碱与内标的峰面积比值为纵坐标，用加权（$w = 1/x^2$）最小二乘法进行回归运算，求得的直线回归方程即为标准曲线。

（2）方法精密度与准确度　取空白血清100μl，按"标准曲线"项下的方法制成低、中、高三个浓度（茶碱浓度分别为2.0、30.0 和 100.0μg/ml）的质量控制（QC）样品，每一浓度进行5样本分析，根据标准曲线，计算QC 样品中茶碱的实测浓度。根据QC 样品的茶碱实测浓度计算本法的精密度与准确度。

（3）回收率　精密吸取空白血清100μl，按"标准曲线"项下方法制成低、中、高三个浓度（茶碱浓度分别为2.0μg/ml、30.0μg/ml 和 100.0μg/ml）的QC 样品，每一浓度进行5样本分析。同时，取空白血清100μl，除不加茶碱标准溶液和内标溶液外，其他按"茶碱血清样品的处理"项下的方法操作，向获得的上清液中加入相应浓度的茶碱标准溶液适量和内标溶液1.0ml，制成茶碱的浓度分别为2.0、30.0 和 100.0μg/ml 的低、中、高浓度的对照样品各两份，5μl 进样分析，获得相应峰面积（三次测定的平均值）。以每一浓度两种处理方法的峰面积比值计算提取回收率。

6. 茶碱血药浓度测定

照高效液相色谱法测定。

（1）色谱条件与系统适用性试验　用十八烷基硅烷键合硅胶为填充剂；流动相为甲醇：水（50：50）；流速1.0ml/min；检测波长254nm。取空白血清样品和"标准曲线"项下标准血清样品（30.0μg/ml）分别测定，茶碱与1，3−二硝基苯的分离度应符合规定，理论板数按茶碱峰计算应不低于3000；在空白血清样品色谱中，在茶碱与内标位置应没有干扰峰。

（2）测定法　取含药血清样品供试液 5μl，注入液相色谱仪，记录色谱图，按内标法用标准曲线计算即得。

四、预习提要

（1）血清和血浆样品有何区别？如何制备血清样品？

（2）在实验前应熟悉抽血技术，如何收集家兔的血样？

（3）血清样品为何要在 38℃ 水浴中保温 30min？在萃取溶剂挥干并用流动相复溶时，为何要离心后进样？

（4）试述血浆样品液液萃取的常用溶剂和注意事项。

五、实验指导

（1）茶碱用于治疗支气管哮喘及其他呼吸不正常的疾病，近代医学用于早产婴儿的窒息。茶碱的治疗血药浓度较窄（5～20μg/ml），血浓高于 25μg/ml 时，常出现中毒症状。服用同剂量茶碱的患者之间的治疗效果有显著差异，与血药浓度有关，因此须进行临床用药监护。血清中茶碱用乙酸乙酯提取、挥干，以流动相复溶后，以 HPLC 分离，以内标法进行定量。

（2）血液采集好之后，由于激活了一系列凝血因子，血中的纤维蛋白原形成纤维蛋白，血液逐渐凝固，上层析出的黄色液体称为血清。血液这种自然凝结的过程在室温高时较快，室温低时则较慢，此时可将其置 37℃ 水浴中加速血清析出。分离血清时，可将凝结后的血液置离心机中离心，上层液即为血清。空白血清可由几只健康家兔的血清混合而得。

（3）色谱系统应符合测定要求，即茶碱、内标物及血清中其他干扰物质应有效分离，其分离度应大于 1.5。定量时，若峰形对称，则可以峰高作为峰响应值。内标溶液亦可使用相同浓度的非那西丁溶液。

（4）液－液萃取法是传统的分离、纯化方法。多数药物是亲脂的，在有机溶剂中的溶解度大于在水相中的溶解度，而血样中的内源性杂质多为强极性的水溶物质，因而用有机溶剂提取可除去大部分内源性杂质。应用液－液提取法时要考虑所选有机溶剂的特性、有机溶剂相和水相的体积及水相的 pH 值等。

（5）液－液提取的浓集方法主要有两种，一种方法是在每次提取时加入的提取液尽量少，使被测组分提取到小体积溶剂中，然后直接吸出适量供测定。另一种方法是挥去提取溶剂法，挥去溶剂时应避免直接加热，防止被测组分破坏或挥发损失。挥去提取溶剂的常用方法是直接通入氮气流吹干；对于易随气流挥发或遇热不稳定的药物，可采用减压法挥去溶剂。

（6）溶剂蒸发所用的试管，底部应为尖锥形，这样可使最后数微升溶剂集中在管尖，便于量取。

（7）在萃取溶剂挥干并用流动相复溶时，常会出现混浊物质（脂肪类物质）。此时，应离心后取上清液进样，以保护色谱柱。

六、讨论

（1）血药浓度测定时，样品预处理方法有哪些？各有何特点？

（2）试述高效液相色谱内标法定量的优点。

（3）在 HPLC 测定血清样品时，应注意哪些基本实验条件及操作注意点？

（4）体内样品的方法学验证主要有哪些内容？

Experiment 17 Determination of Theophylline in Rabbit's Serum by HPLC

1. Purposes

1. 1   To learn the serum sample treatment method and to familiarize with the blood sample collection method.

1. 2   To learn the experiment on the determination of theophylline in rabbit serum.

2. Instruments and chemical Reagents

2. 1   Instruments

HPLC-UV, microliter syringe ($10\mu l$), analytical balance, centrifuge, ultrasonic cleaning instrument, micropipettor($1000\mu l$, $100\mu l$), vortex mixer, volumetric flask(100ml, 10ml), graduated cylinder(500ml), centrifuge tube(5ml, 1. 5ml), pipette tips($1000\mu l$, $100\mu l$), transfer pipette(5ml, 1ml).

2. 2   Chemical reagents

Theophylline aqueous solution (17. 5mg/ml), theophylline reference substance (RS), 1, 3-dinitrobenzene RS, ethyl acetate(AR.), disodium hydrogen phosphate(AR.), hydrochloric acid(AR.), chloroform(AR.), methanol(HPLC), deionized water.

3. Procedures and methods

3. 1   Introduction

Theophylline is 1, 3 – dimethyl – 3, 7 – dihydrogen – 1H – purine – 2, 6 – diketone monohydrate. The molecular formula is $C_7H_8N_4O_2 \cdot H_2O$. The molecular weight is 198. 18. A white crystal powder, is freely soluble in potassium hydroxide solution or ammonia solution, sparingly soluble in ethanol or trichloromethane and mostly dissolved in ethyl ether.

The molecular formula of 1, 3-dinitrobenzene (IS) is $C_6H_4N_2O_4$ and the molecular weight is 168. 11.

3. 2   Sample collection

A 2. 0ml blood sample was drawn from jugular vein(or marginal ear vein)of the healthy rabbits weighing about 2. 5kg. After 15min for complete clotting, blood sample was centrifuged and the blank serum was transferred to a clean glass vial. The rabbits were given quickly a volume of 1ml theophylline aqueous solution (17. 5mg/ml) from marginal ear vein. Blood samples (2. 0ml) were collected at 5min, 15min, 30min and 1h, 2h, 3h, 4h, 6h, 8h, 10h and 12h post dosing, transferred to tubes and standed for 15min. Following centrifugation (3500rpm, 10min), serum samples were transferred to properly labeled tubes and stored at −20℃ prior to analysis.

3. 3　Standard solutions preparation

Standard solutions of theophylline　Weigh about 100mg of theophylline RS, accurately, to a 100ml volumetric flask, dissolve and dilute with water to volume and mix to prepare stock solution of theophylline(1000μg/ml). The stock solution is further diluted with water to obtain standard solutions of 2. 0μg/ml, 5. 0μg/ml, 10. 0μg/ml, 20. 0μg/ml, 30. 0μg/ml, 40. 0μg/ml, 50. 0μg/ml and 100. 0μg/ml. The stock and standard solutions are all stored at 4℃ in the refrigerator.

Standard solutions of 1, 3-dinitrobenzene(IS)　Weigh about 10mg of 1, 3-dinitrobenzene RS, accurately, to a 100ml volumetric flask, dissolve and dilute with ethyl acetate to volume, and mix to prepare stock solution of 1, 3-dinitrobenzene(100μg/ml). The stock solution is further diluted with ethyl acetate to obtain standard solution of 1. 0μg/ml. Keep at 4℃ for further use.

3. 4　Theophylline serum sample preparation

Thaw the frozen serum sample under 37℃ water bath. Transfer accurately 100μl of serum sample to a 10ml centrifuge tube and keep at 38℃ in water bath for 30 minutes. Then, add accurately 1. 0ml of IS standard solution, vortex the mixture for 3 minute and centrifuge at 4000 rpm for 10min. Transfer 0. 8ml of the ethyl acetate phase and evaporate it to dryness in a 50℃ water bath under a gentle stream of nitrogen. The residues are reconstituted in 100μl of the mobile phase and 5μl is injected into the HPLC system after centrifugation.

3. 5　Method validation

Calibration curve　To each of 100μl of blank serum in 10ml centrifuge tubes, add 1. 0ml of a series of theophylline standard solution 2μg/ml, 5μg/ml, 10μg/ml, 20μg/ml, 30μg/ml, 40μg/ml, 50μg/ml and 100. 0μg/ml, respectively. Then, keep them at 38℃ for heat preservation for 30 minutes and process them in the same way as directed under the "Theophylline serum sample preparation" beginning with "add accurately 1. 0ml of IS standard solution". And then 5μl samples are injected and the chromatograms are recorded. The calibration curve is constructed by plotting the peak area ratios of each analyte to the IS versus the concentration using weighed linear least square regression.

Precision and accuracy　To each of the 10ml centrifuge tubes, add accurately 100μl of blank serum. The quality control (QC) samples are prepared according to "Calibration curve" at concentrations of 2. 0μg/ml, 30. 0μg/ml and 100. 0μg/ml(5 replicates at each concentration). The concentrations of theophylline in QC samples are calculated according to calibration curve. The precision and accuracy are determined with the analyzed concentration of the QC samples.

Recovery　QC samples at 2. 0μg/ml, 30. 0μg/ml and 100. 0μg/ml of 5 replicates are prepared according to "Calibration curve". Meanwhile, the corresponding samples are prepared by adding the theophylline standard solutions and IS post extraction (n = 2). The recovery of theophylline is determined by comparing the peak area of the analytes in serum samples that have been spiked with the analytes prior to extraction with those of the samples to which the analytes have been added post-extraction.

3.6 Determination of Theophylline in serum

According to the method of high performance liquid chromatography.

System suitability　The HPLC separations are performed on an ODS C_{18} column. The mobile phase is methanol : water (50 : 50). The flow rate is 1.0ml/min. The wavelength is set up at 254nm. The blank serum sample and the calibration curve solution which contains 30.0μg/ml theophylline are determined, separately, and the peak responses are recorded. The resolution between theophylline and IS complies with the related requirements, and the number of theoretical plates of the column is not less than 3000, calculated with reference to the peak of theophylline. There is no interference in the blank serum sample chromatogram at the retention time of theophylline and IS.

Determination　A portion of the supernatant (5μl) is injected into HPLC system and the chromatogram is recorded. The concentration of theophylline is calculated according to calibration curve by internal standard method.

4. Prepare lessons before class

4.1　What is the difference between serum sample and plasma sample? How to prepare the serum sample?

4.2　How to be familiar with the blood sample collection technique and how to collect rabbit blood sample?

4.3　Why is the serum sample put under 38℃ for heat preservation for 30 minutes? Why are the solutions centrifuged before being injected into the HPLC system when the residues are reconstituted in 100μl of the mobile phase?

4.4　Depict precautions for the liquid-liquid extraction of plasma sample.

5. Guide for experimental

5.1　Theophylline is commonly used in medicine, such as treatment of bronchial asthma and other abnormal respiratory diseases. Premature infant asphyxia is treated with theophylline in modern medicine. Its therapeutic index is very narrow(5 ~ 20μg/ml)and toxic symptom often appears when blood concentrations of theophylline is higher than 25μg/ml. Furthermore, there is significant difference in therapeutic effect between patients with the same dosage, which is related to blood concentration. So, theophylline should be cared and monitored in clinical practice. Theophylline in serum is extracted with ethyl acetate then evaporated and the residues are reconstituted in the mobile phase. The samples are separated and quantified with internal standard method of HPLC.

5.2　Fibrinogen forms in fibrin in blood and blood coagulates gradually because a series of coagulation factors are activated after blood sample collection, the yellow fluid in upper layer precipitate is serum. Spontaneous clotting occures quickly at high temperature but slowly at low temperature. Serum precipitate is accelerated at 37℃ water bath.

5.3　The chromatographic system should meet the determination requirements, that is theophylline, IS and other interferences in serum should be separated effectively and the resolution should be more than 1.5. The peak height is as peak response value if the peak shape is symmetry. The same concentration of phenacetin can also be used as IS.

5.4 Most drugs are lipophilic and more soluble in organic solvent than in water. However, most of the endogenous interferences are water-soluble, so the organic solvent extraction may remove most of the interferences. The properties of organic solvent, the volume of organic solvent and water, and the pH should all be taken into consideration during the process of extraction.

5.5 There are two major methods for the enrichment in liquid-liquid extraction. One method is to use as little volume of solvent as possible in the last extraction so that the determined component could be extracted into a relatively smaller volume. Then the sample may be analyzed directly. The other method is the evaporation of solvent. Direct heating should be avoided in case of destructing or evaporating of the determined components. Stream of nitrogen is a popular choice for solvent evaporation; evaporation under reduced pressure is adopted for components with volatility or thermal instability.

5.6 Tubes with a conical bottom should be used for evaporation in order to concentrate and collect the sample.

5.7 The solution often appears turbidity for containing lipids when extraction solvent is evaporated and reconstituted in the mobile phase. The solution should be centrifuged and the supernatant is injected into HPLC in order to protect the column.

6. Discussion

6.1 What's the method used for pretreatment of samples when determinating the blood concentration? What are the respective characteristics of them?

6.2 What are the advantages of internal standard method of HPLC?

6.3 Which basic experimental conditions and important points of operation should we pay attention to when the concentration of theophylline in serum samples is determined by HPLC?

6.4 What are the contents of methodology validation for biological sample analysis?

(赵云丽)

实验十八 阿司匹林代谢产物水杨酸的血浆浓度测定

一、目的

（1）掌握有机溶剂沉淀法处理血浆的方法。
（2）掌握阿司匹林血浆样品中水杨酸测定的方法和步骤。

二、仪器与试药

1. 仪器

高效液相色谱仪 - 紫外检测器，微量注射器（20μl），分析天平，离心机，超声波清洗器，微量移液器（1000μl、200μl、10μl），涡旋混合振荡器，量瓶（100ml、10ml），量筒

（500ml），离心管（10ml、1.5ml），吸液头（1000μl、200μl、10μl），移液管（5ml、1ml）。

2. 试药

阿司匹林片（500毫克/片）、水杨酸对照品、2-甲基苯甲酸对照品、肝素、磷酸（AR.）、氯化钠（AR.）、盐酸（AR.）、乙腈（HPLC）、去离子水。

三、实验方法

1. 药物简介

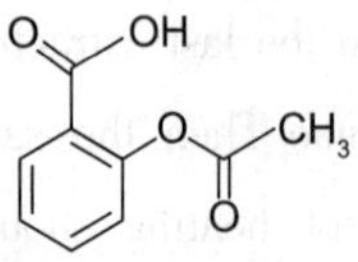

阿司匹林，即2-（乙酰氧基）苯甲酸，又名乙酰水杨酸，分子式为$C_9H_8O_4$，相对分子质量为180.16。白色结晶或结晶粉末，易溶于乙醇，在三氯甲烷或乙醚中溶解，微溶于水或无水乙醚；在氢氧化钠溶液或碳酸钠溶液中溶解，但同时分解。阿司匹林口服后迅速自胃和小肠上段吸收，在吸收过程中水解为水杨酸，从而以水杨酸的形式发挥药效。

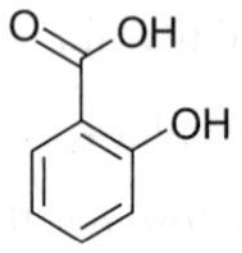

水杨酸，即2-羟基苯甲酸，分子式为$C_7H_6O_3$，相对分子质量为138.12。易溶于乙醇或乙醚中，在沸水中溶解，微溶于水。

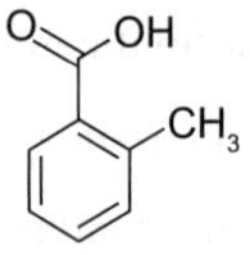

2-甲基苯甲酸（内标），分子式为$C_8H_8O_2$，相对分子质量为136.15。

2. 样本来源及取样方法

受试者隔夜禁食10h，于实验当日晨单次空腹口服阿司匹林片1片，剂量为500mg，200ml温开水送服。试验2h后可适量饮水，4h后进统一清淡午餐。在给药前（0h）及给药后3.0、4.0、5.0、6.0、8.0、10、12、14、16、24、36h分别抽取肘静脉血3ml，置肝素化试管中，混匀，离心（3500 rpm）10min，分离血浆，于-20℃冷冻保存、待测。

3. 标准溶液的制备

（1）水杨酸标准溶液　精密称取水杨酸对照品100mg，置100ml量瓶中，用乙腈溶解，并稀释制成每毫升含1000μg的标准储备液，精密量取水杨酸标准储备液适量，用乙腈稀释制成浓度为0.5、1.0、2.0、5.0、10.0、20.0和50.0μg/ml。水杨酸标准系列溶液，4℃冷藏。

（2）2-甲基苯甲酸内标溶液　精密称取2-甲基苯甲酸对照品10mg，置100ml量瓶中，用乙腈溶解，并定量稀释制成每毫升含100μg的标准储备溶液，4℃冷藏。

4. 样本处理

取冷冻的血浆样品，在冰水浴中解冻，精密吸取200μl，置1.5ml离心管中，精密加入2-甲基苯甲酸内标溶液10μl，加入0.5mol/L盐酸100μl和乙腈400μl，涡旋1min，4℃放置15min后4℃下12000r/min离心10min，分取上清液转移至含有100mg氯化钠的

1.5ml 的塑料离心管中，涡旋 5s，4℃放置 10min 后 12000r/min 离心 10min，取上清液 10μl 进样。

5. 方法学验证

（1）标准曲线　取空白血浆 200μl，分别置 1.5ml 离心管中，精密加入水杨酸标准溶液适量，配制成水杨酸的浓度分别为 0、0.5、1.0、2.0、5.0、10.0、20.0 和 50.0μg/ml 标准系列血浆样品。按"样品处理"项下，自"精密加入 2 - 甲基苯甲酸内标溶液 10μl"起，同法处理，进样 10μl，记录色谱图。以水杨酸血浆浓度为横坐标，水杨酸与内标的峰面积比值为纵坐标，用加权最小二乘法进行回归运算，求得的直线回归方程即为标准曲线。

（2）回收率　精密吸取空白血浆 200μl，按"标准曲线"项下方法制成低、中、高三个浓度（水杨酸浓度分别 0.5、5.0 和 50.0μg/ml）的 QC 样品，每一浓度进行 5 样本分析。同时，取空白血浆 200μl，除不加水杨酸标准溶液和内标溶液外，其他按"样品的处理"项下的方法操作向获得的上清液中加入相应浓度的水杨酸标准溶液适量和内标溶液 10μl，制成水杨酸的浓度分别为 0.5、5.0 和 50.0μg/ml 的低、中、高浓度的对照样品各 2 份，10μl 进样分析，获得相应峰面积（三次测定的平均值）。以每一浓度两种处理方法的峰面积比值计算回收率。

（3）精密度与准确度　取空白市售血浆 200μl，按"标准曲线"项下的方法制成低、中、高三个浓度（水杨酸浓度分别 0.5、5.0 和 50.0μg/ml）的质量控制（QC）样品，每一浓度进行 5 样本分析，根据标准曲线，计算 QC 样品中水杨酸的实测浓度。根据 QC 样品的水杨酸实测浓度计算本法的精密度与准确度。

6. 水杨酸血药浓度测定

（1）色谱条件与系统适用性试验　用十八烷基硅烷键合硅胶为填充剂；流动相为 0.1% 磷酸：乙腈（80：20）；流速 1ml/min；检测波长 237nm。取空白血浆样品和"标准曲线"项下标准血浆样品（50.0μg /ml）分别测定，水杨酸与 2 - 甲基苯甲酸的分离度应符合规定，理论板数按水杨酸峰计算应不低于 3000；在空白血浆样品色谱中，在水杨酸与内标位置应没有干扰峰。

（2）测定法　取含药血浆样品供试液 10μl，注入液相色谱仪，记录色谱图，按内标法，用标准曲线计算即得。

四、预习提要

（1）阿司匹林和水杨酸的化学性质稳定吗？为何在冰水浴中解冻血浆样品？
（2）为何选择测定水杨酸的浓度而不是直接测定阿司匹林的浓度？
（3）试述乙腈直接沉淀法处理血浆样品时注意事项。

五、实验指导

（1）阿司匹林是止痛、抗感染和退热的药物，小剂量的阿司匹林可以作为抗血栓剂。阿司匹林是酯类化合物，不稳定，在人体内能迅速分解为活性代谢物——水杨酸，水杨酸进一步被羟基化代谢为龙胆酸，龙胆酸与体内结合物生成水杨酰甘氨酸或其他结合物。在测定血浆中阿司匹林的浓度时须考虑两个问题：一是阿司匹林在水、甲醇和血浆中能迅速分解为水杨酸，37℃时阿司匹林在血浆中的 $t_{1/2}$ 只为 1h；二是阿司匹林在水中的分解速率取决于溶液的 pH，pH 为 2~3 时阿司匹林的稳定性较好。所以在处理血浆样品时，样品在冰水浴中解冻，加入 0.5mol/L 盐酸 100μl 调节 pH，上清液中加入氯化钠吸收乙腈中的少量水分，都是为了减少阿司匹林的分解量。

（2）传统的分离、纯化方法有直接沉淀法、液–液萃取法和液–固萃取法，阿司匹林在中性溶液或亲质子化的溶剂中易分解为水杨酸，使水杨酸的测定结果偏高，而且在浓缩溶液时水杨酸升华会造成部分损失。水杨酸经乙腈沉淀蛋白后直接进样分析，简便、快速、灵敏度、准确度和精密度较高，而且阿司匹林样品稳定。在分离、纯化样品时，整个操作过程在低温（4℃）下进行，实验中要注意控制温度。操作要迅速，尽量减少阿司匹林的降解量。

六、讨论

（1）同时测定生物样本中的原药和代谢物时，应注意什么问题？

（2）常用于直接沉淀法处理血浆的溶剂有哪些？简述各自的用量和优缺点。

Experiment 18　Determination of Salicylic Acid(SA), Metabolite of Aspirin(ASA) in Human's Plasma by HPLC

1. Purposes

1.1　To learn about the methods for organic solvent precipitation on human plasma processing.

1.2　To learn the experiment on the determination of salicylic acid in human plasma.

2. Instruments and chemical reagents

2.1　Instruments

HPLC-UV, microliter syringe (20μl), analytical balance, centrifuge, ultrasonic cleaning instrument, micropipettor (1000μl, 200μl, 10μl), vortex mixer, volumetric flask (100ml, 10ml), graduated cylinder (500ml), centrifuge tube (10ml, 1.5ml), pipette tips (1000μl, 200μl, 10μl), transfer pipette (5ml, 1ml).

2.2　Chemical reagents

Aspirin tablets (500mg/tablet), salicylic acid reference substance (RS), 2 – methyl benzoic acid RS, heparin, phosphoric acid (AR.), sodium chloride (AR.), hydrochloric acid (AR.), acetonitrile (HPLC), deionized water.

3. Procedures and methods

3.1　Introduction

Aspirin (ASA) is 2 – acetoxybenzoic acid, also known as acetylsalicylic acid. The molecular formula is $C_9H_8O_4$. The molecular weight is 180. 16. As a white crystal or almost white crystal powder, aspirin is freely soluble in ethanol, soluble in trichloromethane or ether, sparingly soluble in water or anhydrous ether. Aspirin is dissolved in sodium hydroxide solution or sodium carbonate solution but hydrolysed to salicylic acid simultaneously. Aspirin is rapidly absorbed from the upper section of the stomach and small intestine after oral and hydrolyzed to salicylic acid in the absorption process, thus playing efficacy in the form of salicylic acid.

Salicylic acid (SA) is 2 – hydroxybenzoic acid. The molecular formula is $C_7H_6O_3$. The molecular weight is 138. 12. Freely soluble in ethanol or ether, soluble in boiling water, sparingly soluble in water.

The molecular formula of 2 – methyl benzoic acid (MBA, IS) is $C_8H_8O_2$ and the molecular weight is 136. 15.

3. 2　Sample collection

Following overnight fasting (at least 10 hours), the subjects should be administered a single dose, 500mg of ASA with 200ml warm water in the morning. Subjects can drink water after 2 hours and have standard meal after 4 hours of administration. Blood samples (3ml) are withdrawn from the forearm vein at 0h, 3. 0h, 4. 0h, 5. 0h, 6. 0h, 8. 0h, 10h, 12h, 14h, 16h, 24h and 36h post dosing, transferred to heparinized tubes and centrifuged. Following centrifugation (3500rpm, 10min), plasma samples are transferred to properly labeled tubes and stored at $-20℃$ prior to analysis.

3. 3　Standard solutions preparation

Standard solutions of SA　Weigh about 100mg of salicylic acid RS, accurately, to a 100ml volumetric flask, dissolve and dilute with acetonitrile to volume and mix to prepare stock solution of SA (1000μg/ml). Keep at 4℃ for future use. The stock solution was further diluted with acetonitrile to obtain standard solutions of 0. 5μg/ml, 1. 0μg/ml, 2. 0μg/ml, 5. 0μg/ml, 10. 0μg/ml, 20. 0μg/ml and 50. 0μg/ml. The standard solutions are stored at 4℃ in the refrigerator.

Standard solutions of MBA (IS)　Weigh about 10mg of 2-methyl benzoic acid RS, accurately, to a 100ml volumetric flask, dissolve and dilute with acetonitrile to volume, and mix to prepare stock solutions of MBA (100μg/ml). Keep at 4℃ for further use.

3. 4　Aspirin plasma sample preparation

Thaw the frozen plasma sample in an ice-water bath. Transfer accurately 200μl of it to a 1. 5ml microcentrifuge tube and add accurately 10μl of MBA standard solution. Then add 100μl of 0. 5mol/L hydrochloric acid and 400μl of acetonitrile. Vortex the mixture for 1 minute and keep at 4℃ for 15 minutes. Then centrifuge at 12000rpm for 10min at 4℃. Add 0. 1g of sodium chloride to the supernatant and vortex for 5s and place at 4℃ for 10min before centrifuging at 12000rpm for 10 min at 4℃. 10μl of the supernatant is injected into the HPLC system for the determination of SA.

3.5 Method validation

Calibration curve   To each of 200μl of blank plasma in 1.5ml microcentrifuge tubes, add a suitable quantity of SA standard solution to make the concentrations of SA to be 0μg/ml, 0.5μg/ml, 1.0μg/ml, 2.0μg/ml, 5.0μg/ml, 10.0μg/ml, 20.0μg/ml and 50.0μg/ml, respectively. Then process them in the same way as directed under the "Aspirin plasma sample preparation" beginning with "add accurately 10μl of MBA standard solution". And then 10μl sample is injected and the chromatograms are recorded. The calibration curve is constructed by plotting the peak area ratios of each analyte to the IS versus the concentration using weighed linear least square regression.

Recovery   QC samples at 0.5μg/ml, 5.0μg/ml and 50.0μg/ml of 5 replicates were prepared according to "Calibration curve". Meanwhile, the corresponding samples were prepared by adding the SA standard solutions and MBA(IS) post extraction($n = 2$). The recovery of SA is determined by comparing the peak area of the analytes in plasma samples that had been spiked with the analytes prior to extraction with those of the samples to which the analytes had been added post-extraction.

Precision and accuracy   To each of the 1.5ml microcentrifuge tubes, add accurately 200μl of blank plasma. The quality control (QC) samples are prepared according to "Calibration curve" at concentrations of 0.5μg/ml, 5.0μg/ml and 50.0μg/ml (5 replicates at each concentration). The concentrations of SA in QC samples are calculated according to calibration curve. The precision and accuracy are determined with the analyzed concentration of the QC samples.

3.6 Determination of SA in plasma

Chromatographic condition and system suitability   The HPLC separations are performed on a C_{18} column. The mobile phase is 0.1% phosphoric acid : acetonitrile(80 : 20). The flow rate was 1.0ml/min. The wavelength is set at 237nm. The blank plasma sample and the calibration curve solution which contains 50.0μg/ml SA, are injected into HPLC separately, recording the peak responses. The resolution between SA and MBA complies with the related requirements, and the number of theoretical plates of the column is not less than 3000, calculated with reference to the peak of SA. There is no interference at the position of SA and MBA in the blank plasma sample chromatogram.

Test mothod   A portion of plasma sample for test solution(10μl) is injected into HPLC system and the chromatogram was recorded. The concentration of SA is calculated according to calibration curve by internal standard method.

4. Prepare lessons before class

4.1   What are the chemical properties of ASA and SA? Why is the frozen plasma sample thawed in the ice-water bath?

4.2   Why determining the concentration of salicylic acid is chosen instead of direct determination of the concentration of aspirin?

4.3   Depict precautions for acetonitrile direct precipitation method of preparation for the plasma sample.

5. Guide for experiment

5.1   Acetylsalicylic acid (ASA) is widely used as an analgesic, anti-inflammatory and antipyretic drug. In addition, low-dose ASA is employed as an anti-thrombotic agent. ASA is rapidly hydrolysed in vivo to salicylic acid (SA) which is also active. SA is further metabolized by hydroxylation to gentisic acid (GA), and by conjugation to salicyluric acid (SUA) and other conjugates. Two problems are associated with the HPLC analysis of ASA and SA in biological fluids. Firstly, ASA hydrolyses to SA in protic solvents such as water or methanol, and also in plasma. The half-life of ASA, when incubated in plasma at 37℃, is about one hour. In water the rate of hydrolysis is dependent on pH with best stability of ASA at pH 2 ~ 3. In order to decrease the degradation of ASA in plasma samples, the samples should be thawed in an ice-water bath, adjust pH to 2 ~ 3 by adding 100μl of 0.5mol/L hydrochloric acid to samples and absorb a little moisture in acetonitrile by adding 100mg sodium chloride to the supernatant.

5.2   The most widely employed biological sample preparation method currently are protein precipitation (PPT), liquid-liquid extraction (LLE) and solid phase extraction (SPE). ASA is hydrolysed easily to SA in neutral aqueous solution or other protic solvents, which has an influence on the determination of SA. Furthermore, partial loss of SA by sublimation is observed during evaporation of the organic solvent. The method described above is outstanding with respect to simplicity in sample treatment and combined with stability of ASA in the samples waiting for injection. The whole operation process should be carried out at 4℃ and the temperature should be controlled. The operation must be fast in order to make less degradation of ASA.

6. Discussions

6.1   What should we pay attention to when the drug and its metabolite are determined simultaneously?

6.2   What are the common solvents used in precipitation pretreatment? And how about their volume ratio, advantage and disadvantage?

(赵云丽)

实验十九　高效液相色谱法测定尿液中苯巴比妥的浓度

一、目的

（1）掌握固相萃取法处理生物样品的方法。

（2）掌握尿液样本的采集方法，以及尿液累积排泄率的计算方法。

（3）掌握高效液相色谱仪测定尿液中苯巴比妥浓度的方法和步骤。

二、仪器与试药

1. 仪器

高效液相色谱仪，C_{18}固相萃取小柱，分析天平，高速离心机，超声波清洗器，微量移液器（1000μl、200μl），涡旋混合振荡器，量瓶（100ml、10ml），量筒（500ml），离心管（5ml、2ml），吸液头（1000μl、100μl）、移液管（5ml、1ml），微量注射器（10μl）。

2. 试药

苯巴比妥片、空白尿液、苯巴比妥对照品、异戊巴比妥对照品、甲醇（AR.）、甲醇（HPLC）、去离子水。

三、实验方法

1. 药物简介

苯巴比妥，即5－乙基－5－苯基－2，4，6（1H，3H，5H）－嘧啶三酮，分子式为$C_{12}H_{12}N_2O_3$，相对分子质量为232.24。为白色或类白色的结晶粉末或无色晶体。在乙醇或乙醚中溶解，在水中极微溶解，在氢氧化钠或碳酸溶液中溶解。

异戊巴比妥（内标），即5－乙基－5－（3－甲基丁基）－2，4，6（1H，3H，5H）－嘧啶三酮，分子式$C_{11}H_{18}N_2O_3$，相对分子质量226.28。白色或类白色结晶粉末。在乙醇或乙醚中易溶，在二氯甲烷中溶解，在水中极微溶解，在氢氧化钠或碳酸钠溶液中溶解。

2. 样本来源及取样方法

受试者隔夜禁食10h，收集给药前的尿液作为空白对照；于实验当日晨单次空腹口服苯巴比妥片一片，剂量为30mg，200ml温开水送服。服药2h后可适量饮水，4h后进统一清淡午餐，收集给药后0～2h，2～4h，4～6h，6～8h，8～12h，12～24h和24～48h尿液，准确测量体积，滤过，于－20℃冷冻保存、待测。

3. 标准溶液

苯巴比妥标准溶液　精密称取苯巴比妥对照品100mg，置100ml量瓶中，用甲醇溶解，并稀释制成每毫升含1000μg的标准储备液，精密量取苯巴比妥标准储备液适量，用水稀释制成浓度分别为1.0、2.0、4.0、10.0、20.0和40.0μg/ml的苯巴比妥标准系列溶液，4℃冷藏。

异戊巴比妥内标溶液　精密称取异戊巴比妥对照品10mg，置100ml量瓶中，用甲醇溶解，并稀释制成每毫升含100μg的储备溶液；精密量取该溶液10ml，置100ml量瓶中，用水稀释至刻度配成10μg/ml的标准溶液，4℃冷藏。

4. 苯巴比妥尿液样品处理

取冷冻的尿液样品，在37℃水浴下解冻，经适当稀释后精密吸取500μl，置10ml离心管中，精密加入内标溶液 50μl，精密加入空白甲醇溶液 50μl（如果是 QC 样品，替换为 50μl 相应浓度的系列对照品溶液），涡旋 10s 混匀待用；另取固相萃取小柱（3ml），用 3ml 甲醇活化，再用 3ml 纯化水清洗，上尿液样品过柱，用 3ml 纯化水清洗血浆内源性杂质，通空气干燥小柱，再用 3ml 甲醇洗脱待测物，收集甲醇洗脱液于 10ml 干燥离心管中，于 50℃ 水浴中氮气流吹干，残渣加 100μl 流动相，涡旋 3min 使溶解，转移至 1.5ml 离心管中，12000rpm 离心 2min，取上清液 20μl 进样，记录色谱图。

5. 方法学验证

标准曲线　取空白尿液 500μl，分别置 10ml 离心管中，精密加入苯巴比妥标准系列溶液各 50μl，制得尿液苯巴比妥浓度为 100、200、400、1000、2000 和 4000ng/ml 的标准曲线样品，按"苯巴比妥尿液样品处理"项下同法处理，进样 20μl，记录色谱图。以苯巴比妥尿液浓度为横坐标，苯巴比妥与内标的峰面积比值为纵坐标，采用线性权重回归标准曲线，权重系数为 $1/C^2$。

方法精密度与准确度　取空白尿液 500μl，按"标准曲线"项下的方法制成高、中、低三个浓度（苯巴比妥浓度分别 200、1000 和 4000ng/ml）的质量控制（QC）样品，每一浓度进行 5 样本分析，根据标准曲线，计算 QC 样品中苯巴比妥的实测浓度。根据 QC 样品的苯巴比妥的实测浓度计算本法的精密度与准确度。

回收率　精密吸取空白尿液 500μl，按"标准曲线"项下方法制成高、中、低三个浓度（苯巴比妥浓度分别 200、1000 和 4000ng/ml）的 QC 样品，每一浓度进行 5 样本分析。同时，空白尿液 500μl，除不加苯巴比妥标准溶液和内标溶液外，其他按"苯巴比妥尿液样品处理"项下的方法操作，向获得的氮气流吹干后的残渣中加入相应浓度的苯巴比妥标准溶液适量和内标溶液 50μl，制成苯巴比妥的浓度分别为 200、1000 和 4000ng/ml 的低、中、高浓度的对照样品各两份，20μl 进样分析，获得相应峰面积（三次测定的平均值）。以每一浓度两种处理方法的峰面积比值计算提取回收率。

6. 未知样品的测定

色谱条件与系统适用性试验　用十八烷基硅烷键合硅胶为填充剂；流动相为甲醇:水（70:30）；流速 1.0ml/min；检测波长 254nm。取空白尿液样品和"标准曲线"项下标准尿液 400ng/ml 分别测定，苯巴比妥与内标巴比妥的分离度应大于 1.5，理论板数按苯巴比妥峰计算应不低 3000；在空白尿液样品色谱中，在苯巴比妥与内标位置应没有干扰峰。

测定法　取待测尿液样品，按"苯巴比妥尿液样品处理"项下同法处理，进样 20μl，记录色谱图。将苯巴比妥与内标的峰面积比值代入标准曲线，按内标法求算未知样品的尿药浓度。尿药累积排泄率的计算公式为

$$排泄率（\%）= \frac{C \times V \times D}{S} \times 100\%$$

式中，C 为测得的一段时间内的尿药浓度（ng/ml）；V 为收集的尿液体积（ml）；D 为尿样的稀释倍数；S 为口服苯巴比妥的量（mg）。

四、预习提要

（1）如何评苯巴比妥在尿中的排泄情况？

（2）尿液样本有何特点，是如何收集和保存的？

（3）固相萃取小柱的种类有哪些？如何根据被测药物选择合适的固定相？

五、实验指导

（1）尿液是一种含有超过95%的水的液体，其次含有9.3g/L的尿素，1.87g/L的氯化物，1.17g/L的钠，0.750g/L的钾，0.670g/L的肌酐，以及其他离子，无机物和有机物。若肾脏的机能正常，在尿液中仅存在极少量的蛋白，但是当肾脏与尿管出现障碍时就会变成蛋白尿。因此尿液不能直接进入色谱系统进行分析，要根据尿液中的药物浓度及分析方法的灵敏度来选择样品前处理方法。如果简单的有机溶剂沉淀法灵敏度不够，可考虑液 – 液萃取法，并增大尿液的取用量，达到"富集"待分析物，提高灵敏度的目的，或者考虑更换更灵敏的检测仪器，比如液质联用。

（2）巴比妥类药物属于中枢神经系统抑制剂，能够产生从中度镇静到失去全部感觉的药理活性。此外，还可作为抗焦虑剂，安眠药，以及抗惊厥药在临床上应用。此类药物具有潜在的生理和心理成瘾性，因此，临床用药有明确管制。巴比妥类药物口服易从肠道吸收，入血后迅速分布全身组织和体液中。巴比妥类药物在体内主要有两种消除方式：一种经肝脏氧化，另一种以原形由肾脏排泄，例如苯巴比妥有48%左右在肝脏氧化，15% ~ 20%以原形由尿液排出。

（3）固相萃取利用溶解或悬浮在液体里溶质在固定相和流动相中的亲和力不同来分离待测物与杂质。将不同填料作为固定相装入微型小柱，当含有药物的生物样品溶液通过时，由于受到吸附、分配、离子交换或其他亲和力作用，药物或杂质被保留在固定相上，用适当溶剂清洗杂质后再用适当溶剂洗脱药物。最常用的 C_{18} 填料的固相萃取实验步骤如下所述。第一步：用6 ~ 10 倍体积甲醇润湿小柱，活化填料；第二步：用6 ~ 10 倍体积水或适当的缓冲液冲洗小柱，除去残留的甲醇；第三步：加样，使样品经过小柱，非极性的待测物吸附在固相上，而弃取废液；第四步：用水或适当的缓冲液冲洗小柱，去除内源性杂质，通空气或 N_2 干燥固相；第五步：选择适当的洗脱溶剂洗脱分析物，收集洗脱液，挥干溶剂。

六、讨论

（1）尿液中药物浓度的测定主要用于哪些方面的研究？

（2）处理生物样品时，固相萃取法与液液萃取法相比有何优点？实验操作时应注意哪些事项？

（3）在用固相萃取法处理苯巴比妥尿样时，甲醇洗脱液为何用氮气吹干？

Experiment 19　　Determination of Phenobarbital in Human's Urine by HPLC

1. Purposes

1.1　　To learn the urine sample preparation method by solid phase extraction(SPE) technique.

1.2　　To learn the urine sample collection method and the calculation of the accumulative urine excretion rate of the sample.

1. 3 To learn the determination of metoprolol in urine samples by HPLC.

2. Instruments and chemical reagents

2. 1 Instruments

HPLC, C_{18} solid phase extraction cartridge, analytical balance, centrifuge, ultrasonic cleaning instrument, micropipettor (1000μl, 200μl), vortex mixer, volumetric flask (100ml, 10ml), graduated cylinder(500ml), centrifuge tube(5ml, 2ml), pipette tips(1000μl, 100μl), transfer pipette(5ml, 1ml), microliter syringe(10μl).

2. 2 Chemical reagents

Phenobarbital tablets, blank urine, phenobarbital reference substance (RS), amobarbital RS, methanol(AR.), methanol(HPLC), deionized water.

3. Procedure and methods

3. 1 Introduction

Phenobarbital is 5 – ethyl – 5 – phenylpyrimidine – 2, 4, 6 (1H, 3H, 5H) – trione. The molecular formula is $C_{12}H_{12}N_2O_3$. The molecular weight is 232. 24. White or almost white, crystalline powder or colourless crystals, it is freely soluble in ethanol and ether, very slightly soluble in water. It forms water-soluble compounds with alkali hydroxides and carbonates.

Amobarbital is 5 – ethyl – 5 – (3 – methylbutyl) pyrimidin – 2, 4, 6 (1H, 3H, 5H) – trione. The molecular formula is $C_{11}H_{18}N_2O_3$. The molecular weight is 226. 28. White or almost white, crystalline powder, it is freely soluble in ethanol and ether, soluble in methylene chloride, very slightly soluble in water, It forms water-soluble compounds with alkalihydroxides and carbonates.

3. 2 Sample collection

Following overnight fasting (at least 10 hours), the blank urine samples are collected before administration. The subject should be administered a single dose, 30mg of phenobarbital tablet with 200ml warm water in the morning. Subjects can drink water after 2 hours and have standard meal after 4 hours of administration. Urine samples are collected for a period of 0 ~ 2h, 2 ~ 4h, 4 ~ 6h, 6 ~ 8h, 8 ~ 12h, 12 ~ 24h and 24 ~ 48h after dosing, volume measured accurately, filtrated and stored at − 20℃ for later analysis.

3. 3 Standard solutions preparation

Standard solutions of phenobarbital Weigh about 100mg of phenobarbital RS, accurately, to a 100ml volumetric flask, then dissolve and dilute with methanol to volume and mix to prepare stock solution of phenobarbital(1000μg/ml). The stock solution is further diluted with methanol to obtain standard solutions of 1.0μg/ml, 2.0μg/ml, 4.0μg/ml, 10.0μg/ml, 20.0μg/ml and 40.0μg/ml. The stock and standard solutions are all stored at 4℃ in the refrigerator.

Standard solutions of bisoprolol hemifumarate(IS)   Weigh about 10mg of amobarbital RS, accurately to a 100ml volumetric flask, then dissolve and dilute with methanol to volume, and mix to prepare stock solutions of amobarbital(100μg/ml). The stock solution is further diluted with water to obtain standard solutions of 10.0μg/ml. Keep at 4℃ for further use.

3.4   Phenobarbital urine sample preparation

Thaw the frozen urine samples at 37℃ water bath. Transfer accurately 500μl of it to a 10ml centrifuge tube after proper dilution. Add accurately 50μl of IS standard solution to the tube, then add accurately 50μl of methanol or the corresponding standard solutions when preparing the calibration curve and quality control(QC) samples, vortex the mixture for 10s. SPE is used for sample pretreatment. A cartridge(3ml) is activated with 3ml of methanol followed by 3ml of water. An urine sample mixture is loaded onto the prepared cartridge. The cartridge is washed with 3ml of water. The analyte is eluted with 3ml of methanol. The eluted solution is transferred to a 10ml glass tube and is evaporated to dryness at 50℃ under a stream of nitrogen. Then, the dried extract is dissolved in 100μl of mobile phase, and then vortex 3 mins, transfer to 1.5ml centrifuge tubes, centrifuge for 2 mins at 12000r/min, and the supernatant of 20μl is injected into the chromatographic system.

3.5   Method validation

Calibration curve   To each of 500μl of blank urine in 10ml centrifuge tubes, add 50μl of a series of phenobarbital standard solution and obtain phenobarbital concerntrations of 100,200,400, 1000,2000 and 4000ng/ml, respectively. Then, process them in the same way as directed under the "Phenobarbital urine sample preparation". And then 20μl samples are injected and the chromatograms are recorded. The calibration curve is constructed by plotting the peak area ratios of each analyte to the IS versus the concentration using weighted least square linear regression with a factor of $1/C^2$.

Precision and accuracy   To each of the 10ml centrifuge tubes, add precisionly 500μl of blank urine. The quality control(QC) samples are prepared according to "Calibration curve" at concentrations of 200ng/ml,1000ng/ml and 4000ng/ml(5 replicates at each concentration). The concentrations of phenobarbital of QC samples are calculated according to calibration curve. The precision and accuracy are determined by analyzed concerntrations of the QC samples.

Recovery   QC samples at 200,1000 and 4000ng/ml of 5 replicates are prepared according to "Calibration curve". Meanwhile, the corresponding samples are prepared by adding the phenobarbital standard solutions and IS after extraction($n = 2$). The recovery of metoprolol tartrate is determined by comparing the peak area of the analytes in urine samples that had been spiked with the analytes prior to extraction with those of the samples to which the analytes have been added after extraction.

3.6   Determination of phenobarbital in urine

Chromatographic condition and system suitability   HPLC separations are performed on an ODS column. The mobile phase is a mixture of methanol-water(70 : 30). The flow rate is 1.0ml/

min. The wavelength is set at 254nm. Chromatograph the blank urine sample and the calibration curve solution which contains 400 ng/ml phenobarbital, separately, and record the peak responses. The resolution between phenobarbital and IS should be not less than 1.5, and the number of theoretical plates of the column is not less than 3000, calculated with reference to the peak of phenobarbital. There is no interference in the blank urine sample chromatogram at the position of phenobarbital and IS.

Determination A portion of the supernatant (20μl) is injected into HPLC system and the chromatogram is recorded. The concentration of phenobarbital is calculated according to calibration curve by internal standard method.

Calculation of the accumulative urine excretion rate is as follows.

$$\text{Accumulative urine excretion rate} = \frac{C \times V \times D}{S} \times 100\%$$

In this formula, C is urine concentration in a period of time (ng/ml), V is volume of urine sample collection (ml), D is dilution fold of urine sample, S is oral administration dose of phenobarbital (mg).

4. Prepare lessons before class

4.1   How to evaluate the excretion of phenobarbital in urine?

4.2   What are the characteristics of the urine samples? How to collect and store urine samples?

4.3   What are the types of SPE cartridge? How to select the appropriate solid phase according to the property of the analyte?

5. Guide for experiment

5.1   Urine is an aqueous solution consisting of more than 95% water, 9.3g/L urea, 1.87g/L chloride, 1.17g/L sodium, 0.750g/L potassium, 0.670g/L creatinine and other dissolved ions, inorganic and organic compounds. If kidney function is normal, there is only a very small amount of protein in urine. However, the urine will become proteinuria if the kidneys and urinary tract was abnormal. So, urine can't be injected directly into the chromatograph system. The selection of sample preparation method bases on the drug concentration in urine and the sensitivity of desired analytical methods. If the sensitivity of organic solvent precipitation method is not enough, liquid-liquid extraction with a larger amount of urine can be employed to enrich analytes and increase sensitivity. Furthermore, more sensitive instruments can also be considered, such as LC – MS.

5.2   Barbiturates are drugs that act as central nervous system depressants, and can therefore produce a wide spectrum of effects, from mild sedation to total anesthesia. They are also effective as anxiolytics, hypnotics, and anticonvulsants. They have addictive potentials, both physically and psychologically, therefore, the clinical application of barbiturates are controlled. Barbiturates can be absorbed easily from the intestinal tract by oral administration, then distributed to body tissues and fluids rapidly. There are two main ways to eliminate in vivo. One is to be oxidized by the liver, the other is to be excreted by the kidneys in form of original drug. For example, about 48% of phenobarbitals are oxidized in the liver, and 15% ~ 20% of them are excreted by urine in the form of prototype drug.

5.3   SPE uses the affinity of solutes dissolved or suspended in a liquid(known as the mobile phase) for a solid through which the sample is passed(known as the stationary phase) to separate a mixture into desired and undesired components. When the biological sample solution containing drugs flow through cartridge which is loaded different packing material as stationary phase, drugs or impurities are retained on the stationary phase because of absorption, distribution, ion exchange or other affinity roles. Elute drugs with suitable solvent after washing the impurities with appropriate solvent. A typical C_{18} solid phase extraction involves five basic steps. First, the cartridge is equilibrated with 6 ~ 8 times volume of methanol, which wets the surface and penetrates the bonded phase. Then 6 ~ 10 times volume of water, or buffer of the same composition as the sample, is typically washed through the column to remove the remaining methanol. Next, the sample is then added to the cartridge. As the sample passes through the stationary phase, the non-polar analytes in the sample will interact and retain on the non-polar sorbent while the solvent, and other polar impurities pass through the cartridge. Then, after the sample is loaded, the cartridge is washed with a polar solvent(water or appropriate buffer) to remove further impurities, and then dry stationary phase with air or nitrogen. Finally, the analyte is eluted with a non-polar solvent or a buffer of the appropriate pH, and the elution solvent is evaporated.

6. Discussions

6.1   What is the purpose to determine the concentration of drug in the urine sample?

6.2   What are the advantages of SPE compared with liquid-liquid extraction? What precautions should be paid to in the experiment?

6.3   Why is the nitrogen used for the dryness of the methanol elute during the SPE procedure?

(赵云丽)

实验二十   LC – MS/MS 法测定比格犬血浆中
阿奇霉素的含量

一、目的

（1）掌握阿奇霉素血浆样品的处理方法和基质效应的考察方法。

（2）掌握阿奇霉素血浆样品直接沉淀法的预处理方法和测定步骤。

（3）熟悉液质联用的原理及优势。

二、仪器与试药

1. 仪器

高效液相色谱－串联质谱联用仪（ESI 离子源），微量注射器（25μl），分析天平，离心机，超声波清洗器，微量移液器（1000μl、100μl），涡旋混合振荡器，量瓶（100ml、10ml），量筒（500ml），离心管（2ml），吸液头（1000μl、100μl），移液管（5ml、1ml）。

2. 试药

阿奇霉素片（500mg），阿奇霉素对照品，罗红霉素对照品，甲醇（色谱纯），乙腈（色谱纯），乙酸铵（分析纯），乙酸（分析纯），超纯水，空白血浆（-20℃冷冻保存）。

三、实验方法

1. 药物简介

阿奇霉素为半合成的十五元环大环内酯类抗生素。分子式 $C_{38}H_{72}N_2O_{12}$，相对分子质量748.98，白色或类白色结晶粉末；无臭，味苦。本品在水中几乎不溶，甲醇、丙酮、三氯甲烷、无水乙醇或稀盐酸中易溶。

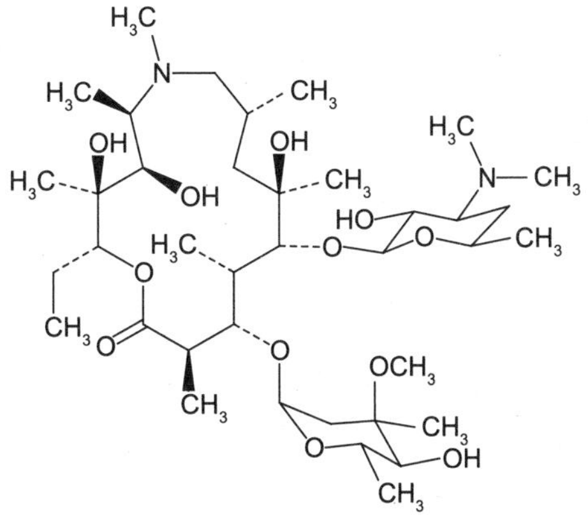

罗红霉素（内标），即 9-［O-（2-甲氧基乙氧基）甲肟］红霉素。红霉素分子式为 $C_{14}H_{76}N_2O_{15}$，相对分子质量为 837.05。

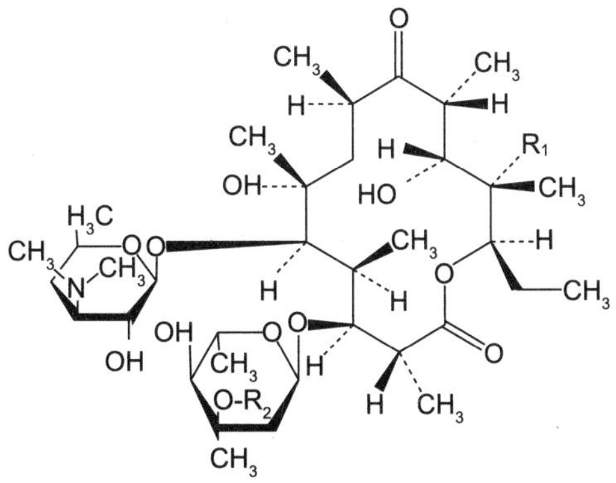

2. 样本来源及取样方法

受试比格犬于受试的前晚起禁食 12h，次日口服给药，剂量为 500 毫克/只，于服药前（0h）及服药后 0.5、1、1.5、2、3、4、6、8h 分别经前肢静脉取血约 3.0ml，置肝素化离心管中，3000r/min 离心 10min 分取血浆，血浆立即放入 -20℃ 的冰箱保存。

3. 标准溶液的制备

（1）阿奇霉素对照品溶液的配制　精密称取阿奇霉素对照品，用甲醇溶解并稀释制成含阿奇霉素 200μg/ml 的标准储备液。精密量取阿奇霉素标准储备液适量至合适的容量瓶中，用流动相稀释分别配成 0.2、0.4、2.0、10.0、20.0、80.0 和 100μg/ml 的阿奇霉素标准系列溶液。以上各种溶液均置4℃保存。

（2）内标溶液的配制　精密称取罗红霉素对照品适量，用甲醇溶解并稀释至刻度，摇匀，制成每毫升中含200μg的储备液，精密吸取适量，用甲醇稀释制成4.0μg/ml的内标溶液。4℃保存，备用。

4. 血浆样品处理

精密吸取血浆样品200μl，置2ml塑料离心管中，精密加入甲醇10μl（标准曲线和质控样品加入相应浓度的阿奇霉素10μl对照品溶液），精密加入内标溶液10μl，旋涡30s混匀；加0.8ml乙腈沉淀蛋白，旋涡3min，15000r/min高速离心3min，取上清液10μl进行LC-MS/MS分析。

5. 方法学验证

（1）标准曲线　分别精密吸取系列浓度的阿奇霉素对照溶液10μl和内标溶液10μl，置2ml塑料尖头离心管中，精密加入空白血浆200μl，涡旋30s混匀，配制成阿奇霉素血浆浓度分别为10、20、100、500、1000、4000和5000ng/ml的血浆样本，按上述"血浆样品处理"处理，进样分析，分别记录阿奇霉素的色谱峰面积（A_s）与内标罗红霉素的色谱峰面积（A_i）。以阿奇霉素与内标的峰面积比值为纵坐标（y），阿奇霉素血浆浓度为横坐标（x），标准曲线采用线性权重回归，权重系数为$1/C^2$。

（2）基质效应

基质样品的制备　分别取来源于6个不同个体的空白血浆适量，加入4倍量的乙腈，涡旋3min，15000r/min离心3min，得空白基质，备用；取干净10ml离心管，分别精密加入阿奇霉素对照品溶液（0.4、10和80μg/ml）10μl和内标溶液10μl，加入空白基质0.9ml，涡旋3min混匀，制成低、中、高三个浓度的基质样品，即得。

对照样品的制备　取干净10ml离心管，分别精密加入阿奇霉素对照溶液（0.4、10和80μg/ml）10μl和内标溶液10μl，加入空白流动相0.9ml，涡旋3min混匀，制成低、中、高三个浓度的对照样品，每个浓度两份，即得。

计算基质效应的公式为

$$基质效应（\%）=\frac{基质样品峰面积}{对照样品峰面积}\times100\%$$

6. 测定法

（1）色谱条件　色谱柱为Kromasil C_6H_6（250mm×4.6mm，5μm，江苏汉邦科技有限公司），流动相为乙腈∶水溶液［70∶30（V/V），水相中含10mmol/L醋酸铵和0.1%醋酸］，流速：1ml/min；柱温为30℃。

（2）质谱条件　离子化方式：ESI；扫描方式：选择反应监测（SRM）；离子极性：正离子；检测离子：阿奇霉素选择性反应检测离子［$M+H$］$^+$ m/z 749.9→m/z 592.0（33eV），内标罗红霉素选择性反应检测离子［$M+H$］$^+$ m/z 837.2→m/z 679.1（23eV）；喷雾电压4500eV；鞘气压力35psi；辅助气压力5psi；毛细管温度350℃。

（3）血浆中阿奇霉素浓度的测定　取待测血浆样品，按"血浆样品处理"项下同法处理，进样10μl，记录色谱图。将阿奇霉素与内标的峰面积比值代入标准曲线，按内标法求算未知样品的血药浓度。

四、预习提要

（1）了解阿奇霉素的化学性质和高效液相色谱–串联质谱联用仪的使用方法。

（2）了解阿奇霉素血浆样品液液萃取的步骤和注意事项。

（3）什么是基质效应？在何种情况下要考察基质效应？

五、实验指导

1. 阿奇霉素

阿奇霉素（azithromycin）是一种属于大环内酯的抗生素，于1980年发现，1981年推出。阿奇霉素是在红霉素结构基础上修饰后得到的一种广谱抗生素，同罗红霉素一样属大环内酯类第二代抗生素，适用于敏感菌所致的呼吸道、皮肤软组织感染和衣原体所致的传播性疾病。

2. LC‑MS 的使用注意事项

流动相一般选择甲醇∶水，乙腈∶水或甲醇∶乙腈∶水，水相比例若过高，会降低离子化效应，有机相有利于离子化效率提高，因此在实际操作过程中要优先使用较高比例有机相的溶液作为流动相；一般正离子方式有机相用甲醇，负离子方式用乙腈。有时为了获得更好的离子化效率，也会加入些低浓度挥发性电解质，如乙酸铵、甲酸铵、甲酸、乙酸、氨水等，而磷酸盐、枸橼酸盐等非挥发性盐和离子对试剂与 LC‑MS 不相匹配，故须用上述挥发性的缓冲剂代替。离子化程度主要与待测组分的 pK_a 和流动相的 pH 有关，待测组分在流动相中成为离子状态，可以提高生成气相离子效率以提高检测灵敏度。当待测组分为碱性物质时，可以在流动相中添加乙酸或甲酸使其 pH 值在待测组分的（$pK_a - 2$）左右，使待测组分在流动相中形成正离子，采用正离子检测方式。当待测组分为酸性物质时，可以选择加氨水使流动相的 pH 值在待测组分的（$pK_a + 2$）左右，常添加少量的乙酸（0.05%以下），使流动相保持微弱的酸性，待测组分在流动相中形成负离子，采用负离子检测方式。

HPLC 流动相流速的选择对分析的成功有十分重要的影响，流速主要由柱子内径和流动相的组成等因素共同决定，较小的流速和内径小的色谱柱，可获得较好的离子化效率。一般样品分析常采用 2.1mm 内径的色谱柱，300～400μl/min 的流速作为分析选择。

3. 基质效应的评价方法

基质效应（matrix effect，ME）是由于样品中存在干扰物质，对响应造成直接或间接的影响。LC‑MS 分析时，内源性物质使待测物的离子化效率降低或者增强，影响定量分析结果准确率。基质效应的评价方法有两种，绝对基质效应评价和相对基质效应评价，本实验采用的是绝对基质效应的评价。绝对基质效应配制两组不同的标准曲线，每组包括5条标准曲线。第一组用流动相配制，制成含系列浓度待测组分的标准曲线，本实验中每条曲线含有7个浓度，每一浓度进行5样本分析（共35个样品）。第二组标准曲线将6种不同来源的空白生物样品经提取后加入与第一组相同系列浓度的待测组分后制得。第二组测定结果同第一组测定结果相比，若待测组分响应值的相对标准偏差明显增加，表明存在基质效应的影响。如果将第一组和第二组各浓度水平测得的相应的响应值（峰面积）分别用 A、B 表示，可按下列公式计算基质效应。

$$ME（\%）= \frac{B}{A} \times 100\%$$

一般的 ME 值在 85%～115% 之间，基质效应可以忽略。在实际工作中常采用高、中、低三种浓度的质控点来考察基质效应。

六、讨论

（1）液质联用仪测定阿奇霉素的原理是什么？质谱检测器的特点是什么？

（2）LC – MS 的流动相选择时应注意什么？

（3）如何评价绝对基质效应？消除基质效应有哪些措施？

Experiment 20　Determination of Azithromycin in Beagle Dog Plasma by LC – MS/MS

1. Purposes

1.1　To learn the method of plasma sample preparation and investigation of matrix effect.

1.2　To learn about the protein precipitation and determination of azithromycin in plasma samples.

1.3　To be familiar with the principles and advantages of LC – MS/MS.

2. Instruments and chemical reagents

2.1　Instruments

HPLC – MS/MS（ESI），microliter syringe（25μl），analytical balance，centrifuge，ultrasonic cleaning instrument，micropipettor（1000μl，100μl），vortex mixer，volumetric flask（100ml，10ml），graduated cylinder（500ml），centrifuge tube（2ml），pipette tips（1000μl，100μl），transfer pipette（5ml，1ml）.

2.2　Chemical reagents

Azithromycin tablet（500mg），azithromycin reference substance，roxithromycin reference substance，methanol（HPLC），acetonitrile（HPLC），ammonium acetate（AR.），acetic acid（AR.），ultra-pure grade water，blank beagle dog plasma（store at −20℃）.

3. Procedure and methods

3.1　Introduction

Azithromycin is a semi-synthetic macrolide antibiotic of the erythromycin group with a 15-

membered azalactone ring. Molecular formula：$C_{38}H_{72}N_2O_{12}$. Molecular weight：748.98. It is a white or almost white crystalline powder, odourless, bitter taste; practically insoluble in water, freely soluble in methanol, acetone, chloroform, anhydrous ethanol and in diluted hydrochloric acid.

Roxithromycin, erythromycin 9 － [O － [(2 － methoxyethoxy) methyl] oxime]；molecular formula：$C_{41}H_{76}N_2O_{15}$；molecular weight：837.05.

3.2　Sample collection

After an overnight fast (12 h), beagle dog was given a 500mg single dose of azithromycin tablet. About 3.0ml blood samples were collected from the forelimb vein at 0h, 0.5h, 1h, 1.5h, 2h, 3h, 4h, 6h, 8h respectively after the drug administration. Plasma was separated by centrifugation at 3000rpm for 10min and kept at －20℃ until analysis.

3.3　Standard solutions preparation

3.3.1　Standard solutions of azithromycin

Weigh azithromycin accurately. Dissolve and dilute it with methanol to volume and mix to prepare stock solution of azithromycin(200μg/ml). The stock solution is further diluted with mobile phase to obtain standard solutions of 0.2μg/ml, 0.4μg/ml, 1.0μg/ml, 2.0μg/ml, 10.0μg/ml, 20.0μg/ml, 80.0μg/ml and 100μg/ml. The stock and standard solutions are all stored at 4℃ in the refrigerator.

3.3.2　Standard solutions of IS

Weigh roxithromycin accurately, to a volumetric flask, and then dissolve and dilute it with methanol to volume, and mix to prepare stock solutions of IS(200μg/ml). The stock solution is further diluted with methanol to obtain standard solutions of 4.0μg/ml. Keep at 4℃ for further use.

3.4　Sample preparation

An aliquot of 200μl plasma sample in 2ml Eppendorf tube is spiked with 10μl of IS solution and 10μl of methanol or of the corresponding standard solutions when preparing the calibration and quality control(QC) samples. After vortex mixing for 30s, 0.8ml acetonitrile is added and vortexed for 3min, and then centrifuged at 15000r/min for 3min. An aliquot of 10μl of the supernatant obtained is then injected for the LC－MS/MS analysis.

3.5　Method validation

3.5.1　Calibration curve

Calibration curves (10ng/ml, 20ng/ml, 100ng/ml, 500ng/ml, 1000ng/ml, 4000ng/ml and 5000ng/ml)for azithromycin in plasma are prepared by spiked 10μl of IS solution and 10μl of the corresponding standard solutions into an aliquot of 200μl plasma sample in 2ml Eppendorf tube. The linearity of each calibration curve is determined by plotting the peak area ratios (y) of azithromycin versus IS with the nominal concentrations (x) of azithromycin in plasma, respectively. The calibration curves is constructed by weighted least square linear regression with a factor of $1/C^2$.

3.5.2　Matrix effect

Matrix sample preparation　Blank samples from six subjects are processed by adding 4 – fold acetonitrile, and vortexed for 3min, and then centrifuged at 15000r/min for 3min. Secondly, 10μl of azithromycin standard solution(three concentration levels of 0.4μg/ml, 10μg/ml and 80μg/ml, respectively) and 10μl of IS solution are transferred to 10ml test tube, next 0.9ml of above-mentioned processed blank solution(from six subjects) is added, and then mixed well by vortexing for 3min.

Reference solutions preparation　Reference solutions of azithromycin are prepared by mixing 10μl of azithromycin standard solution(three concentration levels of 0.4μg/ml, 10μg/ml and 80μg/ml, respectively, $n=2$), 10μl of IS solution and 0.9ml of mobile phase, and mixed well by vortexing for 3min.

The matrix effect of azithromycin is evaluated using the ratio ($A/B \times 100$)%, where A is the corresponding peak areas of matrix sample and B is the corresponding peak areas of reference solutions.

3.6　Determination of azithromycin in plasma

3.6.1　Chromatographic conditions

A Kromasil C_6H_6 column(250mm × 4.6mm, 5μm, Jiangsu Hanbon Science & Technology Co., Ltd) is used for the chromatographic separation using a mixture of acetonitrile : water solution(70 : 30, containing 10mmol/L ammonium acetate and 0.1% acetic acid) as the mobile phase pumped at a flow-rate of 1.0ml/min. The column temperature is maintained at 30℃.

3.6.2　MS conditions

All analyses are carried out in positive-ion ESI and monitored in SRM mode. Based on the full-scan MS and MS/MS spectra of the analytes, the most sensitive ion transitions are selected for the monitoring with m/z 749.9→592.0(33eV) for azithromycin and 837.2→679.1(23eV) for the IS with the collision energy 33eV and 23eV, respectively. The MS/MS conditions are optimized as follows: the spray voltage is set at 4500eV with the capillary temperature at 350℃. Nitrogen is used as sheath(35psi) and auxiliary(5psi) gases.

3.6.3　Determination

A portion of the aqueous phase (10μl) is injected into LC – MS/MS system and the chromatogram is recorded. The concentration of azithromycin is calculated according to the calibration curve by internal standard method.

4. Prepare lessons befor class

4.1　What are the chemical properties of azithromycin? How to use LC – MS/MS instrument?

4.2　Depict the process and precautions for the liquid-liquid extraction of azithromycin in plasma samples.

4.3　What does matrix effect mean? Under what conditions should matrix effect be investigated?

5. Guide for experiment

5.1　Azithromycin

Azithromycin is a macrolide antibiotic belonging which was discovered in 1980 and launched in 1981. Azithromycin is a broad spectrum antibiotic erythromycin after the structure has been modified in the same genus as roxithromycin second-generation macrolide antibiotics, applied to goods caused by the respiratory tract, skin and soft tissue infections and chlamydia are diseases caused by the spread.

5.2　Precautions of LC – MS

Mobile phase often consists of methanol-water, acetonitrile-water or methanol-acetonitrile-water. Ionization effect decreases if aqueous phase ratio is too high while organic phase is favorable to increase ionization effect. So, high proportion of organic phase is preferable to use as mobile phase in practical operation. Methanol is used as organic phase in positive mode while acetonitrile is used as organic phase in negative mode in general cases. Sometimes low concentration of volatile weak electrolyte, for example, ammonium acetate, ammonium formate, formic, acetic acid and ammonia etc, is added to mobile phase in order to obtain better ionization effect. However, involatile salts, such as phosphate, citrate etc and ion-pair reagent do not match LC-MS system and should be replaced by the above volatile buffer.

Degree of ionization is mainly related to the pK_a value of determined components and pH value of mobile phase. Generation of gas phase ion effect and the detection sensitivity are improved if determined components exist as ionic state in mobile phase. Acetic acid or formic acid are added to mobile phase, which makes pH value of mobile phase nearly pK_a value subtract 2 of determined components when the determined components are basic substance. So, the determined components are detected in positive mode for forming positive ion in the mobile phase. Ammonia is added to mobile phase, which makes pH value of mobile phase nearly pK_a value plus 2 of determined components when the determined components are acid substance. Small amount of acetic acid is usually added to mobile phase, whose concentration is below 0.05%, keeping weak acid of mobile phase. So, the determined components are detected in negative mode for forming negative ion in the mobile phase.

Flow selection of mobile phase has an important effect on analytical success. Flow is mainly dependent on column internal diameter and mobile phase composition. The column internal diameter is as small as possible at lower flow in order to obtain better ionization efficiency. The 2.1mm internal diameter of column is often used for sample analysis and flow rate is set at $300 \sim 400\mu l/min$ for analysis and selection.

5.3　Strategies for the assessment of matrix effect

Matrix effect(ME) caused by the sample matrix and interferences from metabolites have direct or indirect impact on responses. The endogenous substance in biological fluid interferes with the determination of the samples for ion suppression or enhancement of compounds analyzed by LC –

MS. This effect may reduce or increase the intensity of analyte ions and affect the accuracy of the assay. There are two methods for quantitative assessment of the matrix effect, absolute versus relative matrix effect. Absolute matrix effect is used in the experiment. Two sets of five standard lines were prepared to evaluate the absence or presence of matrix effect. In the first set(set 1), standards of the analytes present in the neat reconstitution solvent(HPLC mobile phase used in the assay) were analyzed directly at seven concentrations and analyses were repeated five times at each concentration (35 samples). In the second set(set 2), five different blank biological samples were first extracted and spiked after extraction with the analytes in the same solvent(mobile phase) as in set 1. Any additional variability of the peak areas for the analytes than those observed in set 1, as demonstrated by an increase in the coefficients of variation(CV) at each concentration, would be indicative of an effect of sample matrix since analytes at the same concentrations were spiked into plasma extracts. If one depicts the peak areas obtained in neat solution standards in set 1 as A, the corresponding peak areas for standards spiked after extraction into plasma extracts as B(set 2), the ME values can be calculated as follows.

$$ME(\%) = \frac{B}{A} \times 100\%$$

A ME value from $85\% \sim 115\%$ indicated that the responses for analytes in the mobile phase and in the plasma extracts were the same and that no ME was observed. Low, medium and high concentrations of QC samples are usually used for evaluating matrix effect in practice.

6. Discussion

6.1　What is the principle of determining azithromycin in plasma by LC – MS? What are the characteristics of MS detector?

6.2　What are the precautions for mobile phase selection of LC – MS?

6.3　How to evaluate the absolute matrix effect? Which methods are used for eliminating matrix effect?

(赵云丽)

第六章 设计性实验

Chapter 6　Designing Experiment

实验二十一　兰索拉唑的鉴别实验

一、目的

（1）掌握药物鉴别试验的目的和意义。

（2）掌握药物鉴别试验的内容，如性状、一般鉴别试验、专属鉴别试验。

（3）掌握药物常用的鉴别方法（化学、光谱、色谱）和原理。

二、药品简介

中文名称：兰索拉唑。

英文名称：Lansoprazole。

化学名称：2－［［［3－甲基－4－（2，2，2－三氟乙氧基）－2－吡啶基］甲基］－亚硫酰基］－1H－苯并咪唑。

分子式：$C_{16}H_{14}F_3N_3O_2S$。

相对分子质量：369.37。

三、实验方法

（1）根据兰索拉唑的结构、理化特性与鉴别方法的关系，结合自己的实验设计进行讨论，然后根据实验室条件和实验时数选择合适的鉴别实验内容。

（2）写出性状（外观、溶解度、物理常数）鉴别试验操作方法和理论依据。

（3）写出一般鉴别试验操作方法和理论依据。

（4）写出专属鉴别试验操作方法和理论依据。

（5）进行实际操作，对兰索拉唑进行鉴别。

四、实验指导

（1）设计实验前须充分了解兰索拉唑的结构与理化特性，与同类药物的个性与共性，即一般鉴别试验与特殊鉴别试验的内容。选择最具该类药物结构特征的鉴别试验来判断药物的类型；选择兰索拉唑最具特征的专属反应来确证该药物。

（2）应对被检样品进行某一实验，由反应结果作出结论，通过一般鉴别试验将未知样品进行初步分类，然后再用专属鉴别试验进行确证。

Experiment 21　Identification of Lansoprazole

1. Purposes

1.1　To understand the aims and purposes of the identification tests.

1.2　To learn about the contents of the identification tests, such as the characteristics of drugs, common and special identification tests.

1.3　To study the principles and methods of the identification of Lansoprazole.

2. Drug

Lansoprazole：

$$(C_{16}H_{14}F_3N_3O_2S, M_w = 369.37)$$

3. Procedures and methods

3.1　Discuss the experimental design according to the structure, physicochemical properties and the identification tests, and then select proper tests according to the laboratory conditions and time.

3.2　Write down the procedure, theoretical basis and reaction principles of characteristic identification tests.

3.3　Write down the procedure, theoretical basis and reaction principles of common identification tests.

3.4　Write down the procedure, theoretical basis and reaction principles of special identification tests.

3.5 Do the actual operation, confirm the Lansoprazole.

4. Guide for experiment

4.1 Fully understand the structure and physicochemical properties of Lansoprazole beforehand, as well as common and special identification tests. Select the suitable tests to distinguish the type of the drug and then the special tests to identify the drug among one type.

4.2 The sample should be tested and distinguished by the results. During the general identification test, classification of unknown sample would be made, which should be confirmed by special identification tests.

（高晓霞）

实验二十二　兰索拉唑的杂质检查实验

一、目的

（1）通过兰索拉唑的生产工艺和储藏条件了解其杂质来源。
（2）掌握药物中一般杂质的检查方法。
（3）掌握药物中特殊杂质的检查方法。
（4）掌握杂质限量的计算方法。

二、药品简介

药品简介同实验二十一。

三、实验方法

（1）针对兰索拉唑设计其一般杂质和特殊杂质的检查方法，写出实验操作方法、理论依据和反应原理。

（2）结合自己的实验设计进行讨论，然后根据初步设计方案考虑实验室条件和实验时数，并选择合适的实验方法。

（3）进行实际操作。对兰索拉唑进行一般杂质和特殊杂质的检查，制订合理的杂质检查方法和限度。

四、实验指导

（1）设计实验前须充分了解药物的结构与理化特性，分析其可能存在的杂质。
（2）可选择两种或两种以上的方法进行比较，最后确定最佳的杂质检查的质量标准。
（3）注意方法的专属性和灵敏度。
（4）注意各种杂质检查方法和限度控制方法的优缺点。

Experiment 22　Examination for Impurities in Lansoprazole

1. Purposes

1. 1　To know the impurity source of Lansoprazole from its production process and storage conditions.

1. 2　To master the methods for the examination of ordinary impurities in drugs.

1. 3　To master the methods for the examination of special impurities in drugs.

1. 4　To master the calculation of impurity limits.

2. Drug

See Experiment 21.

3. Procedures and methods

3. 1　Independently design a method to examine the impurities in lansoprazole, and write down the procedure, theorical basis and reaction principle.

3. 2　Discuss the experimental design and then select proper tests according to the laboratory conditions and time.

3. 3　Do the actual operation, examine the ordinary impurities and special impurities in lansoprazole, and establish the proper methods and limits.

4. Guide for experimental

4. 1　Have a better understanding of the structure and physicochemical properties of drugs beforehand, and analyze potential impurities.

4. 2　Compare two or more ways to determine the best way to examine the impurities and their quality standards.

4. 3　Pay attention to specificity and sensitivity.

4. 4　Pay attention to the advantages and disadvantages of various methods of impurity examination and limits control.

（高晓霞）

实验二十三　兰索拉唑的含量测定实验

一、目的

（1）掌握兰索拉唑定量分析方法的分类和特点。

（2）掌握样品分析的预处理方法。

（3）掌握含量测定方法验证的内容。

二、药品简介

药品简介同实验二十一。

三、实验方法

（1）查阅有关兰索拉唑的文献资料，写出简短综述文章。

（2）对文献内容进行交流、讨论，结合实验室条件初步确定几个分析方法并探讨其可行性。

（3）分配任务，根据各自的任务进一步查阅有关文献，记录实验内容，写出实验方案和实验用仪器、试剂、试药及样品的制备方法。

（4）完成兰索拉唑的含量测定工作（包括供试品溶液的制备、对照品的配制、仪器选用与调试、测定与计算），并对分析方法进行验证（包括准确度、精密度、专属性、检测限等），写出分析报告。

四、实验指导

（1）设计实验前须充分了解兰索拉唑的组成与生产工艺。

（2）特别关注样品预处理对测定的影响。

（3）可选择两种或两种以上的方法进行比较，最后确定最佳的含量测定方法。

（4）特别注意方法验证中的专属性和准确度指标。

Experiment 23　Content Determination of Lansoprazole

1. Purposes

1. 1　To master the classification and characteristics of the quantitatively analytical methods of Lansoprazole.

1. 2　To master the pretreatment methods of sample analysis.

1. 3　To master the validation of the content determination methods.

2. Drug

See Experiment 21.

3. Procedures and methods

3. 1　Retrieve the relevant literature about lansoprazole and write a short review.

3. 2　Discuss the literature, establish several analytical methods according to the laboratory conditions, and study their feasibility.

3. 3　Further retrieve related literature after task distribution, write down the experimental scheme, selected instruments, reagents, drugs and sample preparation methods.

3. 4　Complete the content determination of lansoprazole（including the preparation of sample

solution and reference, equipment selection and commissioning, the determination and calculation), validate the analytical methods (including accuracy, precision, specificity, detection limit and so on) and write a report.

4. Guide for experiment

4.1　Have a better understanding of the composition and production process of lansoprazole before designing the experiment.

4.2　Pay attention to the pretreatment of drugs and determination of their effects.

4.3　Prepare two or more methods upon comparison, and select the best one to finish the content determination.

4.4　Be particularly attentive to the specificity and accuracy in the validation of the methods.

（高晓霞）

实验二十四　酮康唑的血药浓度测定

一、目的

（1）掌握药物血浆浓度测定的常用分析方法。

（2）学会根据药物的性质设计生物样品预处理方法。

（3）学会生物样本检测的分析方法优化。

二、药品简介

$$（C_{26}H_{28}Cl_2N_4O_4，\quad M_w = 531.44）$$

中文名称：酮康唑。

英文名称：Ketoconazole。

化学名称：（±）－顺－1－乙酰基－4［4－［［2－（2,4－二氯苯基）－2－（1－咪唑－1－甲基）－1,3－二氧戊－4－环基］甲氧基］苯基］哌嗪。

性状：本品为类白色结晶粉末；无臭。本品在三氯甲烷中易溶，在甲醇中溶解，在乙醇中微溶，在水中几乎不溶。

三、可选实验内容

（1）不同预处理方法对血浆中酮康唑浓度测定的提取回收率影响。

（2）不同分析检测方法对血浆中酮康唑浓度测定的灵敏度影响，如 HPLC － UV 和 HPLC － FLD 等。

（3）血浆中酮康唑浓度测定的分析方法学验证，如线性、回收率、精密度等。

（4）实验动物灌胃酮康唑片后酮康唑的血药浓度测定。

四、实验方法

（1）根据酮康唑的结构、理化性质结合血浆样品的特点进行讨论，然后根据实验室条件和学时数，选择合适的实验内容。

（2）设计血浆中酮康唑测定的样品预处理方法及步骤和理论依据。

（3）设计血浆中酮康唑测定的分析方法的选择和条件优化的步骤和理论依据。

（4）写出实验所需的仪器、试剂和试药。

（5）进行实际操作，测定血浆中酮康唑的浓度。

五、实验指导

（1）掌握血浆样本中药物预处理方法有哪些，分别适用于具有什么性质的药物。

（2）掌握各分析检测方法的优缺点，特别是专属性、灵敏度和准确度方面的差异。

（3）掌握动物的给药方法和取样手段。

（4）了解药代动力学参数的计算过程。

Experiment 24　Determination of Ketoconazole Concentration in Plasma

1. Purposes

1.1　To learn the common analysis method for drug plasma concentration determination.

1.2　To learn how to design a pretreatment procedure in bioanalysis according to the character of analytes.

1.3　To learn optimization of analysis method.

2. Drug

Ketoconazole：

$$(C_{26}H_{28}Cl_2N_4O_4, Mw = 531.44)$$

1 － [4 － [4 － [[2 － (2 , 4 － dichlorophenyl) － 2 － (imidazol － 1 － ylmethyl) － 1 , 3 － dioxolan － 4 － yl] methoxy] phenyl] piperazin － 1 － yl] － ethanone

Description：An almost white crystalline powder；odorless. Free soluble in chloroform，soluble in methanol，slightly soluble in ethanol，practically insoluble in water.

3. Optional contents

3.1 Extraction recovery experiments in different pretreatment processes.

3.2 Sensitivity experiments in different detection methods, such as HPLC-UV and HPLC-FLD.

3.3 Analysis method validation, such as linearity, recovery and precision.

3.4 Determination of ketoconazole in plasma samples after an oral administration of ketoconazole tablet to experiment animal.

4. Procedures and methods

4.1 Discuss the experimental design according to the structure, physicochemical properties and feature of bioanalysis, and then select proper experiment contents according to the laboratory conditions and time.

4.2 Write down the proper pretreatment method, the procedure, and theoretical basis.

4.3 Write down the proper detection method and the procedure of optimization, and theoretical basis.

4.4 Write down the equipment, reagents and drugs.

4.5 Perform the experiment procedure.

5. Guide for experiment

5.1 To learn what the common pretreatment processes in bioanalysis are, and how to choose a proper pretreatment method according to the character of analyte.

5.2 To learn the advantage and disadvantage of common detection methods, especially in term of specificity, sensitivity and accuracy.

5.3 To learn the administration and sampling method.

5.4 To be familiar with the pharmacokinetic calculation.

(宋　敏)

实验二十五　清开灵口服液的质量分析

一、目的

(1) 掌握中药制剂质量控制方法选择的依据。

(2) 掌握中药制剂鉴别和含量测定方法的建立过程。

(3) 掌握中药制剂含量测定方法验证的内容。

二、药品简介

1. 处方

胆酸　　　　　珍珠母

猪去氧胆酸　　　栀子

水牛角　　　　　板蓝根

黄芩苷　　　　　金银花

2. 制法

以上八味，水牛角磨粉；板蓝根、栀子、金银花加水煎煮两次，每次 1h，合并煎液，滤过，滤液浓缩至相对密度为 1.15～1.20（50℃）的清膏，放冷，加乙醇适量，静置，滤过，回收乙醇，加水适量，静置。将水牛角粉、珍珠母加硫酸适量，水解，滤过，滤液用 15% 氢氧化钙溶液调节 pH 值至 4，滤过，滤液浓缩至相对密度为 1.05～1.10（50℃），放冷，加乙醇适量，静置，滤过，回收乙醇，加水适量，静置。胆酸、猪去氧胆酸加乙醇适量溶解。将上述药材提取液与水解液合并，混匀，加至胆酸、猪去氧胆酸乙醇液中，加乙醇适量，静置，滤过，滤液回收乙醇，加水适量，静置，加入黄芩苷，调节 pH 值使之溶解，加入矫味剂适量并加水至 1000ml，用氢氧化钠调节 pH 值至 7.2～7.5，搅匀，静置，滤过，即得。

3. 性状

本品为棕红色的液体；味甜、微苦。

三、可选实验内容

（1）清开灵口服液的鉴别：猪去氧胆酸、胆酸、栀子中栀子苷或黄芩苷的鉴别。

（2）清开灵口服液中胆酸、栀子苷或黄芩苷的含量测定。

（3）含量测定方法学验证，如专属性、加样回收率实验。

四、实验方法

（1）查阅相关文献资料，写出简短的综述文章。

（2）根据清开灵口服液中指标性成分的理化性质结合中药制剂的特点进行讨论，然后根据实验室条件和学时数，选择合适的实验内容。

（3）写出实验所需的仪器、试剂和试药。

（4）根据选择的实验对象，设计清开灵口服液鉴别实验的样品处理方法、鉴别方法及实验步骤和理论依据。

（5）根据选择的实验对象，设计清开灵口服液含量测定的样品处理方法、检测方法、实验步骤和理论依据。

（6）含量测定方法学验证，如专属性、加样回收率实验，比较不同样品处理方式和检测方法对结果的影响。

五、实验指导

（1）掌握中药制剂分析样品预处理方法及其特点。

（2）掌握中药制剂鉴别实验的常用方法、特点，与化学药品鉴别实验常用方法和手段的异同。

（3）掌握中药制剂含量测定常用方法的建立和优化，特别是中药复方制剂可采用多指标成分同时定量分析。

（4）掌握中药制剂含量测定方法学验证的内容，特别是专属性和准确度的考察。

Experiment 25　Analysis of Qingkailing Koufuye

1. Purposes

1. 1　To learn how to choose a proper method for Traditional Chinese Medicine quality control.

1. 2　To learn how to establish an analysis method for the identification and determination of Traditional Chinese Medicine.

1. 3　To learn the validation of the content determination method.

2. Drug

2. 1　Ingredients

Cholic acid; Margaritifera Concha; Hyodeoxycholic acid; Gardeniae Fructus Bubali Cornu; Isatidis Radix; Baicalin; Lonicerae Japonicae Flos.

2. 2　Procedure

Grind Bubali Cornu to fine powder. Decoct Isatidis Radix, Gardeniae Fructus and Lonicerae Japonicae Flos with water for 2 times, 1 hour for each time, combine the decoctions, filter, concentrate to a thin extract with a relative density of 1. 15 ~ 1. 20 (50℃), stand to cool, add a quantity of ethanol, stand, filter, recover ethanol, add a quantity of water and stand. Hydrolyze Bubali Cornu powder and Margaritifera Concha Sulfuric acid, filter and adjust to pH 4 with 15% solution of calcium hydroxide. Filter, concentrate the filtrate to a thin extract with a relative density of 1. 05 ~ 1. 10 (50℃), allow to cool, add a quantity of ethanol, stand, filter, recover ethanol, add a quantity of water and stand. Dissolve cholic acid, and hyodeoxycholic acid with a quantity of ethanol. Combine the above extracts and hydrolyzate, mix well and add to ethanol solution of cholic acid and hyodeoxycholic acid. Add a quantity of ethanol, stand and filter. Recover ethanol, add a quantity of water, stand, add baicalin, dissolve by adjusting pH, add an appropriate quantity of flavoring agents, dilute to 1000ml with water, and adjust to pH 7. 2 ~ 7. 5 with sodium hydroxide. Stir thoroughly, stand, and filter.

Description: A clear, brownish red liquid; taste, sweet and slightly bitter.

3. Optional contents

3. 1　Identification of Qingkailing Koufuye, such as hyodeoxycholic acid, cholic acid, geniposide in Gardeniae Fructus and baicalin.

3. 2　Determination of the contents of cholic acid, geniposide, and baicalin in Qingkailing Koufuye.

3. 3　Analysis method validation, such as specificity, recovery.

4. Procedures methods

4. 1　Retrieve the relevant literature about the targeted drug and write a short review.

4.2 Discuss and design the experiment on the basis of the physicochemical properties of marker components in Qingkailing Koufuye and the feature of Traditional Chinese Medicine, and then select proper experiment contents according to the laboratory conditions and time.

4.3 Write down the equipment, reagents and drugs.

4.4 According to the analytes, design the proper pretreatment process, identification method, procedure, and theoretical basis.

4.5 According to the analytes, design the proper pretreatment process, determination method, procedure, and theoretical basis.

4.6 Validation of the determination method, such as specificity and recovery, and comparison the results from different pretreatment and detection methods.

5. Guide for experiment

5.1 To learn what the common pretreatment processes are and their features in Traditional Chinese Medicine analysis.

5.2 To learn the common identification methods and their features, and difference between chemical drug and Traditional Chinese Medicine.

5.3 To learn how to establish and optimize determination method, especially multiple-marker qualification in Traditional Chinese Medicine.

5.4 To learn the validation of determination for Traditional Chinese Medicine, especially the test of specificity and accuracy.

（宋　敏）

第七章 分析方法验证

Chapter 7 Validation of Analysis Method

第一节 药品质量标准分析方法验证指导原则

药品质量标准分析方法验证的目的是证明采用的方法适合相应的检测要求。在建立药品质量标准时，分析方法须经验证；在药品生产工艺变更、制剂的组分变更、原分析方法进行修订时，则质量标准分析方法也须进行验证。方法验证理由、过程和结果均应记载在药品质量标准起草说明或修订说明中。

须验证的分析项目：鉴别试验、限度或定量检查、原料药或制剂中有效成分含量测定，以及制剂中其他成分（如防腐剂等，中药中其他残留物、添加剂等）的测定。在药品溶出度、释放度等检查中，其溶出量等的测定方法也应进行必要验证。

验证指标：准确度、精密度（包括重复性、中间精密度和重现性）、专属性、检测限、定量限、线性、范围和耐用性。在分析方法验证中，须采用标准物质进行实验。由于分析方法具有各自的特点，并随分析对象而变化，因此需要具体方法拟订验证的指标，表 7 – 1 列出的分析项目和相应的验证指标可供参考。

表 7 – 1　检验项目和验证指标

项目内容	鉴别	杂质测定		含量测试及溶出量测定
		定量	限度	
准确度	–	+	–	+
精密度	–	–	–	+
重复性	–	+	–	+
中间精密度	–	+[1]	–	+[1]
专属性[2]	+	+	+	+
检测限	–	–[3]	+	–
定量限	–	+	–	–
线性	–	+	–	+
范围	–	+	–	+
耐用性	–	+	+	+

注：①已有重现性验证，无须验证中间精密度；②如一种方法不够专属，可用其他分析方法予以补充；③视具体情况予以验证。

一、准确度

准确度系指采用该方法测定的结果与真实值或参考值接近的程度，一般用回收率（%）

表示。准确度应在规定的范围内测试。

1. 化学药含量测定方法的准确度

原料药可用已知纯度的对照品或供试品进行测定，或用本法所得结果与已知准确度的另一个方法测定的结果进行比较。制剂可在处方量空白辅料中加入已知量被测物对照品进行测定。如不能得到制剂辅料的全部组分，可向待测制剂中加入已知量的被测物对照品进行测定，或用所建立方法测得结果与已知准确度的另一种方法测定结果进行比较。

准确度也可由所测定的精密度、线性和专属性推算出来。

2. 化学药杂质定量测定的准确度

可向原料药或制剂处方量空白辅料中加入已知量杂质进行测定。如不能得到杂质或降解产物对照品，可用所建立方法测定结果与另一成熟的方法进行比较，如药典标准方法或经过验证的方法。在不能测得杂质或降解产物的校正因子或不能测得对主成分的相对校正因子的情况下，可用不加校正因子的主成分自身对照法计算杂质含量。应明确表明单个杂质和杂质总量相当于主成分的重质比（%）或面积比（%）。

3. 中药化学成分测定方法的准确度

可用对照品进行加样回收率测定，即向已知被测成分含量的供试品中再精密加入一定量的被测成分对照品，依法测定。用实测值与供试品中含有量之差，除以加入对照品量计算回收率。

$$回收率\% = \frac{(C - A)}{B} \times 100\%$$

式中，A 为供试品所含被测成分量；B 为加入对照品量；C 为实测值。

在加样回收试验中须注意对照品的加入量与供试品中被测成分含有量之和必须在标准曲线线性范围之内。加入对照品的量要适当，过小则引起较大的相对误差；过大则干扰成分相对减少，真实性差。

4. 校正因子的准确度

对色谱方法而言，绝对（或定量）校正因子是指单位面积的色谱峰代表的待测物质的量。待测定物质与所选定的参照物质的绝对校正因子之比即为相对校正因子。相对校正因子计算法常应用于化学药有关物质的测定、中药材及其复方制剂中多指标成分的测定。校正因子的表示方法很多，本指导原则中的校正因子是指气相色谱法和高效液相色谱法中的相对质量校正因子。

相对校正因子可采用替代物（对照品）和被替代物（待测物）标准曲线斜率比值进行比较获得；采用紫外吸收检测器时，可将替代物（对照品）和被替代物（待测物）在规定波长和溶剂条件下的吸收系数比值进行比较、计算获得。

5. 数据要求

在规定范围内，取同一浓度（相当于 100% 浓度水平）的供试品，用至少测定 6 份样品的结果进行评价，或设计 3 种不同浓度，每种浓度分别制备 3 份供试品溶液进行测定，用 9 份样品的测定结果进行评价。对于化学药，一般中间浓度加入量与所取供试品中待测定成分量之比控制在 1:1 左右，建议高、中、低浓度对照品加入量与所取供试品中待测定成分量之比分别控制在 1.2:1，1:1，0.8:1 左右，应报告已知加入量的回收率（%），或测定结果平均值与真实值之差及其相对标准偏差或置信区间（置信度一般为 95%）。对于中药，一般中间浓度加入量与所取供试品中待测成分量之比分别控制在 1:1 左右，建议高、中、低浓度对照品加入量与所取供试品中待测定成分量之比分别控制在 1.5 : 1，1 : 1，0.5 : 1 左右，应报告供试品取样量、供试品中含有量、对照品加入量、测定结果和回收率（%）计算值，以及回收率（%）的相对标准偏差（RSD%）或置信区间。对于校正因子，应报告测定方法、测定结果和 RSD%。样品中待测定成分含量和回收率限度关系可参考表 7-2。在基质复杂、组分含量低于 0.01% 及多成分等分析中，回收率限度可适当放宽。

表 7-2　样品中待测定成分含量和回收率限度

待测定成分含量	回收率限度/%
100%	98 ~ 101
10%	95 ~ 102
1%	92 ~ 105
0.1%	90 ~ 108
0.01%	85 ~ 110
10μg/g（ppm）	80 ~ 115
1μg/g	75 ~ 120
10μg/kg（ppb）	70 ~ 125

二、精密度

精密度系指在规定的条件下，同一个均匀供试品，经多次取样测定所得结果之间的接近程度。精密度一般用偏差、标准偏差或相对标准偏差表示。

在相同条件下，由同一个分析人员测定所得结果的精密度称为重复性；在同一个实验室，不同时间由不同分析人员用不同设备测定结果之间的精密度称为中间精密度；在不同实验室由不同分析人员测定结果之间的精密度称为重现性。

含量测定和杂质的定量测定应考虑方法的精密度。

1. 重复性

在规定范围内，取同一浓度（相当于 100% 浓度水平）的供试品，用至少测定 6 份的结果进行评价，或设计 3 种不同浓度，每种浓度分别制备 3 份供试品溶液进行测定，用 9 份样品的测定结果进行评价。采用 9 份测定结果进行评价时，对于化学药，一般中间浓度加入量与所取供试品中待测定成分量之比控制在 1 : 1 左右，建议高、中、低浓度对照品加入量与所取供试品中待测定成分量之比分别控制在 1.2 : 1，1 : 1，0.8 : 1 左右。对于中药，一般中间浓度加入量与所取供试品中待测定成分量之比控制在 1 : 1 左右，建议高、中、低浓度对照品加入量与所取供试品中待测定成分量之比分别控制在 1.5 : 1，1 : 1，0.5 : 1 左右。

2. 中间精密度

为考察随机变动因素，如不同日期、不同分析人员、不同仪器对精密度的影响，应设计方案进行中间精密度试验。

3. 重现性

国家药品质量标准采用的分析方法应进行重现性试验，如通过不同实验室检验获得重现性结果。协同检验的目的、过程和重现性结果均应记载在起草说明中。应注意重现性试验用样品质量的一致性及贮存运输中的环境对该一致性的影响，以免影响重现性结果。

4. 数据要求

均应报告偏差、标准偏差、相对标准偏差或置信区间。样品中待测定成分含量和精密度可接受范围参考表 7 - 3。在基质复杂、含量低于 0.01% 及多成分等分析中，精密度接受范围可适当放宽。

表 7 - 3 样品中待测定成分含量和精密度 RSD 可接受范围

待测定成分含量	重复性/RSD%	重现性/RSD%
100%	1	2
10%	1.5	3
1%	2	4
0.1%	3	6
0.01%	4	8
10μg/g（ppm）	6	11
1μg/g	8	16
10μg/kg（ppb）	15	32

三、专属性

专属性系指在其他成分（如杂质、降解产物、辅料等）存在的情况下，采用的分析方法能正确测定出被测物的能力。鉴别反应、杂质检查和含量测定方法均应考察其专属性。如方法专属性不强，应采用多种不同原理的方法予以补充。

1. 鉴别反应

应能区分可能共存的物质或结构相似化合物。不含被测成分的供试品，以及结构相似或组分中的有关化合物应均呈阴性反应。

2. 含量测定和杂质测定

采用色谱法和其他分离方法时应附图谱，以说明方法的专属性，并应标明各成分在图中的位置，色谱法中的分离度应符合要求。

在杂质对照品可获得的情况下，对于含量测定，试样中可加入杂质或辅料，考察测定结果是否受干扰，并可与未加杂质或辅料的试样比较测定结果。对于杂质检查，也可向试样中加入一定量的杂质，考察各成分包括杂质之间能否得以分离。

在杂质或降解产物不能获得的情况下，可将含有杂质或降解产物的试样进行测定，与另一个经验证的方法或药典方法比较结果。可用强光照射、高温、高湿、酸（碱）水解或氧化的方法进行加速破坏，以研究可能存在的降解产物和降解途径对含量测定和杂质测定的影响。含量测定方法应比对两种方法的结果，杂质检查应比对检出的杂质个数，必要时可采用光二极管阵列检测法和质谱检测法，进行峰纯度检查。

四、检测限

检测限系指试样中被测物能被检测出的最低量。药品的鉴别试验和杂质检查方法，均应通过测试确定方法的检测限。检测限仅作为限度试验指标和定性鉴别的依据，没有定量意义。常用的方法如下。

1. 直观法

用已知浓度的被测物试验出能被可靠地检测出的最低浓度或量。

2. 信噪比法

用于能显示基线噪声的分析方法，即把已知低浓度试样测出的信号与空白样品测出的信号进行比较，计算出能被可靠地检测出的被测物质最低浓度或量。一般以信噪比为 3∶1 或 2∶1 时相应浓度或注入仪器的量确定检测限。

3. 基于响应值标准偏差和标准曲线斜率法

按照 LOD = 3.3δ/S 公式计算。其中，LOD：检测限；δ：响应值的偏差；S：标准曲线的斜率。

δ 可以通过下列方法测得：①测定空白值的标准偏差；②标准曲线的剩余标准偏差或截距的标准偏差来代替。

4. 数据要求

上述计算方法获得的检测限数据须用含量相近的样品进行验证。应附测定图谱，说明试验过程和检测限结果。

五、定量限

定量限系指试样中被测物能被定量测定的最低量，其测定结果应符合准确度和精密度要求。对微量或痕量药物分析、定量测定药物杂质和降解产物时，应确定方法的定量限。常用方法与检测限类似，为直观法和信噪比法，后者一般以信噪比为 10∶1 时相应的浓度或注入仪器的量确定定量限。

1. 基于响应值标准偏差和标准曲线斜率法

按照 LOQ = 10δ/S 公式计算。其中，LOQ：定量限；δ：响应值的偏差；S：标准曲线的斜率。

δ 可以通过下列方法测得：①测定空白值的标准偏差；②标准曲线的剩余标准偏差或截距的标准偏差来代替。

2. 数据要求

上述计算方法获得的定量限数据须用含量相近的样品进行验证。应附测定图谱，说明试验过程和定量限结果，包括准确度和精密度验证数据。

六、线性

线性系指在设计的范围内，测试响应值与试样中被测物浓度呈比例关系的程度。

应在规定的范围内测定线性关系。可用一对照品贮备液经精密稀释，或分别精密称取对照品，制备一系列对照品溶液的方法进行测定，至少制备 5 份不同浓度的对照品溶液。以测得的响应信号作为被测物的浓度作图，观察是否呈线性，再用最小二乘法进行线性回归。必要时，响应信号可经数学转换，再进行线性回归计算，或者可采用描述浓度 – 响应关系的非线性模型。

数据要求：应列出回归方程、相关系数和线性图（或其他数学模型）。

七、范围

范围系指分析方法能达到一定精密度、准确度和线性要求时的高低限浓度或量的区间。

范围应根据分析方法的具体应用及其线性、准确度、精密度结果和要求确定。原料药和制剂含量测定，范围一般为测定浓度的 80% ~ 120%。制剂含量均匀度检查，范围一般为测试浓度的 70% ~ 130% ；特殊剂型，如气雾剂和喷雾剂，范围可适当放宽。溶出度或释放度中的溶出量测定，范围一般为限度的 ±30% ；如规定了限度范围，则应为下限的 −20% 至上限的 +20% 。杂质测定，范围应根据初步实测数据，拟订为规定限度的 ±20% 。如果含量测定与杂质检查同时进行，用峰面积归一化法进行计算，则线性范围应为杂质规定限度的 −20% 至含量限度（或上限）的 +20% 。

在中药分析中，范围应根据分析方法的具体应用和线性、准确度、精密度结果及要求确定。对于有毒、具特殊功效或药理作用的成分，其验证范围应大于被限定含量的区间。

校正因子测定时，范围一般应根据其应用对象的测定范围确定。

八、耐用性

耐用性系指在测定条件有小的变动时，测定结果不受影响的承受程度，为所建立方法用于日常检查提供依据。开始研究分析方法时，就应考虑其耐用性。如果测试条件要求苛刻，则应在方法中写明，并注明可以接受变动的范围，可以先采用均匀设计确定主要影响因素，再通过单因素分析等确定变动范围。典型的变动因素有：被测溶液的稳定性，以及样品的提取次数、时间等。高效液相色谱法中典型的变动因素有：流动相的组成和 pH 值，以及不同品牌或不同批号的同类型色谱柱、柱温、流速等。气相色谱法中典型的变动因素有：不同品牌或批号的色谱柱、固定相，以及不同类型的担体、载气流速、柱温、进样口和检测器温度等。

经试验，测定条件小的变动应能满足系统适用性试验的要求，以确保方法可靠。

Section 1　A Guideline for the Validation of Analytical Method Adopted in Pharmaceutical Quality Specification

The purpose of validation of analytical method is to ensure that the adopted method meets the requirements for the intended analytical applications. In the course of drafting of the drug quality specification, the analytical method must be validated. In case of changing of pharmaceutical synthetic processes or the components of preparation, or revising of the original analytical method, the analytical method of the specification must also be validated. Both process and results of the method validation must be recorded in the description of draft and revision of pharmaceutical quality specification.

The analytical items that should be validated include identification, limit or quantification test, content determination of the active ingredient in drug substance or preparation as well as other components in the preparation, such as antiseptic, residues in Traditional Chinese Medicine, additives etc. In the dissolution test and drug release test of pharmaceuticals, the analytical method of dissolution amount must also be validated.

The validation indexes include accuracy, precision (including repeatability, intermediate - precision and reproducibility), specificity, detection limit, quantitation limit, linearity, range and robustness. Because of intrisic characteristics of validation method and possible influences from analytes, the parameters to be validated should be decided depending on specific analytical method involved. The analytical items and the corresponding parameters to be validated are listed in the table 7 – 1, which can be used as a reference.

Table 7 – 1   Analytical items and parameters of validation characteristics

Type of analytical procedure characteristics	Identification	Testing for impurities		Assay-dissolution (measurement only) -content/potency
		Quantitation	limit	
Accuracy	–	+	–	+
Precision	–	–	–	+
Repeatability	–	+	–	+
Inter mediate Precision	–	+[1]	–	+[1]
Specificity[2]	+	+	+	+
Detection limit	–	–[3]	+	–
Quantitation limit	–	+	–	–
Linearity	–	+	–	+
Range	–	+	–	+
Robustness	+	+	+	+

– signifies that this characteristic is not normally evaluated. + signifies that this characteristic is normally evaluated. [1] It is not necessary to validate the intermediate precision when the reproducibility has been developed. [2] Lack of specificity of an individual analytical method may be compensated by other supporting analytical methods. [3] It depends on the specific condition.

1. Accuracy

The accuracy of an analytical method is the closeness of test results obtained by that method to the true value or the reference value. Accuracy is often represented as percent recovery and should be determined in the specified range.

1. 1   Accuracy of the method for content determination of chemical medicine

The accuracy for drug substance may be determined with a reference substance, or by comparing the result obtained by this method with the result obtained by another method of which the accuracy has been established. For drug preparation, its accuracy may be determined by spiking the exact amount of blank excipient in prescription dosage with known quantity of reference substance. If it is not possible to obtain all the components of excipient, the accuracy may be determined by adding known amounts of analyte to the preparation, or by comparing the result obtained by this established method with the result obtained by another method with known accuracy. The accuracy can be calculated by the precision, linearity and specificity of the method.

1. 2   Accuracy of quantitative determination of impurity for chemical medicine

The accuracy may be determined by spiking the drug substance or blank excipients of prescription dosage with known quantity of impurity. When the reference substance is not available for impurity or degradation product, the accuracy may be determined by comparing the result obtained by this established method with the result obtained by another matured method, such as pharmacopoeia method or validated method. Peak areas of impurities compared with that produced by the main peak of a diluted solution of substance being examined, if the correction factor of the impurity and degradation product or the relative correction factor to the drug substance cannot be determined. The percent ratio of weight or area of a single impurity and total impurities to that of the active ingredient should be testified definitely.

1. 3　Accuracy of determination of ingredients for Traditional Chinese Medicine

The accuracy could be determined by recovery test, accurately adding known amount of reference to analyte whose amount is known. The recovery ratio is calculated by dividing the difference between measured value and known quantity of analyte by added amount of reference. It is noticed that the sum of added amounts of reference and the quantity of analyte should be covered in the linear range. The amount of the added reference substance should be proper. A very low amount of reference substance will cause a large relative error while a high amount of reference substance will reduce the relative amount of the interference substances, so the authenticity is poor.

$$\text{Recovery}\% = \frac{(C - A)}{B} \times 100\%$$

Where, A is the amount of the analyte in the substance being examined; B is the amount of the added reference substance; C is the determined value.

1. 4　Accuracy of correction factor

For a chromatography method, the absolute (or quantitative) correction factor refers to the quotient of the content of analyte divided by the chromatographic peak area. Relative correction factor is the ratio between absolute correction factor of analyte and reference substance. Relative correction factor is normally used in the determination of related substance for chemical drug, or multiple – index substance in crude drugs and compound preparations. Correction factor has a lot of expressions, in this guideline it refers to the relative weight correction factor in gas chromatography and high performance liquid chromatography.

The relative correction factor can be obtained by the ratio of slopes of standard curves of the substitution (reference substance) and the substance (test substance). When using UV – absorbance detector, relative correction factor can be calculated by comparing the absorption coefficients of the substitute (reference substance) and substance (test substance) under specified wavelength and solvent.

1. 5　Requirements for the data

In specified range, the accuracy should be evaluated by using results from at least 6 samples of test substance at the same concentration (equivalent to 100% concentration level), or 9 samples with 3 different concentration of test substance and 3 test solutions at each concentration. For chemical drug, the ratio between the amount of reference substance added and test substance to be determined in the sample is recommended to be controlled around 1. 2 : 1, 1 : 1 and 0. 8 : 1 for the high, middle and low concentration, respectively. The percent recovery of the added amount, or the difference between the average value of testing results and nominal value and its relative standard deviation or confidence interval (normally at 95% confidence level) should be reported. For Traditional Chinese Medicine, the ratio between the amount of reference substance added and test substance to be determined in the sample is recommended to be controlled around 1. 5 : 1, 1 : 1 and 0. 5 : 1 for the high, middle and low concentration, respectively. The amount of sample used, the content of test substance in the sample, the amount of reference substance added, the testing results and calculated percent recovery, and the relative standard deviation (RSD, %) or confidence interval of percent recovery should be reported. For correction factor, the testing method, testing result and RSD should be reported.

The acceptable range of recovery varies according to the content of analyte (Table 7 – 2), which can be used for reference. The acceptable limitation could be relaxed when the analyte is in complex matrix, with content blow 0.01% or multiple-component analysis.

Table 7 – 2   The acceptable range of recovery and the content of analyte

Content of analyte	Recovery(%)
100%	98 ~ 101
10%	95 ~ 102
1%	92 ~ 105
0.1%	90 ~ 108
0.01%	85 ~ 110
$10\mu g/g$(ppm)	80 ~ 115
$1\mu g/g$	75 ~ 120
$10\mu g/kg$(ppb)	70 ~ 125

2. Precision

The precision of an analytical method is the closeness of agreement between a series of measurements obtained from multiple sampling of the same homogeneous sample under the prescribed conditions. The precision of an analytical method is usually expressed as deviation, standard deviation or relative standard deviation.

Repeatability is the precision obtained by the same analyst within a laboratory over a short period of time with the same equipment. Intermediate-precision is the precision obtained by different analysts within the same laboratory on different days with different equipment. Reproducibility is the precision obtained by different analysts in different laboratories using the same analytical procedure.

Precision of the method should be considered when the content of the active ingredient or impurity is determined.

2.1   Repeatability

In specified range, the repeatability of the precision study should be evaluated using results from at least 6 samples of test substance at the same concentration (equivalent to 100% concentration level), or 9 samples with 3 different concentration of test substances and 3 test solutions at each concentration. When the repeatability is evaluated by 9 testing results, the ratio between the amount of reference substance added and test substance to be determined in the sample is recommended to be controlled around 1.2 : 1, 1 : 1 and 0.8 : 1 for chemical drugs and 1.5 : 1, 1 : 1 and 0.5 : 1 for Traditional Chinese Medicine, for the high, middle and low concentration, respectively.

2.2   Intermediate-precision

A scheme should be designed to inspect the effect of random variable factors on the precision.

The variable factors include different dates, different analysts and different equipments.

2.3 Reproducibility

Reproducibility should be tested when an analytical method is adopted as the national drug quality standard, for example, reproducibility should be inspected by collaborative study when pharmacopoeial. Both the process of the collaborative study and result of the reproducibility should be recorded in the description of draft file. Where a reproducibility testing is to be conducted, the sample should be uniform, properly stored and transported to obtain reliable result.

2.4 Requirement for data

Deviation, standard deviation, relative standard deviation and confidence interval should be reported. Acceptable range of precision varies according to the content of analyte (Table 7 – 3), which can be used for reference. The acceptable limitation could be relaxed when the analyte is in complex matrix, the content of component lower than 0.01% and multiple – components analysis.

Table 7 – 3 The acceptable range of precision and the content of analyte

Content of analyte	Repeatability/RSD%	Reproducibility/RSD%
100%	1	2
10%	1.5	3
1%	2	4
0.1%	3	6
0.01%	4	8
10μg/g(ppm)	6	11
1μg/g	8	16
10μg/kg(ppb)	15	32

3. Specificity

The specificity of an analytical method is the ability to measure the analyte accurately and specifically in the presence of components that may be expected to be present in the sample matrix, such as impurities, degradation product and excipients. Specificity concerns should be investigated on identification, impurity test and content determination will be done. If the specificity of the method is not enough, other methods with different principles should be adopted for supplementation.

3.1 Identification

The compounds that may coexist or have closely related structures should be distinguished from the active ingredient. All the samples without the tested ingredient, compounds with closely related structures and related chemical compounds should produce a negative response.

3.2 Assay and test for impurity

The representative graphs should be recorded for verifying specificity when chromatography or other separation methods are used. The position of each component should be marked in the graph. The resolution of the chromatographic method should meet the requirements. If the reference substances of impurities are available, the impurities or excipients may be added to the sample for assay to inspect whether the result is interfered, and the result can be compared with that from the sample without adding impurities or excipients. As to test for impurity, a certain amount of the impurity may be added to the sample to inspect whether all ingredients including the impurity can be separated from other ingredients.

If the impurities or degradation products are not available, the sample with impurities or degradation products may be used for determination, and the result may be compared with that obtained by the pharmacopoeia method or other validated method. Accelerating decomposition may be done for studying degradation products, such as irradiation with strong light, high temperature, high humidity, acidic or alkaline hydrolysis, oxidation etc. The results of two methods should be compared for content determination and the number of impurities should be compared with that obtained in test for impurity. Diode array detector and mass spectrometer may be used for purity test when necessary.

4. Detection Limit

Detection limit is the lowest concentration of the analyte in a sample that can be detected. The detection limit for identification and impurity test should be determined by experiment. The detection limit can only be used as the reference for limit test and qualitative identification, which is not applicable to quantitative analysis. The methods in common use are as follows.

4.1 Noninstrumental Method

The detection limit is generally determined by the analysis of samples with known concentrations of analyte and by establishing the minimum level at which the analyte can be reliably detected.

4.2 Signal – to – Noise Ratio Method

For the instrumental method recording the noise at the baseline, the lowest concentration or content of test substance that is reliably detected can be calculated by comparing the signal of sample at a known low concentration and the signal of the blank. The concentration or the amount injected into the instrument corresponding to the signal – to – noise ratio of 2 : 1 or 3 : 1 is generally accepted.

4.3 Method of Standard Deviation and Slope of Standard Curve Based on Response Value

The detection limit is calculated by the following formula:

$$LOD = 3.3\delta/S$$

In the formula, LOD is the detection limit, δ is the standard deviation of the response value, and S is the slope of standard curve.

The estimate of δ may be carried out in a variety of ways, for example: ① determining the standard deviation of blank; ② substituting by the residue standard deviation or the standard deviation of intercept of standard curve.

4.4 Requirement for data

Detection limit obtained by above methods must be validated by samples with similar content of test substance. The test graphs should be attached and the test procedures and the results of detection limit should be reported.

5. Quantitation Limit

Quantitation limit is the lowest concentration of the analyte in a sample that can be determined with acceptable precision and accuracy under the stated experimental conditions. The quantitation limit should be determined for the analytical method of micro or trace substance or the quantitative determination for impurities and degraded products.

Analogous to LOD, visual evaluation and signal – to – noise ratio are common approaches to determine the limit of quantitation. The concentration or the amount injected into the instrument corresponding to the signal – to – noise ratio of 10 : 1 is generally accepted.

5.1　Based on the standard deviation of the response and the slope

The limit of quantitation(LOQ) may be expressed as follows.

$$LOQ = 10\delta/S$$

where δ is the standard deviation of response value, and S is the slope of standard curve.

The estimate of δ may be carried out in a variety of ways, for example: ① determining the standard deviation of blank; ② substituting by the residue standard deviation or the standard deviation of intercept of standard curve.

5.2　Requirements for data

Quantitation limit obtained by above methods must be validated by samples with similar content of test substance. The test graphs should be attached and the test procedures and the results of quantitation limit, including validation data of precision and accuracy, should be reported.

6. Linearity

The linearity of an analytical method is its ability to elicit test results that are directly proportional to the concentration of analyte in samples within a given range.

Linea relationship should be determined over the claimed range of the method. The samples with varying concentrations of analyte for linearity determination are prepared by diluting accurately a stock solution, or by measuring accurately an amount of analyte separately. At least 5 portions samples should be prepared. The treatment is normally a calculation of a regression line by the method of least squares of test results versus analyte concentrations. In some cases, the test data may have to be subjected to mathematical transformation prior to the linearity regression analysis. It is acceptable to use a non – linear model for concentration – response relation.

Requirement for data: regression equation, correlation coefficient and the linear graph should be listed (or other mathematical models).

7. Range

The range of an analytical method is the concentration or quantity interval between the upper and lower levels of analyte (including these levels) that have been demonstrated to be determined with precision, accuracy, and linearity using the method as written.

The range of the analytical method should be determined based on specific application of the method, its linearity, accuracy and precision, and related requirement. For content determination of drug substance and preparation, the range should be 80% to 120% of the test concentration. For content uniformity of preparation, the range should be 70% to 130% of test concentration and this range may be widened appropriately for special dosage forms, such as aerosol and sprays. For dissolution test and drug release test, the range should be ±30% of the limit. If the range of limit is provided, it should be −20% of lower limit to +20% of upper limit. For impurity determination, the range should be stipulated from −20% to +20% of the provided limit on the basis of preliminary actual determination. If the content determination and impurities test are performed simultaneously with peak area normalization method, the linear range should be −20% of the provided limit of impurity to +20% of the provided limit of content (or upper limit).

For Traditional Chinese Medicine, the range of analytical method should be determined based on specific application linearity, accuracy and precision of the method, and related requirement. For toxic ingredients or those with unique efficacy or pharmacological effect, the range to be validated should be wider than the range of content.

For correction factor, its range should be determined on the basis of the range of test object.

8. Robustness (Ruggedness)

Robustness of an analytical method is the degree of tolerance that the determining result is not affected when there is small change in the operational condition. The robustness of the method should be taken into account at the beginning to develop an analytical method. If the requirement for test condition is strict, it should be recorded clearly in the method and the acceptable range of variations should be indicated. Uniform design can be used for determination of primary influencing factor then the changing range can be confirmed by single factor analysis. The typical variable factors are stability of the test solution, times and duration of sample extraction, and so on. The variable factors of liquid chromatography are composition and pH value of the mobile phase, same type of chromatographic column from different manufacturers or batches, column temperature, flow rate, etc. The variable factors of GC are column and stationary phase with different brands or batches, different types of support, carrier gas flow rate, column temperature, temperature of injection port and detector, etc.

To ensure reliability of the method, the testing conditions with slight change should be confirmed to meet the requirements for system suitability.

第二节　生物样品分析方法的基本要求

准确测定生物基质（如全血、血清、血浆、尿液或其他组织）中的药物浓度，对于药物和制剂研发非常重要，可被用于支持药品的安全性和有效性，或根据毒动学、药动学和生物等效性试验的结果做出关键的决定。由于生物样品具有取样量少、药物浓度低、干扰物质多（如无机盐、脂质、蛋白质、代谢物）及个体差异大等特点，因此必须根据待测物的结构、生物基质和预期的浓度范围建立适宜的生物样品定量分析方法，并完整地对方法进行验证，以获得可靠的结果。首选色谱法，如 HPLC、GC 及 GC - MS、LC - MS、LC - MS/MS 联用技术，一般应采用内标法定量。必要时也可采用生物学方法或生物化学方法。

1. 选择性

必须证明该分析方法能够区分目标分析物和内标与基质的内源性组分或样品中其他组分。应该使用至少 6 个受试者适宜的空白基质来证明选择性（动物空白基质可以不同批次混合），它们被分别分析并评价干扰。当干扰组分的响应低于分析物定量下限响应的 20%，并低于内标响应的 5% 时，通常即可以接受。

应该考察药物代谢物、经样品预处理生成的分解产物及可能的同服药物引起干扰的程度。在适当情况下，也应该评价代谢物在分析过程中回复转化为母体分析物的可能性。

色谱法至少要提供空白生物样品色谱图、空白生物样品外加对照物质色谱图（注明浓度）及用药后的生物样品色谱图。对于 LC - MS 和 LC - MS/MS 方法，应着重考察基质效应。

2. 残留物

应该在方法建立中考察残留物并使之最小。残留物可能不影响准确度和精密度。应通过在注射高浓度样品或校正标样后注射空白样品来估计残留物。高浓度样品之后在空白样品中的残留物应不超过定量下限的 20%，并且不超过内标的 5%。如果残留物不可避免，应考虑特殊措施，在方法验证时检验并在试验样品分析时应用这些措施，以确保不影响准确度和精密度。这可能包括在高浓度样品后注射空白样品，然后分析下一个试验样品。

3. 定量下限

定量下限（LLOQ）是标准曲线上的最低浓度点，要求至少满足测定 3 ~ 5 个半衰期时样品中的药物浓度，或 C_{max} 的 1/10 ~ 1/20 时的药物浓度，其准确度应在真实浓度的 80% ~ 120% 范围内，RSD 应小于 20%，信噪比应大于 5。

4. 标准曲线与线性范围

根据所测定物质的浓度与响应的相关性，用回归分析方法获得标准曲线，标准曲线高低浓度范围为线性范围。当线性范围较宽时，推荐采用加权的方法对标准曲线进行计算，以使低浓度点计算比较准确。校正标样回算的浓度一般应该在标示值的 ±15% 以内，定量下限处应该在 ±20% 以内。至少 75% 校正标样，含最少 6 个有效浓度，应满足上述标准。标准曲线不包括零点。如果某个校正标样结果不符合这些标准，应该拒绝这一标样，不含这一标样的标准曲线应重新评价，包括回归分析。

线性范围要能覆盖全部待测浓度，不允许在线性范围外推求算未知样品的浓度。

5. 准确度与精密度

要求选择以下 4 个浓度的质控样品，通过单一分析批（批内）和不同分析批（批间）获得质控样品值来评价方法的精密度和准确度：定量下限 LLOQ 的 3 倍以内、低浓度在 LLOQ 的 3 倍以内、中浓度在标准曲线中部附近的质控样品、高浓度设置于标准曲线的上限约 75% 处。每一浓度至少测定 5 个样品。

准确度是指用特定方法测得的生物样品浓度与真实浓度的接近程度，一般应在 85% ~ 115% 范围内，在 LLOQ 准确度应在 80% ~ 120% 范围内。

精密度用质控样品的日内和日间相对标准差（RSD）表示，RSD 一般应小于 15%，在 LLOQ 的 RSD 应小于 20%。

6. 稀释可靠性

样品稀释不影响准确度和精密度。应通过向基质中加入分析物至高于定量上限浓度，并用空白基质稀释该样品（每个稀释因子至少 5 个测定值），来证明稀释的可靠性。准确度和精密度应在 ±15% 之内，稀释的可靠性应覆盖试验样品所用的稀释倍数。

7. 基质效应

采用质谱方法时，应该考察基质效应。使用至少 6 批来自不同供体的空白基质，不应使用合并的基质。如果基质难以获得，则使用少于 6 批基质，应说明理由。

对于每批基质，应该通过计算基质存在下的峰面积（由空白基质提取后加入分析物和内标测得），与不含基质的相应峰面积（分析物和内标的纯溶液）比值，计算每一分析物和内标的基质因子。进一步通过分析物的基质因子除以内标的基质因子，计算经内标归一化的基质因子。从 6 批基质计算的内标归一化的基质因子的变异系数不得大于 15%。该测定应分别在低浓度和高浓度下进行。

如果不能适用上述方式，如采用在线样品预处理的情况，则应该通过分析至少 6 批基质，分别加入高浓度和低浓度，来获得批间响应的变异系数。其验证报告应包括分析物和内标的峰面积，以及每一样品的计算浓度。这些浓度计算值的总体变异系数不得大于 15%。

8. 样品稳定性

采用低浓度和高浓度质控样品，在预处理后及在所评价的条件储存后立即分析。由新鲜制备的校正标样获得标准曲线，根据标准曲线分析质控样品，将测得浓度与标示浓度相比较，每一浓度的均值与标示浓度的偏差应在 ±15% 范围内。

根据具体情况，通常应该进行下列稳定性考察：①分析物和内标的储备液稳定性和工作溶液的稳定性；②从冰箱储存条件到室温或样品处理温度，基质中分析物的冷冻和融化稳定性；③基质中分析物在冰箱储存的长期稳定性；④处理过的样品在室温下或在试验过程储存条件下的稳定性；⑤处理过的样品在自动进样器温度下的稳定性。

应特别关注受试者采血时，以及在储存前预处理的基质中分析物的稳定性，以确保由分析方法获得的浓度反映受试者采样时刻的分析物浓度。可能须根据分析物的结构，按具体情况证明其稳定性。

9. 质控样品

质控样品系将已知量的待测药物加入到生物介质中配制的样品，用于质量控制。

10. 质量控制

应在生物样品分析方法确证完成之后开始测试未知样品。每个未知样品一般测定一次，必要时可进行复测。生物样品每个分析批测定时应建立新的标准曲线，并随行测定高、中、低 3 个浓度水平质控样本（低、中、高浓度双重样品，或至少试验样品总数的 5%，两者中取数目更多者），以及被分析的试验样品。质控样品应分散到整个分析批中，以保证整个分析批的准确度和精密度。质控样品测定结果的偏差一般应小于 15%，低浓度点偏差一般应小于 20%，最多允许 33% 的质控样品结果超限，且不得均在同一浓度。如不合格，则该分析批样品测试结果作废。

11. 测试结果

应详细描述所用的分析方法，引用已有的参考文献，提供每天的标准曲线、质控样品及未知样品的结果计算过程。还应提供全部未知样品分析的色谱图，包括全部相关的标准曲线和质控样品的色谱图，以供审查。

Section 2　The Basic Requirements for Analytical Methods of Biological Specimen

The specificity and the sensitivity of quantitative analytical methods for native ingredient and metabolites in biological specimen are the key points for performing successful bioavailability and bioequivalence studies.

The drug concentration in biological matrix (such as blood, serum, plasma, urine or other tissue else) are of great importance in medicine and preparation development, which can support the safety and effectivity of the medicine, or make critical decision according to the results of toxicokinetics, pharmacokinetics and bioequivalence studies. Because there are various factors, which can affect biological specimens analysis, e. g., less specimen, low concentration of active ingredient, endogenous substances (such as inorganic salt, lipide, protein and metabolite) and individual difference, analytical methods of biological specimen must be established on the basis of the structure of the substance being examined, biological matrix and predicted concentration range and the methods must be validated to assure the reliability of the methods.

The chromatography, such as HPLC, GC and the combination techniques, e. g., GC – MS, LC – MS, LC – MS/MS, are best recommended, and internal standard method is usually used for quantitative analysis. Biological or biochemical methods can also be used if necessary.

1. Selectivity

By this analytical method, the analytes of interest and IS should be differentiated from endogenous components in the matrix or other components in the samples. Selectivity should be demonstrated using appropriate blank matrix from at least 6 test subjects (different batches of blank matrix of animals can be mixed), which are analysed separately and evaluated for interference. It is generally acceptable that responses of interfering components are less than 20% of the lower limit of quantification for analytes and 5% for the responses of IS.

It is necessary to investigate the extent of any interference caused by metabolites of the drugs, degradation products through sample preparation, and possible co – administrated drugs. Under certain conditions, the possibility of back – conversion of a metabolite into parent analyte should be taken into consideration during the analysis.

It is necessary to submit the chromatograms of blank, biological matrix, standard substance (indicated with its concentration) combined with blank biological matrix and the biological sample taken after administration. For LC – MS and LC – MS/MS methods, matrix effect should be emphasized on inspection.

2. Residues

Residues should be addressed and minimized during development of analytical methods. Residues may not affect the accuracy and precision. Residue should be assessed by blank samples administrated after high concentration samples or calibration standards. Residue in the blank sample following the high concentration standard should not be greater than 20% of the lower limit of quantification and less than 5% for the IS. If it appears that a residue is unavoidable, specific measures that are validated during method development should be considered to be applied to sample analysis in order to prevent possible influences on accuracy and precision, such as performance analysis of test sample after the injection of blank samples following administration of high concentration samples.

3. Lower limit of quantitation

The lower limit of quantitation (LLOQ) is the lowest concentration on the standard curve. At least, it should meet analysis of the concentration of specimen at the time of three to five times the half-life or one tenth to one twentieth of the C_{max} of the active ingredient concentration. Its accuracy should be within 80% to 120% of the true concentration RSD should be less than 20%, and signal-to-noise ratio should be more than 5.

4. Standard curve and linear range

Standard curve should be obtained by the method of regression analysis on the basis of the relationship between responses and concentrations of measured analyte. Linear range is the interval between the upper and lower concentration in a standard curve. The simplest model that adequately describes the concentration-response relationship should be used. Selection of weighting and use of a complex regression equation should be justified. The standard calibrator concentrations should be within 20% of the nominal concentration at LLOQ and within 15% of the nominal concentration at all other concentrations. The acceptance criterion for the standard curve is that at least 75% of non-zero standards should meet the above criteria, including the LLOQ. Values falling outside these limits should be discarded, provided they do not change the established model. A calibration curves should consist of a zero sample, at least six non-zero samples covering the expected range, including LLOQ. Estimation of unknown concentrations by extrapolations of linear range is not recommended.

5. Precision and accuracy

It is required that precision and accuracy should be determined intra-batch and inter-batch using 4 concentrations of the quality control samples: LLOQ, low concentration (approaching LLOQ and within 3-fold of LLOQ), high concentration (about 75% of the upper limit of the standard curve), and one concentration near the center. At least 5 samples per concentration should be measured.

Accuracy refers to the closeness of the concentration of biological specimen to the true value determined by a special method. It should be within 85% to 115%, but within 80% to 120% for near the lower limit of quantitation.

The precision can be interpreted as the relative standard deviation (RSD) intra-day and inter-day by determining the quality control sample. In general, RSD should not exceed 15%, except for near the lower limit of quantitation where it should not exceed 20%.

6. Reliability of dilution

Sample dilution may not affect the accuracy and precision. The reliability of dilution should be demonstrated by blank matrix diluted solutions (at least 5 measurements per dilution factor) from the sample prepared by spiking the matrix with an analyte concentration above the ULOQ. Accuracy and precision should be ±15%. The reliability of dilution should cover the dilution factors applied to the test samples.

7. Matrix effect

Matrix effects should be investigated for mass spectrometric methods using at least 6 batches of blank matrix from various vendors. Pooled matrix should not be used. If the matrix is difficult to obtain, it is acceptable to use less than 6 batches of matrix and the reason should be stated.

For each matrix, the matrix factor (MF) for each analyte and IS should be calculated by the ratio of the peak area in the presence of matrix (measured by the blank matrix spiked with analyte and IS) to the peak area in absence of matrix (pure solution of the analyte and IS). The IS – normalized MF should also be calculated by the division of the MF of the analyte by the MF of the IS. The coefficient of variation (CV%) of the IS normalized MF calculated from 6 batches of matrix should not be greater than 15%. The determination of matrix effect should be performed at a low and a high concentration level separately.

If some cases where the above method is not applicable, for instance on – line sample pretreatment, the batch – to – batch variability of the response should be assessed by analyzing at least 6 batches of matrix spiked with a low (less than 3 times the concentration of LLOQ) and high concentration (close to the ULOQ) level. The validation report should include the peak areas of the analyte and IS and the calculated concentration for each individual sample. The overall CV of calculated concentrations should not be greater than 15%.

8. Stability

Stability samples should be compared to freshly made calibrators and/or freshly made QCs. At least three replicates at each of the low and high concentrations should be assessed. All stability determinations should use samples prepared from a freshly made stock solution. Stability sample results should be within 15% of nominal concentrations.

Conditions used in stability experiments should reflect situations likely to be encountered during actual sample handling and analysis (e. g. , long-term, bench top, and room temperature storage, and freeze-thaw cycles). If, during sample analysis for a study, storage conditions changed and/or exceed the sample storage conditions evaluated during method validation, stability should be established under the new conditions. Stock solution stability also should be assessed.

The chemical stability of an analyte in a given matrix under specific conditions for given time intervals is assessed in several ways. Pre-study stability evaluations should cover the expected sample handling and storage conditions during the conduct of the study, including conditions at the clinical site, during shipment, and at all other secondary sites.

9. Quality control samples

The quality control samples, which are used for quality control, are biological matrix spiked with known quantities of the drug substance to be analyzed.

10. Quality control

The unknown biological specimen is determined after the analytical method is validated. Analysis of unknown samples can be done by single determination, or replicate analysis if necessary. A new standard curve should be generated for analysis of each batch of biological specimen and the duplicate quality control samples at three concentrations (upper, middle and lower) should be incorporated in each run. The number of quality control samples for each analytical batch should not be less than 5% unknown samples. In general, the deviation from the results of the quality control samples is not more than 15%, and the deviation from the low concentration is not more than 20%. Not more than 33% quality control samples in different concentrations, whose results exceed the limit, are allowed. If not, the test results that batch are invalid.

11. Test result

The analytical methods in detail, published references, every standard curves, and the calculating process of results of quality control samples and unknown samples should be included in the test results. The chromatograms of all unknown samples, including the chromatograms of all correlated standard curve and quality control samples should be available for regulatory authorities.

（宋　敏）

附录　实验室常用英语

Appendix　Laboratory Commonly Used in English

容器类

白细口 flint glass solution bottle with stopper

表面皿 watch glass

玻棒 glass rod

搅拌棒 stirring rod

玻璃活塞 stopcock

不锈钢杯 stainless-steel beaker

称量瓶 weighing bottle

瓷器 porcelain

滴定管 burette

滴瓶 dropping bottle

小滴管 dropper

碘量瓶 iodine flask

分析天平 analytical balance

坩埚 crucible, crucible pot, melting pot

搅拌装置 stirring device

酒精灯 alcohol burner

酒精喷灯 blast alcohol burner

刻度移液管 graduated pipettes

冷凝器 condenser

量杯 measuring glass

量筒 measuring flask/measuring cylinder/graduated flask

漏斗 funnel

分液漏斗 separating funnel

滤管 filter tube

容量瓶 volumetric flask/measuring flask

塞子 stopper

烧杯 beaker

烧瓶 flask

试管 test tube rack

试管架 test tube holder

试剂瓶 reagent bottles

台秤 platform balance

天平 balance/scale

吸液管 pipette

洗耳球 rubber suction bulb

洗瓶 plastic wash bottle

研磨钵 mortar

研磨棒 pestle

玛瑙研钵 agate mortar

移液管（one-mark）pipette

游码 sliding poise

蒸发皿 evaporating dish

蒸发器 evaporator

蒸馏烧瓶 distilling flask

蒸馏装置 distilling apparatus

锥形瓶 conical flask

试验用器材

pH 计 pH meter

pH 试纸 universal pH indicator paper

pH 值指示剂，氢离子（浓度的）负指数指示剂

pH indicator

白滴定管（碱）flint glass burette for alkali

白滴定管（酸）flint glass burette with glass stopcock

比重瓶 specific gravity bottle

擦镜纸 wiper for lens

称量纸 weighing paper

磁力搅拌器 magnetic stirrer

打孔器 stopper borer

滴定管 burette

电动搅拌器 power basic stirrer

电炉 heater

电炉丝 wire coil for heater

防毒面具 respirator, gasmask

沸石 boiling stone

坩埚钳 crucible tong/crucible clamp

烘箱 oven

蝴蝶夹 double-buret clamp

化学反应产物 product

剪刀 scissor

烤钵 cupel

口罩 respirator

冷热浴 bath

离心机 centrifuge

滤纸 filter paper

卵形瓶 matrass

马弗炉 Muffle furnace

秒表 stopwatch

镊子 forceps

闪点仪 flash point tester

设备 apparatus

升降台 lab jack

石棉网 asbestos-free wire gauze

石蕊试纸 litmus paper

双顶丝 clamp regular holder

水银温度计 mercurial thermometer

铁架台 iron support

脱脂棉 absorbent cotton

万能夹 extension clamp

电热套 heating mantle

橡胶管 rubber tubing

药匙 lab spoon

移液管架 pipet rack

圆形漏斗架 cast-iron ring

折光仪 refractometer

真空泵 vacuum pum

棕色滴定管（碱）brown glass burette for alkali

棕色滴定管（酸）brown glass burette with glass
　　stopcock

化学反应

碱性 alkalinity

碱化 alkalinization

阳极，正极 anode

催化作用 catalysis

催化剂 catalyst

阴极，负极 cathode

燃烧 combustion

分解 decomposition

蒸馏 distillation

电极 electrode

电解 electrolysis

吸热反应 endothermic reaction

放热反应 exothermic reaction

发酵 fermentation

分馏 fractionation

熔解 fusion, melting

水解 hydrolysis

同分异物现象 isomerism, isomery

氧化 oxidization, oxidation

沉淀 precipitation

还原剂 reducer

可逆的 reversible

溶解 solution

合成 synthesis

煅烧 to calcine

脱水 to dehydrate

蒸馏 to distill

水合，水化 to hydrate

氢化 to hydrogenate

中和 to neutralize

氧化 to oxidize

脱氧 to deoxidize

沉淀 to precipitate

仪器

原子吸收光谱仪 Atomic Absorption Spectro – scopy

原子发射光谱仪 Atomic Emission Spectro – meter

原子荧光光谱仪 Atomic Fluorescence Spe – ctroscopy

自动滴定仪 Automatic Titrator

离心机 Centrifuge

CO_2 培养箱 CO_2 Incubators

恒温循环泵 Constant Temperature Circulator

电泳 Electrophoresis

傅里叶变换红外光谱仪 FT – IR Spectrometer

气相色谱仪 Gas Chromatograph

气相色谱 – 质谱联用仪 GC – MS

凝胶渗透色谱仪 Gel Permeation Chromato- graph

高压/效液相色谱仪 High Pressure/Perform-ance Liquid Chromatography

PCR 仪 Instrument for Polymerase Chain Reaction/
　　PCR Amplifier

倒置显微镜 Inverted Microscope

液相色谱 – 质谱联用仪 LC – MS

质谱仪 Mass Spectrometer

核磁共振波谱仪 Nuclear Magnetic Resonan-ce
　　Spectrometer

光学显微镜 Optical Microscopy

粒度分析仪 Particle Size Analyzer

PCR 仪 PCR Amplifier

pH 计 pH Meter

摇床 Shaker

体积排阻色谱 Size Exclusion Chromatograph

热分析仪 Thermal Analyzer

超滤器 Ultrahigh Purity Filter

超低温冰箱 Ultra-low Temperature Freezer

超声破碎仪 Ultrasonic Cell Disruptor

紫外检测仪 Ultraviolet Detector

紫外观察灯 Ultraviolet Lamp

紫外 – 可见光分光光度计 UV – Visible Spectro –
　　photometer

黏度计 Viscometer

X 射线衍射仪 X – Ray Diffractometer